Handbook of Diversity Issues in Health Psychology

THE PLENUM SERIES IN CULTURE AND HEALTH

SERIES EDITORS:

Richard M. Eisler and Sigrid Gustafson
Virginia Polytechnic Institute and State University, Blacksburg, Virginia

---

HANDBOOK OF DIVERSITY ISSUES IN HEALTH PSYCHOLOGY
    Edited by Pamela M. Kato and Traci Mann

Handbook of Diversity Issues in Health Psychology

Edited by
Pamela M. Kato and
Traci Mann

Stanford University
Stanford, California

Plenum Press • New York and London

Library of Congress Cataloging-in-Publication Data

Handbook of diversity issues in health psychology / edited by Pamela
M. Kato and Traci Mann.
        p.   cm. -- (Plenum series in culture and health)
    Includes bibliographical references and index.
    ISBN 0-306-45325-8
    1. Clinical health psychology. 2. Clinical health psychology-
-United States--Cross-cultural studies. 3. Minorities--United
States--Health and hygiene. 4. Minorities--United States--Medical
care.   I. Kato, Pamela M. II. Mann, Traci. III. Series.
    R726.7.H356 1996
    610'.8'693--dc20   96-32564
                                                               CIP

ISBN 0-306-45325-8

© 1996 Plenum Press, New York
A Division of Plenum Publishing Corporation
233 Spring Street, New York, N. Y. 10013

Printed in the United States of America

For my godfather, Joseph C. Mancuso

—PMK

For my brother, Dr. Barry Mann

—TM

Contributors

MARC H. BORNSTEIN, National Institute of Child Health and Human Development, 9000 Rockville Pike, Bethesda, Maryland 20892

FELIPE G. CASTRO, Department of Psychology and Hispanic Research Center, Arizona State University, Tempe, Arizona 85287

MARGARET A. CHESNEY, School of Medicine, University of California, San Francisco, San Francisco, California 94061

CHI-AH CHUN, Department of Psychology, University of California at Los Angeles, Los Angeles, California 90095

KATHRYN COE, Hispanic Research Center, Arizona State University, Tempe, Arizona 85287

MICHAEL M. COPENHAVER, Department of Psychology, Virginia Polytechnic Institute and State University, Blacksburg, Virginia 24060

RICHARD M. EISLER, Department of Psychology, Virginia Polytechnic Institute and State University, Blacksburg, Virginia 24060

KANA ENOMOTO, Department of Psychology, University of California at Los Angeles, Los Angeles, California 90095

TIFFANY M. FIELD, Touch Research Institute, University of Miami School of Medicine, Miami, Florida 33101

GARY GROSSMAN, 2150 Sutter Street, San Francisco, California 94115

SARA GUTIERRES, Department of Social and Behavioral Sciences and Hispanic Research Center, Arizona State University, Tempe, Arizona 85287

JAMES S. JACKSON, Institute for Social Research, University of Michigan, Ann Arbor, Michigan 48106

BETTY R. KASSON, Departments of Nursing and Pediatric Surgery, Lucile Salter Packard Children's Hospital at Stanford, Palo Alto, California 94304

PAMELA M. KATO, Department of Psychiatry and Behavioral Sciences, Stanford University School of Medicine, Stanford, California 94305

HELENA CHMURA KRAEMER, Department of Psychiatry and Behavioral Sciences, Stanford University School of Medicine, Stanford, California 94305

ELLEN LANGER, Department of Psychology, Harvard University, Cambridge, Massachusetts 02138

NANCY LEFFERT, Search Institute, 700 South Third Street, Suite 210, Minneapolis, Minnesota 55915

BECCA LEVY, Division on Aging, Harvard Medical School, Boston, Massachusetts 02115

PETER M. LEWINSOHN, Oregon Research Institute, 1715 Franklin Boulevard, Eugene, Oregon 97403

KEH-MING LIN, Research Center on the Psychobiology of Ethnicity, Harbor–UCLA Research and Education Institute, Torrance, California 90502

TRACI MANN, Health Risk Reduction Projects, UCLA Neuropsychiatric Institute, 10920 Wilshire Boulevard, Suite 1103, Los Angeles, California 90024

LINDA C. MAYES, Child Study Center, Yale University, New Haven, Connecticut 06510

JILL B. NEALEY, Department of Psychology, University of Utah, Salt Lake City, Utah 84112

KATHERINE A. O'HANLAN, Gynecologic Cancer Section, Stanford University School of Medicine, Stanford, California 94305

MONISHA PASUPATHI, Department of Psychology, Stanford University, Stanford, California 94305

ANNE C. PETERSEN, Institute of Child Development, University of Minnesota, Minneapolis, Minnesota 55455

PAUL ROHDE, Oregon Research Institute, 1715 Franklin Boulevard, Eugene, Oregon 97403

Toni Rucker, Department of Sociology, University of Michigan, Ann Arbor, Michigan 48109

Delia Saenz, Department of Psychology and Hispanic Research Center, Arizona State University, Tempe, Arizona 85287

Steven Schinke, Columbia University School of Social Work, New York, New York 10025

Sherrill L. Sellers, Institute for Social Research, University of Michigan, Ann Arbor, Michigan 48106

Sandra K. Sentivany, Departments of Nursing and Pain Management, Lucile Salter Packard Children's Hospital at Stanford, Palo Alto, California 94304

Michael Smith, Research Center on the Psychobiology of Ethnicity, Harbor–UCLA Research and Education Institute, Torrance, California 90502

Stanley Sue, Department of Psychology, University of California at Los Angeles, Los Angeles, California 90095

David R. Williams, Department of Sociology and Survey Research Center, Institute for Social Research, University of Michigan, Ann Arbor, Michigan 48106

Antonette M. Zeiss, Geriatric Research Education and Clinical Center, Veterans Affairs Palo Alto Health Care System, Palo Alto, California 94304

Foreword

The field of health psychology has grown dramatically in the last decade, with exciting new developments in the study of how psychological and psychosocial processes contribute to risk for and disease sequelae for a variety of medical problems. In addition, the quality and effectiveness of many of our treatments, and health promotion and disease prevention efforts, have been significantly enhanced by the contributions of health psychologists (Taylor, 1995). Unfortunately, however, much of the theorizing in health psychology and the empirical research that derives from it continue to reflect the mainstream bias of psychology and medicine, both of which have a primary focus on white, heterosexual, middle-class American men. This bias pervades our thinking despite the demographic heterogeneity of American society (U.S. Bureau of the Census, 1992) and the substantial body of epidemiologic evidence that indicates significant group differences in health status, burden of morbidity and mortality, life expectancy, quality of life, and the risk and protective factors that contribute to these differences in health outcomes (National Center for Health Statistics, 1994; Myers, Kagawa-Singer, Kumanyika, Lex, & Markides, 1995). There is also substantial evidence that many of the health promotion and disease prevention efforts that have proven effective with more affluent, educated whites, on whom they were developed, may not yield comparable results when used with populations that differ by ethnicity, social class, gender, or sexual orientation (Cochran & Mays, 1991; Castro, Coe, Gutierres, & Saenz, this volume; Chesney & Nealey, this volume).

The *Handbook of Diversity Issues in Health Psychology* makes a strong case for the need for more systematic research that investigates possible differences in health between and within groups along the dimensions of age, gender, social class, race/ethnicity, and sexual orientation. The chapters provide the reader with critical, scholarly reviews of the extant knowledge about differences as a function of each of these dimensions, and point out some of the major lacunae as a guide to future research. Three strong themes emerge throughout the book that are important to highlight and to reiterate. First, a number of differences between the groups are identified and discussed. Group differences are salient for some disorders and not for others, and not all differences are disadvantageous to the socially marginalized group (e.g., lesbians are at lower risk for HIV/AIDS than heterosexual women; Latinas have comparable or better obstetrical outcomes than white women when SES differences are controlled; very old African Americans are often healthier than their white counterparts). Authors also note that these differences are not attributable to any single set of factors, but are more likely the result of the interplay of biological, sociocultural, and psychological factors. Further, these factors exert their effects through social class, life stresses, health beliefs and behaviors, and access to and utilization of quality health services.

Second, it is important to note, however, that the merits of between-group comparisons should be tempered by an appreciation of the substantial heterogeneity and behavioral variability that characterizes these groups. For example, in arguing for ethnic group differences in health behaviors, some investigators have erroneously treated sociopolitical descriptors such as "racial/ethnic minorities" as if they were scientifically meaningful groups that differ in meaningful and systematic ways from whites. While it is true that people of color do differ in important ways from whites, the groups that are usually subsumed under this heading are extremely heterogeneous on a number of important dimensions, and often differ as much from each other as they do from whites. Similarly, even meaningful groups such as Hispanics/Latinos and Asian/Pacific Islanders evidence significant within-group differences on a number of health-relevant factors as a function of national origin, language, and level of acculturation.

Appreciation of these within-group differences also adds a second level of complexity to our analysis. For example, while it is clear that there are significant differences in health status and related predictors between African Americans and white Americans, there is also substantial evidence of health differentials among the subgroups that differ by social class, gender, and sexual orientation. Thus, low-SES African American gay and bisexual men evidence different health-risk profiles than African American heterosexuals and than white gay and heterosexual men (Cochran & Mays, 1988; Johnson, 1993). As in other cases of cross-ethnic comparisons, social class is an important contributor to these differences (Kessler & Neighbors, 1986; Williams & Collins, 1995). There is also growing evidence that similar differences may be observed between subgroups of women (Wyatt, 1991; Nyamathi, Bennett, Leake, Lewis, & Flaskerud, 1993).

The research on diversity issues in health psychology is still in its infancy, and formal theoretical models that integrate the findings and give them conceptual coherence are still not available. This is the next step in the development of this research. The field must now struggle to try to understand what attributes of these groups are the most important in shaping health outcomes, how these factors interact to predict health outcomes, and what interventions can be used to reduce risk and to enhance resilience in each of the groups. Such developments should stimulate growth in the field of health psychology generally by improving the generalizability and applicability of current theories and methodologies.

Finally, while there continues to be debate and doubts in some circles about the scientific merit of research on group differences, especially with respect to ethnicity and sexual orientation, the case for this work is quite compelling. The third point made by the authors in this book is that perhaps the most important reason for pursuing this line of inquiry is ultimately to inform the design and implementation of more effective intervention and prevention programs that are tailored to the unique needs of each of these groups. Not only does this offer the field the opportunity to enhance our intervention science, but more important, it gives us the information we need to enhance the health and well-being of all segments of our society. With the shift in health care policy toward managed care, the need to develop effective health promotion, disease prevention, treatment, and rehabilitation services—especially with the most vulnerable segments of society—is becoming more acute. The *Handbook of Diversity Issues in Health Psychology* makes a significant contribution toward this end.

REFERENCES

Castro, F. G., Coe, K., Gutierres, S., & Saenz, D. (1996). Designing health promotion programs for Latinos. In P. M. Kato & T. Mann (Eds.), *Handbook of diversity issues in health psychology* (pp. 319–345). New York: Plenum Press.

Chesney, M. A., & Nealey, J. B. (1996). Smoking and cardiovascular disease risk in women: Issues for prevention and women's health. In P. M. Kato & T. Mann (Eds.), *Handbook of diversity issues in health psychology* (pp. 199–218). New York: Plenum Press.

Cochran, S. D., & Mays, V. M. (1988). Epidemiologic and sociocultural factors in the transmission of HIV infection in Black gay and bisexual men. In M. Shernoff & W. A. Scott (Eds.), *A sourcebook of gay/lesbian health care. 2nd edition* (pp. 202–211). Washington, DC: National Gay and Lesbian Foundation.

Cochran, S. D., & Mays, V. M. (1991). Psychosocial HIV interventions in the second decade: A note on social support and social networks. *The Counseling Psychologist, 19(4)*, 551–557.

Johnson, E. (1993). Multiple sex partners and risky sexual behavior. *Risky sexual behaviors among African Americans.* Westport, CT: Praeger Press.

Kessler, R. C., & Neighbors, H. W. (1986). A new perspective on the relationships among race, social class, and psychological distress. *Journal of Health & Social Behavior, 27*, 107–115.

Myers, H. F., Kagawa-Singer, M., Kumanyika, S. K., Lex, B. W., & Markides, K. S. (1995). Panel III: Behavioral risk factors related to chronic diseases in ethnic minorities. *Health Psychology, 14(7)*, 613–621.

National Center for Health Statistics. (1994). *Health United States, 1993*. Hyattsville, MD: U.S. Department of Health and Human Services.

Nyamathi, A., Bennett, C., Leake, B., Lewis, C., & Flaskerud, J. (1993). AIDS-related knowledge, perceptions, and behaviors among impoverished minority women. *American Journal of Public Health, 83*, 65–71.

Taylor, S. E. (1995). *Health psychology*, 3rd edition. New York: McGraw-Hill.

U.S. Bureau of the Census. (1992). Population projections of the United States, by age, sex, race and Hispanic origins: 1992–2050. Washington, DC: U.S. Government Printing Office.

Williams, D. R., & Collins, C. (1995). U.S. socioeconomic and racial differences in health: Patterns and explanations. *Annual Review of Sociology, 21*, 349–386.

Wyatt, G. E. (1991). Ethnic and cultural differences in women's sexual behavior. In S. Blumenthal, A. Eichler, & G. Weissman (Eds.), *Women & AIDS: Promoting healthy behavior*. DHHS publication, 174–182.

HECTOR F. MYERS

University of California at Los Angeles
Los Angeles, California

Preface

The field of health psychology has grown rapidly in the past 20 years. This growth is largely the result of the increased incidence in the United States of chronic illnesses that are managed not only with the wisdom of the traditional biomedical model but also with unique contributions from the field of psychology. Along with the growth of health psychology, it is necessary to address the needs of members of our society that differ from the "norm" in terms of their age, gender and orientation, and ethnicity. As teachers of an undergraduate course on health psychology and as researchers with particular interests in health psychology and special populations, we created this volume because we became keenly aware of a void in the literature. Although much work has been done relating issues of age, gender and orientation, and ethnicity to health psychology, there are virtually no volumes that bring this work together. All of these research areas, however, share a common theme: To create more effective health-promoting interventions for all people, issues of age, gender and orientation, and ethnicity must be considered.

The *Handbook of Diversity Issues in Health Psychology* brings together the fields of psychology and medicine to provide a valuable resource for understanding the diverse population that exists in the United States. Experts on each issue describe the profound impact the variables of age, gender and orientation, and ethnicity have on both physical and mental health. The research of these experts shows that customized interventions that are sensitive to issues of age, gender and orientation, and ethnicity promote better health for all people.

The volume begins with a section on methodology that provides a rationale for embracing the study of heterogeneity in our population. Each of the following three parts covers one of the variables of age, gender and orientation, and ethnicity. Each part begins with a general chapter that defines relevant terms and describes ways in which people's health may differ based on that variable. Then each chapter within the sections considers the unique health problems faced by people of one particular group or, in a few cases, multiple groups (e.g., the chapters on touch therapies across the life span, on ethnicity and psychopharmacology, and on socioeconomic status and health).

The section on age shows that developmental psychologists and aging researchers can contribute to the clinical skills of pediatricians and geriatricians. The section on gender shows that attention to psychological issues faced by patients with AIDS and patients who are lesbians can improve their care and that health-promoting interventions can be more effective if researchers incorporate gender issues into their work. The section on ethnicity argues that attention to issues of ethnicity can reduce ethnic differences in health outcomes in the United States. Because only one chapter is devoted to a specific issue of diverse populations, the book can only be considered an overview of the type of work that can be done with special populations.

This book will appeal to students, teachers, and researchers of health psychology, social psychology, clinical psychology, and the psychology of gender, life-span, and ethnicity. It will be a valuable resource for doctors and medical students; nurses and nursing students; and public health workers, researchers, and policymakers.

Many people helped to make this volume possible, and we would like to thank them. First of all, we must give special thanks to Laura Carstensen, who believed in the project from the beginning and who gave us endless amounts of wisdom and help. In addition, we would like to acknowledge Al Bandura, Susan Nolen-Hoeksema, David Rosenhan, Lee Ross, Stanley Sue, and Phil Zimbardo for their invaluable advice and encouragement. We also owe Nancy Adler and G'dali Braverman a debt of gratitude for their help. We thank the following people who read and commented on various drafts: Laura Carstensen, Trudie Engel, Steve Engel, James Gross, Derek Isaacowitz, Jennifer Kelsey, Hazel Markus (and her cultural psychology lab group), Andrew Mirhej, Monisha Pasupathi, Rebecca Perkins, John Pinto, Brian Roddy, and Yuval Rottenstreich. Larry Alvarado, Robin Higashi, Kivy Rodriguez, and Phyllis Yang provided invaluable editorial help as well. The students from our health psychology classes in the summers of 1993 and 1994 at Stanford deserve thanks for questioning the existing health psychology research and prodding us to locate work that was more inclusive of people of different groups. We also must thank the anonymous reviewers who gave us important feedback on this project. And we owe enormous thanks to Eliot Werner at Plenum, who has helped us in every aspect of the project. Lastly, we would like to thank all of the contributors to this volume, not only for their interesting and informative chapters but also for the thoughtful research that they do on a daily basis.

Contents

PART II. LIFE-SPAN ISSUES IN HEALTH PSYCHOLOGY

Chapter 5. The Context of Development for Young Children from Cocaine-Abusing Families 69

Linda C. Mayes and Marc H. Bornstein

Chapter 6. The Problem of Pediatric Pain ....

Betty R. Kasson, Sandra K. Sentivany, and Pamela M. Kato

PART III. GENDER AND SEXUAL ORIENTATION ISSUES IN HEALTH PSYCHOLOGY

Chapter 10. Why Do We Need a Health Psychology of Gender or Sexual Orientation? 187

Traci Mann

Chapter 11. Smoking and Cardiovascular Disease Risk in Women: Issues for Prevention and Women's Health 199

Margaret A. Chesney and Jill B. Nealey

Chapter 12. Masculine Gender Role Stress: A Perspective on Men's Health **219**

Michael M. Copenhaver and Richard M. Eisler

PART IV. ETHNICITY ISSUES IN HEALTH PSYCHOLOGY

Chapter 15. On Nothing and Everything: The Relationship between Ethnicity and Health 287

Pamela M. Kato

Chapter 16. African-American Health over the Life Course: A Multidimensional Framework 301

James S. Jackson and Sherrill L. Sellers

Chapter 19. Behavioral Approaches to Illness Prevention for Native Americans 367

Steven Schinke

Chapter 20. A Biological, Environmental, and Cultural Basis for Ethnic Differences in Treatment 389

Michael Smith and Keh-Ming Lin

Chapter 21. Socioeconomic Status and the Health of Racial Minority Populations 407

David R. Williams and Toni Rucker

PART I

INTRODUCTION AND METHODOLOGY

CHAPTER 1

Diversity Issues in Health Psychology

TRACI MANN AND PAMELA M. KATO

As medicine and psychology join forces in the rapidly growing field of health psychology, the opportunity arises for each to benefit from the other. Research in medicine has typically focused on white males in their 30s, while research in psychology has focused on upper-middle-class college sophomores. Both approaches tend to neglect issues of populations that differ from these norms by age, gender, sexual orientation, or ethnicity in the United States. The aim of this book is to bring together the work of physicians, nurses, epidemiologists, sociologists, social workers, and psychologists who specialize in these populations so that we can learn how to approach these issues in research and clinical practice.

Health psychology focuses on psychological and behavioral factors related to health maintenance, disease prevention, and treatment of illness. Because different groups of people may have different health problems, people of different ages, genders, sexual orientations, and ethnic groups need to be included in research and investigated separately. We need to learn which behaviors specific to a certain group put members of that group at risk for illness. We need to learn how characteristics of certain groups or stereotypes about members of these groups lead them

TRACI MANN • Health Risk Reduction Projects, UCLA Neuropsychiatric Institute, 10920 Wilshire Boulevard, Suite 1103, Los Angeles, California 90024.   PAMELA M. KATO • Department of Psychiatry and Behavioral Science, Stanford University School of Medicine, Stanford, California 94305.

Handbook of Diversity Issues in Health Psychology, edited by Pamela M. Kato and Traci Mann. Plenum Press, New York, 1996.

to be misunderstood by the medical community, resulting in the mismanagement of their health care. We also need to learn about the different pressures faced by members of these groups and the ways in which these pressures impact their health.

In order to incorporate diversity issues, health psychology must focus on groups that differ from the norm and that have traditionally been excluded from mainstream research on health psychology. In some cases, findings from mainstream research are overgeneralized to members of these groups. For example, the medical community once believed that females had abnormally low levels of blood sugar. In actuality, the levels only seemed abnormally low because females were not included in the samples researchers used to determine "normal" blood sugar levels. In terms of blood sugar levels, then, research on males cannot be accurately generalized to females (Tavris, 1992). In other cases, researchers assume that differences between members of particular groups and members of the majority group are much larger than they actually are. For example, it is often thought that as people age they suffer inevitable and irreversible declines in muscle tone. One study, however, found that resistance weight training among elderly volunteers led to significant gains in muscle tone (Fiatarone et al., 1994; see Levy & Langer in this volume for a more complete description of the study).

If our research samples are not adequately diverse, we are in danger of coming to false conclusions about particular groups and subsequently providing them with ineffective health care interventions. The goal of focusing on diversity issues in health psychology is to find ways to provide effective health care for all people. In this chapter, we first describe ways in which certain populations have been marginalized. We then talk about shifting conceptions of health and how psychological variables can affect health. In the next part of the chapter, we describe some health differences between people of various groups and propose psychological explanations for them. We conclude this chapter by describing the risks and benefits of acknowledging diversity issues in health psychology.

MARGINALIZING POPULATIONS

There are two main ways in which populations have been marginalized: (1) They have not been included in samples, or (2) they have been included in samples, but data have not been analyzed separately for each group. We will examine these methods in turn.

Some researchers set up inclusion and exclusion criteria that specifically exclude certain age, gender, sexual orientation, or ethnic groups. The rationale for this practice is to have more "control" over the outcomes in the study. Researchers fear that including both males and females or people of numerous ethnic groups or age categories will add extra variability—extra "noise"—to the questions being studied. This fear is what Kraemer calls "fear of heterogeneity" (Kraemer, this volume). Since all populations are heterogeneous, we need to include heterogeneous populations in our initial research and then focus on the sources of heterogeneity in follow-up research. We will ultimately have more control over our outcomes by uncovering the ways in which they are heterogeneous in the first place.

Populations may also be inadequately represented in studies because of recruitment problems. Members of some groups are difficult to locate and thus difficult to include in studies. Researchers at large universities and medical centers often must recruit subjects from among their own population, which may not be diverse. People of low socioeconomic status (SES) groups may not read newspapers, and therefore may not see advertisements for subjects, or may not have phones to receive random recruitment calls.

Even when members of these groups are located, they do not necessarily participate in research. For example, publicized incidents of unethical research involving some ethnic groups may make members of these groups hesitant to participate (Jones, 1993). People who work at an hourly wage may not wish to take time off without pay to participate in research or may not be able to get permission to do so. Women are often caretakers of young children and the elderly and may not be able to participate in research unless special provisions are made. Adolescents, particularly those living in poverty, may lead chaotic lives in which participation in a longitudinal study is not a priority. Finally, language barriers may keep members of some ethnic groups from participating in studies.

In many studies, members of a variety of populations are included in samples, but the different populations are still not studied. Sometimes this occurs because researchers do not adequately assess or report the characteristics of the sample. Differential outcomes based on group membership therefore cannot be examined, even though members of diverse populations were included in the research. If characteristics of the sample are not assessed and reported, readers may falsely conclude that the sample is homogeneous.

At other times, researchers include diverse populations in their samples, and do adequately report the characteristics of their samples, but still fail to analyze and report differences between these diverse groups of people. Researchers often fail to analyze these differences because they do not have a large enough sample or adequate power to examine age, sex, or ethnicity differences in their study design. However, if researchers include diverse populations in their samples but fail to analyze the outcomes by group membership, we learn nothing about these groups and nothing about whatever group the researchers are considering the norm.

When researchers fail to plan for, analyze, and report these differences, we do not learn whether it is necessary to address the needs of one group differently from that of another or whether the same intervention will be effective for all groups.

SHIFTING CONCEPTIONS OF HEALTH

Conceptions of health have been changing over the last 20 years (Engel, 1977). The biomedical model, which still prevails in the field of medicine, reduces health and disease to the basic components of organs and biochemicals. According to this model, health is the absence of disease, and disease, in turn, is a biochemical imbalance of bodily functions, the presence of faulty organs, or the presence of harmful pathogens. In order to rid the body of the state of disease, doctors create a biochemical balance of bodily functions by treating the organs that caused the biochemical imbalance or by removing the pathogens from the body.

Pneumonia, tuberculosis, and influenza were the leading causes of death in 1900. The biomedical model was so effective in addressing those illnesses (and others like them) that it is rare today for people to die of them. Life expectancy has grown since that time from approximately 50 years in 1900 to more than 70 years today.

The biomedical model, however, does not adequately explain how to treat or prevent the diseases that people most frequently die of today. Today, the leading causes of death are chronic illnesses: cardiovascular disease, cancer, and stroke. Instead of striking suddenly, these diseases are characterized by a slow accumulation of damage, often brought about by lifestyle factors. Medications and surgical procedures are not always sufficient to cure these diseases, and treatment often requires a change in lifestyle in addition to medication or surgery. In addition, treatment may take many months and have psychologically and physically unpleasant side effects. The biomedical model is inadequate because it fails to address the psychological aspects of modern illnesses.

To be successfully treated for these diseases, patients need to learn techniques to help them comply with their treatment schedules, as well as coping behaviors that can help them to endure the pain of their treatments, as well as methods for changing their lifestyles. The biomedical model does not stress the importance of these behaviors. In addition, heart disease, cancer, and stroke are largely preventable by changing the behaviors of high-risk people. In fact, in one study of ischemic heart disease (Rothenberg, Ford, & Vartiainen, 1992), researchers found that positive health behaviors, such as reducing cholesterol intake and cigarette smoking, accounted for a greater decline in heart disease mortality than did medical interventions (e.g., prehospital resuscitation and care, coronary artery bypass surgery). Since the focus of the biomedical model is on organ systems and biochemicals, it does not stress the importance of health behaviors.

Techniques for treating heart disease, for example, illustrate the shortcomings of the biomedical model. Prevention goals include lowering lipid profiles, decreasing obesity, and controlling hypertension. These preventive treatments require behavior changes that are difficult to accomplish, such as following complex medication schedules, quitting smoking, and exercising.

A diagnosis of heart disease also includes conferral of a stigma. Patients often first notice the stigma when they learn that their insurance status has changed. They also have to cope with families that take a patronizing nursing attitude toward them. In addition, heart disease patients often become "cardiac cripples," afraid to engage in strenuous activities, including regular exercise, for fear of inducing a heart attack. Dealing with all of these psychological issues is a part of being treated for heart disease; however, the biomedical model does not include them.

As it has become increasingly clear that the biomedical model is inadequate for the diseases we are faced with today, the biopsychosocial model has emerged (Engel, 1977). The biopsychosocial model acknowledges biological disease processes of disordered cells and chemical imbalances, but it also emphasizes psychosocial factors that determine the presence or absence of illness. The psychosocial factors include social support, lifestyle, and cognitive processes. According to a biopsychosocial definition of health, health is compromised not only when people have identifiable illnesses but also when they have symptoms that compromise their overall well-being. The biopsychosocial model, then, would require patients to cope with the stigma associated with their illness, make the necessary lifestyle changes to prevent further problems, and cope with the other stresses associated with being ill. In the next section, we discuss some of the psychosocial factors that affect health and describe how they might account for health differences between people of different groups.

PSYCHOLOGICAL EXPLANATIONS FOR DIFFERENCES IN GROUP HEALTH

Psychological variables can explain many differences in health between groups, and therefore it is not always necessary to point to biological distinctions between people of different ages, ethnic groups, or genders to explain the health differences between them. For example, health can be significantly impacted by whether people use the medical system, by the stress associated with social roles and by the practice of high-risk behaviors. These types of explanations for health differences between groups will be examined in turn.

Use of the Medical System

People vary in their use of the medical system in terms of whether they are willing to see physicians when necessary, whether they are able to see physicians when necessary, and, if they see physicians, whether they comply with recommendations that are made. Beliefs or biases within the medical community may also affect adequate health care delivery to diverse populations. These factors play an important role in determining people's health.

Whether or not sick people go to the doctor is based partly on whether they are willing to consider themselves sick. It may be more socially acceptable for some people to accept the sick role than for other people to do so. For instance, the sick role is more compatible with traditional female gender roles than with male roles, so females may feel less constrained than males in defining and reporting mild symptoms as illness (Marcus & Seeman, 1981). Masculine gender role proscriptions, on the other hand, are contrary to the requirements of health maintenance (David & Skidmore, 1976). Even routine medical visits may threaten males who adhere to masculine gender roles. They may have to disclose intimate feelings, give up control to a doctor, reveal their vulnerabilities, or depend on others for their care.

In general, females seek medical care more than males do. Once females become sexually active, they tend to have yearly gynecologic checkups. There is no such yearly doctor visit for males. Even if gynecologic visits are not counted, however, females still go to the doctor more than males (Verbrugge, 1989). If females have young children, they are particularly likely to see doctors, since they tend to see the pediatrician one or more times a year for the child's health. During these visits, the mother's health may also be attended to, which may result in medical advice, direct medical care, or referrals to other physicians.

Another reason why some people are unwilling to see a doctor is because they do not feel comfortable with doctors. Patients who do not speak English have trouble being understood and understanding doctors. Physicians may not take the health complaints of Asian patients seriously because of the stereotype that when Asian patients have psychological symptoms, they tend to describe them as physical symptoms. Homosexuals may feel uncomfortable with doctors because they feel stigmatized by the medical community (Kass, Faden, Fox, & Dudley, 1992). Finally, elderly patients may feel uncomfortable because physicians treat them like young children (Greene, Adelman, Charon, & Hoffman, 1986).

Compliance with doctors' orders is crucial in dealing with the illnesses that are common today. Whether doctors recommend bed rest, a change in diet, or medication, adhering to the recommendations is important for recovery. Compliance with doctors does not seem to be related to ethnic group, although it has been shown to increase with age (Daniels, Rene, & Daniels, 1994).

Many patients who are willing to see a doctor are simply not able to see one. Females are less likely to have insurance than males, especially if they are unemployed or single. Lesbians are less likely to have insurance than heterosexual females, partly because, compared to heterosexual females, they are more likely to be unemployed, and partly because they do not have access to a spouse's insurance. Mexican-Americans are less likely to be insured than any other ethnic group. Native Americans, on the other hand, see doctors more than any other group (including whites), most likely because of their access to health insurance (National Center for Health Statistics [NCHS], 1991).

The ability to see a doctor impacts health particularly in terms of prenatal care. Asians and Caucasians have more access to prenatal care than African-Americans and Mexican-Americans. Not surprisingly, Caucasians and Asians show better outcomes on measures of infant birth weight, infant mortality rates, and even death rates than African-Americans and Hispanics (NCHS, 1991). These differences are probably not based on ethnic group per se, but rather on the availability of prenatal care.

Stress and Roles

The negative effects of stress on virtually every system of the body are well documented (see, for an overview, Sapolsky, 1994). If people of any particular group have more stress than people of other groups, then their health will be correspondingly compromised. Does stress vary by age, gender, orientation, or ethnicity? This question is difficult to answer, partly because the stresses associated with gender roles, minority status, and age are hard to measure and partly because these stresses are chronic rather than acute. We can only surmise that stress plays a role in the health differences between groups.

According to research on the concept of masculine gender role stress, males will find situations more stressful than females when the imperatives of the male role are beyond their coping abilities and when they perceive the coping behaviors required of a situation as "unmanly" or "feminine" (Eisler, 1990). Other research, however, points to the stresses females encounter when either filling a traditional female gender role by being a homemaker (Gove, 1972) or coping with the multiple demands of combining work and a family (Wortman, Biernat, & Lang, 1991).

When stressed, females are more likely than males to mobilize social support (Belle, 1991). They are more likely to seek out support, receive support, and to be pleased with the support they receive (Belle, 1991). Males under stress, on the other hand, are more likely to engage in behaviors that put their health at risk, such as drinking alcohol or using drugs (Eisler, Skidmore, & Ward, 1988).

The stress of being a member of a minority group may negatively affect health. While being a target of racism puts people at increased risk for poor health, other factors, such as group identity, spirituality, and kinship ties, may buffer these risks (Barbarin, 1993). Some of the impact of minority status on health disappears when researchers control for SES. (Kessler & Neighbors, 1986). SES, however, cannot always be used as a proxy for ethnicity (Williams, 1990), as important differences still exist between ethnic groups even after controlling for SES.

The techniques that adolescent males and females use to cope with stress are similar to those employed by adult males and females (Frydenberg & Lewis, 1993). If adolescents do engage in maladaptive coping habits, however, continuing these habits throughout their lives will be particularly detrimental. In old age, these people will then be left to deal with the consequences of a lifetime of maladaptive coping habits.

Risk Factors

Lifestyle factors such as cigarette smoking, drug and alcohol use, diet, and exercise have an enormous impact on the health of all people (Hamburg, Elliot, & Parron, 1982). Groups will differ in health to the extent that they differ in the practice of these behaviors. If these behaviors explain group differences, interventions that focus on modifying these behaviors may help improve the health of certain groups. This is not to suggest that we can improve the health of all groups merely by intervening at the behavioral level. All of these behavioral interventions should be implemented in conjunction with regular medical interventions.

Cigarette Smoking. Smoking is a significant risk factor for cancer of the lung, larynx, oral cavity, and esophagus, and it contributes to cancer of the kidney, urinary bladder, and pancreas (Department of Health and Human Services [DHHS], 1982). Smoking is also related to the development of cardiovascular diseases (DHHS, 1984). Males smoke more than females, but male rates are decreasing over time, while female rates are increasing (Chesney, 1991). Female smoking rates may be increasing because of a shift in social norms portraying female smokers as glamorous and independent (Gilchrist, Schinke, & Nurius, 1989). In addition, Asians smoke less (NCHS, 1991) and Native Americans and African-Americans smoke more than members of other ethnic groups (Beauvais & LaBoueff, 1985). For Native Americans, tobacco use has cultural meanings, which may partially explain the high levels of smoking for members of that group (Weibel-Orlando, 1985).

Alcohol Use. Alcohol affects numerous areas of the body. Since it is distributed by the bloodstream, it does most of its damage to organs with the highest rates of circulation, as well as to highly specialized organs.

Thus the brain, liver, peripheral nerves, pancreas, and endocrine glands show early and serious impairment from alcohol (Selzer, 1980). Alcohol is metabolized mostly in the liver, and cirrhosis of the liver is commonly associated with heavy alcohol use. Cirrhosis of the liver is the ninth leading cause of death in the United States (NCHS, 1991). When broken down by gender and ethnicity, however, the story changes somewhat. Males are more likely to abuse alcohol than females. For females of most ethnic groups, cirrhosis of the liver is not one of the top ten causes of death. For Native American females, however, cirrhosis is the sixth leading cause of death (NCHS, 1991). In fact, the rate of alcohol abuse and alcohol-related illness is higher in Native Americans than in any other ethnic group (May, 1989). Asians have a particularly low incidence of alcoholism, possibly due to a deficiency in one of the enzymes that metabolizes alcohol, making the digestion of alcohol more difficult for them (Mendoza, Smith, Poland, Lin, & Strickland, 1991).

Diet. The typical American diet is associated with obesity, heart disease, cancer, and cerebrovascular diseases (Sheridan & Radmacher, 1992). In general, it is too high in calories, fat, cholesterol, sugar, protein, and sodium. A diet that is low in fat can help reduce the risk of cancer of the breast, colon, rectum, and prostate, as well as the risk of heart disease and stroke. While the American Cancer Society and the American Heart Association recommend limiting fat calories to 30%, Americans consume about 44% of their calories from fat.

A diet high in fiber can help prevent cancer of the rectum and colon by providing roughage that prevents constipation (Anderson, Smith, & Gustofson, 1994). Some fibers have even been found to shrink polyps in the colon (Raub, 1989). Soluble fibers dissolve in water and absorb fat and are important in preventing heart disease and some cancers. A diet with protein within an acceptable range can help prevent osteoporosis (Schaafsma, 1992) and gout (Star & Hochberg, 1993). Obesity is more prevalent in African-Americans than in Caucasians and more prevalent in African-American females than African-American males (Rand & Kuldau, 1990), placing African-American females at high risk for diabetes, heart disease, and hypertension. In addition, obesity is also more prevalent in Hispanics than in Caucasians (Furukawa & Harris, 1986). Finally, the prevalence of obesity is lowest among the youngest and oldest people and highest among middle-aged people (Rand & Kuldau, 1990).

Exercise. Regular exercise can result in enhanced cardiovascular fitness by decreasing resting heart rate and increasing maximum oxygen consumption (Haskell, 1984). Exercise is associated with reduced risk for heart attacks (Paffenbarger, Hyde, Wing, & Steinmetz, 1984), lower cholesterol levels, and a trend toward increases in bone mineral content among those at risk for bone fractures (Blumenthal et al., 1989). Only 15%

of adults in the United States participate in a regular exercise program that results in a health-enhancing energy expenditure (Oldridge, 1984). In general, Caucasians exercise more than people of other ethnic groups, although this phenomenon may have more to do with socioeconomic status than with ethnicity (Fitzgerald, Singleton, Neale, & Prasad, 1994). The lack of exercise among the elderly is strongly related to illness and mortality (Kaplan, Seeman, Cohen, Knudsen, & Guralnik, 1987).

RISKS AND BENEFITS OF ACKNOWLEDGING DIVERSITY ISSUES IN HEALTH PSYCHOLOGY

Possible Negative Consequences of Studying Group Differences

Acknowledging diversity issues in health psychology has the potential to bring enormous rewards. There are, however, several risks to the undertaking. Focusing on differences between groups can have several negative consequences if it is not done carefully and by sensitive researchers. Studying differences between groups can (1) lead to negative generalizations about groups, and (2) mask the heterogeneity that exists within groups. These two types of risks will be examined in turn.

When researchers look at differences between groups, they may find differences they would rather not know about. Revealing these differences may serve to stigmatize members of one or the other of the groups. For instance, suppose research revealed that females got ulcers more often than males did. This information could be used by people as evidence that females are physically weaker than males—that their bodies are less able to fight off the pathogens that cause ulcers. This information could also be used to argue that women are psychologically weaker than males—that they are unable to cope with stress in healthy ways or that they cannot handle the same problems that males handle. While it is true that this difference can be used to make a case about gender and weakness, it is also possible to use this difference to argue about the pressures that society places on people of different groups. Perhaps the role of being female is more stressful than the role of being male. It could also be argued that females are more likely to be living in poverty, so they are more susceptible to all kinds of stress-related illnesses.

The point being made here should be clear: For any one difference between groups, multiple explanations can be proposed. Some explanations will stigmatize the group; some will not. Some explanations will be based on biology, some will be based on psychology, and still others will be based on an interaction between the two. The cause of the difference will be important only to the extent that it can help lead to an effective solution to the problem. In the case of ulcers, effective interventions may or may not be based on any of the above explanations, but these interventions cannot be designed at all unless the difference is discovered. Researchers should not use differences to stigmatize groups, nor should they use differences to praise groups. Instead, researchers should simply use the knowledge of differences as a way to better target interventions and thereby promote health for all people. As expressed by Sandra Scarr, "There should be no qualms about the forthright study of racial and gender differences; science is in desperate need of good studies that highlight race and gender variables, unabashedly, to inform us of what we need to do to help underrepresented people to succeed in this society" (Scarr, 1988, p. 56).

The second type of risk that comes from focusing on differences between groups is that this focus may cause researchers to ignore, or to forget, the differences that exist within groups. Returning to the ulcer example, we need to remember that even if women are more likely to get ulcers than men, not all women are equally likely to get ulcers nor is any particular woman more likely to get an ulcer than any particular man. The existence of a group difference does not say anything about the difference between any two individuals.

As researchers study a specific population, they must keep in mind that not all members of the population have that particular health problem or are at risk for it. In many cases, membership in a particular population is only a proxy indicator of a particular risk factor. For instance, although it cannot be stated conclusively, lesbians appear to be more likely to have breast cancer than heterosexual women (O'Hanlan, this volume). This difference is most likely due to differences between lesbians and heterosexual women on another variable: whether or not they have carried a pregnancy to term, as nulliparous females are at higher risk for breast cancer than parous females (Kvale, Heuch, & Nilssen, 1994). While many lesbians have carried a pregnancy to term, as a group they are less likely to have done so than heterosexual women. In sum, being a lesbian is only a proxy indicator of being at risk for breast cancer.

Interventions that target people with a particular risk factor (e.g., women who have never been pregnant) will be more effective than interventions that target a particular population (e.g., lesbians) because not all members of that population will have the risk factor. Membership in the population is only a proxy indicator for the risk factor, and it is not as precise an indicator as the actual circumstance. The proxy indicator, however, is usually the only information that health promotion workers have. It is much more difficult to locate, for example, all 40-year-old women who have never been pregnant than to simply target the lesbian community for interventions designed to increase mammogram use.

When it is relatively easy to target a set of people with a particular risk factor, doing so is clearly the best way to proceed, but this option is not always available. In many cases, the circumstance that leads to a health problem is unknown, and the only information researchers have is the group difference. Studying diverse populations is simply an easy way to target groups of people that are at higher risk for a health problem than the population in general. In addition, identifying group differences may help researchers pinpoint risk factors, which may then lead to further understanding of the health problem. The result will be the creation of more effective interventions to treat and prevent the problem.

Benefits of Studying Group Differences

The potential rewards from studying group differences in health psychology can easily outweigh the risks, particularly if researchers are sensitive to the groups they are studying. One reason to study groups separately is to gain detailed knowledge about those groups. The groups considered in this volume are understudied, and a health psychology that acknowledges diversity can serve them by uncovering valuable information about them. In the past, even when members of these groups were included in research samples, the results were not frequently analyzed based on group membership. We are, therefore, faced with a scarcity of information about the health of various groups of people.

Knowledge about the health and health behaviors of a variety of different groups can help to dispel generalizations about these groups by clarifying societal causes for certain health problems. For example, the notion that homosexuals abuse alcohol more than heterosexuals could lead to negative generalizations about homosexuals. However, the knowledge that bars are virtually the only acceptable social outlets for homosexuals should help to explain why homosexuals drink. The enormous stress placed on homosexuals by a society that discriminates against them can also help to explain why homosexuals drink. These facts should lead to fewer negative generalizations about homosexuals rather than to more generalizations.

If data are collected on a large group of people—combined across various groups—and then analyzed without looking at the groups separately, the results will not be valid for anybody. For example, suppose a researcher does a study to see if a social support intervention helps cancer patients live longer. The researcher compares patients who were randomly assigned to attend support groups to patients who were randomly assigned to a no-intervention control group and finds that there is no difference between the two groups. The researcher concludes that social support interventions do not help. However, since there are both male and female patients in the study, another researcher decides to analyze the results by gender. When analyzed this way, the hypothetical data reveal that females in the social support condition lived longer than females in the control condition but that males show the opposite effect:

Males in the control condition live longer than males in the social support condition. The researchers hypothesized that the social support condition promoted stress for males but reduced stress for females. When the results are analyzed without taking gender into account, the conclusion (that the intervention has no effects) is not valid for males or for females.

Perhaps the most important reason to study diverse populations is to create interventions that are expressly tailored to particular groups. As virtually every chapter in this book demonstrates, targeted interventions are more effective than nontargeted interventions. Continuing with our hypothetical social support and cancer example, social support will make an appropriate intervention for female cancer patients, but not for male patients. Without analyzing the data for the two groups separately, researchers would not be able to create effective interventions for cancer patients.

A real example of the importance of targeting interventions to specific groups involves Native Americans and smoking. Native Americans are at high risk for smoking-related illnesses, but prevention strategies that are effective in the general population have not been successful with Native Americans (Schinke, this volume). Part of the reason for this problem is that tobacco use has a spiritual meaning among Native Americans and is associated with positive attributes in some tribes. In addition, among Native Americans tobacco use is considered a rite of passage into adulthood, and refusing tobacco is seen as rude and confrontational (Schinke, this volume). Clearly, an intervention targeted at Native Americans, which takes into account these cultural issues, will be most effective with this population.

This volume is a first attempt to integrate research on the health psychology of diverse populations. Because it is a first attempt, it cannot include every issue that is relevant to every group. For example, we have not included research on middle-aged people, on the Nepalese, or on people of various religious groups. We believe, however, that one must begin the process of inclusion somewhere. We have chosen age, gender, and ethnicity because they are common dimensions in which group differences are often found in important health variables and because traditional research commonly ignores them. In this volume we provide examples of the kinds of research that can be done, and the kinds of interventions that can be devised, when studying diverse populations. We intend this book to be the first of many attempts to understand and include groups that mainstream research has traditionally ignored.

REFERENCES

Anderson, J. W., Smith, B. M., & Gustofson, N. J. (1994). Health benefits and practical aspects of high-fiber diets. *Journal of Clinical Nutrition, 59,* 1242S–1247S.

Barbarin, O. (1993). Emotional and social development of African American children. *Journal of Black Psychology, 19,* 381–390.

Beauvais, F., & LaBoueff, S. (1985). Drug and alcohol abuse intervention in American Indian communities. *International Journal of the Addictions, 20,* 139–171.

Belle, D. (1991). Gender differences in the social moderators of stress. In A. Monat & R. Lazarus (Eds.), *Stress and coping* (pp. 258–274). New York: Columbia University Press.

Blumenthal, J. A., Emery, C. F., Madden, D. J., Geouge, L. K., Coleman, R. E., Riddle, M. W., McKee, D. C., Reasoner, J., & Williams, R. S. (1989). Cardiovascular and behavioral effects of aerobic exercise training in healthy older men and women. *Journal of Gerontology, 44,* M147–M1157.

Chesney, M. (1991). Women, work-related stress, and smoking. In M. Frankenhaeuser, U. Lundberg, & M. Chesney (Eds.), *Women, work, and health* (pp. 139–155). New York: Plenum Press.

Daniels, D., Rene, A., & Daniels, V. (1994). Race: An explanation of patient compliance: Fact or fiction? *Journal of the National Medical Association, 86,* 20–25.

David, D. S., & Skidmore, J. R. (1976). *The forty-nine percent majority: The male sex role.* Reading, MA: Addison-Wesley.

Department of Health and Human Services. (1982). *The health consequences of smoking— Cancer, a report of the surgeon general* (DHHS Publication No. PHS 82-50179). Washington, DC: U.S. Government Printing Office.

Department of Health and Human Services. (1984). *The health consequences of smoking— Cardiovascular disease, a report to the surgeon general* (DHHS Publication No. PHS 84-50204). Washington, DC: U.S. Government Printing Office.

Eisler, R. M. (1990). Gender role issues in the treatment of men. *The Behavior Therapist, March,* 57–60.

Eisler, R. M., Skidmore, J. R., & Ward, C. H. (1988). Masculine gender role stress: Predictor of anger, anxiety, and health-risk behaviors. *Journal of Personality Assessment, 52,* 133–141.

Engel, G. (1977). The need for a new medical model: A challenge for biomedicine. *Science, 196,* 129–136.

Fiatarone, M., O'Neill, E., Ryan, N., Clements, K., Solares, G., Nelson, M., Roberts, S., Kehayias, J., Lipsitz, P., & Evans, L. (1994). Exercise training and nutritional supplementation for physical frailty in very elderly people. *New England Journal of Medicine, 330,* 1769–1775.

Fitzgerald, J., Singleton, S., Neale, A., & Prasad, A. (1994). Activity levels, fitness status, exercise knowledge, and exercise beliefs among healthy, older African American and white women. *Journal of Aging and Health, 6,* 296–313.

Frydenberg, E., & Lewis, R. (1993). Boys play sport and girls turn to others: Age, gender, and ethnicity as determinants of coping. *Journal of Adolescence, 16,* 253–266.

Furukawa, C., & Harris, M. (1986). Some correlates of obesity in the elderly: Hereditary and environmental factors. *Journal of Obesity and Weight Regulation, 5,* 55–76.

Gilchrist, L., Schinke, S., & Nurius, P. (1989). Reducing onset of habitual smoking among women. *Preventative Medicine, 18,* 235–248.

Gove, W. (1972). The relationship between sex roles, marital status, and mental illness. *Social Forces, 51,* 34–44.

Greene, M., Adelman, R., Charon, R., & Hoffman, S. (1986). Ageism in the medical encounter: An exploratory study of the doctor-elderly patient relationship. *Language and Communication, 6,* 113–124.

Hamburg, D., Elliot, G., & Parron, D. (1982). *Health and behavior: Frontiers of research in the biobehavioral sciences.* Washington, DC: National Academy Press.

Haskell, W. L. (1984). Overview: Health benefits of exercise. In J. D. Matarazzo, S. M. Weiss, J. A. Herd, N. E. Miller, & S. M. Weiss (Eds.), *Behavioral health: A handbook of health enhancement and disease prevention* (pp. 490–423). New York: John Wiley & Sons.

Jones, J. (1993). *Bad blood: The Tuskegee syphilis experiment* (New and expanded ed.). New York: Free Press.

Kaplan, G., Seeman, T., Cohen, R., Knudsen, L., & Guralnik, J. (1987). Mortality among the elderly in the Alameda County study: Behavioral and demographic risk factors. *American Journal of Public Health, 77*, 307–312.

Kass, N., Faden, R., Fox, R., & Dudley, J. (1992). Homosexual and bisexual men's perceptions of discrimination in health services. *American Journal of Public Health, 82*, 1277–1279.

Kessler, R., & Neighbors, H. (1986). A new perspective on the relationships among race, social class, and psychological distress. *Journal of Health and Social Behavior, 27*, 107–115.

Kessler, R., Price, R., & Wortman, C. (1985). Social factors in psychopathology: Stress, social support, and coping processes. *Annual Review of Psychology, 36*, 531–572.

Kvale, G., Heuch, I., & Nilssen, S. (1994). Parity in relation to mortality and cancer incidence: A prospective study of Norwegian women. *International Journal of Epidemiology, 23*, 691–699.

Marcus, A. C., & Seeman, T. E. (1981). Sex differences in reports of illness and disability: A preliminary test of the "Fixed Role Obligations" hypothesis. *Journal of Health and Social Behavior, 22*, 174–182.

May, P. (1989). Alcohol abuse and alcoholism among American Indians: An overview. In T. Watts & R. Wright (Eds.), *Alcoholism in minority populations*. Springfield, IL: Charles C. Thomas.

Mendoza, R., Smith, M., Poland, R., Lin, K., & Strickland, T. (1991). Ethnic psychopharmacology: The Hispanic and Native American perspective. *Psychopharmacology Bulletin, 27*, 449–461.

National Center for Health Statistics. (1991). *Health, United States, 1990*. Hyattsville, MD: Public Health Service.

Oldridge, N. B. (1984). Adherence to adult exercise fitness programs. In J. D. Matarazzo, S. M. Weiss, J. A. Herd, N. E. Miller, & S. M. Weiss (Eds.), *Behavioral health: A handbook of health enhancement and disease prevention* (pp. 467–487). New York: John Wiley & Sons.

Paffenbarger, R., Hyde, R. T., Wing, A. L., & Steinmetz, C. H. (1984). A natural history of athleticism and cardiovascular health. *Journal of the American Medical Association, 222*, 491–495.

Rand, C., & Kuldau, J. (1990). The epidemiology of obesity and self-defined weight problem in the general population: Gender, race, age, and social class. *International Journal of Eating Disorders, 9*, 329–343.

Raub, W. (1989). High-fiber diet may inhibit large bowel neoplasia. *Journal of the American Medical Association, 262*, 2359.

Rothenberg, R., Ford, E., & Vartiainen, E. (1992). Ischemic heart disease prevention: Estimating the impact of interventions. *Journal of Clinical Epidemiology, 45*, 21–29.

Sapolsky, R. (1994). *Why zebras don't get ulcers*. New York: W.H. Freeman.

Scarr, S. (1988). Race and gender as psychological variables: Social and ethical issues. *American Psychologist, 43*, 56–59.

Schaafsma, G. (1992). The scientific basis of recommended dietary allowances for calcium. *Journal of Internal Medicine, 231*, 187–194.

Selzer, M. (1980). Alcoholism and alcoholic psychoses. In H. I. Kaplan, A. M. Freedman, & B. L. Sadock (Eds.), *Comprehensive textbook of psychiatry/III* (Vol. 2, pp. 1629–1644). Baltimore: Williams and Wilkins.

Sheridan, C. L., & Radmacher, S. A. (1992). *Health psychology: Challenging the biomedical model*. New York: John Wiley & Sons.

Star, V., & Hochberg, M. C. (1993). Prevention and managment of gout. *Drugs, 45*, 212–222.

Tavris, C. (1992). *The mismeasure of woman*. New York: Simon and Schuster.

Verbrugge, L. (1989). The twain meet: Empirical explanations of sex differences in health and mortality. *Journal of Health and Social Behavior, 30*, 282–304.

Weibel-Orlando, J. (1985). Indians, ethnicity, and alcohol: Contrasting perceptions of the ethnic self and alcohol use. In L. A. Bennett & G. M. Ames (Eds.), *The American experience with alcohol* (pp. 201–226). New York: Plenum Press.

Williams, D. (1990). Socioeconomic differentials in health: A review and redirection. *Social Psychology Quarterly, 53,* 81–99.

Wortman, C., Biernat, M., & Lang, E. (1991). Coping with role overload. In M. Frankenhaeuser, U. Lundberg, & M. Chesney (Eds.), *Women, work, and health* (pp. 85–110). New York: Plenum Press.

CHAPTER 2

Fear of Heterogeneity in the Study of Human Populations and the Statistical Artifacts It Produces

HELENA CHMURA KRAEMER

INTRODUCTION

There are few absolute statements worth risking in characterizing bio-behavioral research with living human populations. One exception might be: Whatever the population, whatever the response, living human populations are heterogeneous.

Populations comprise male and female subjects whose responses are not uniform. Subjects of either gender are likely to differ from each other in age, and frequently responses are age dependent. The trajectories of age-related changes may well be different for male and female subjects. To focus on a single age of assessment, say female subjects who are 25 years old, does not solve the problem of heterogeneity, for females born in 1940 might well respond quite differently at the age of 25 from females born in 1950, 1960, or 1970. Birth cohorts may have very different life

HELENA CHMURA KRAEMER • Department of Psychiatry and Behavioral Sciences, Stanford University School of Medicine, Stanford, California 94305.

Handbook of Diversity Issues in Health Psychology, edited by Pamela M. Kato and Traci Mann. Plenum Press, New York, 1996.

experiences that may induce heterogeneity of response, even among age- and gender-matched subjects.

Many other factors may influence response. These factors may include the ethnic or racial group of the subjects, the strength of the connection to that ethnic or racial group subjects feel, the socioeconomic class to which they belong, the area of the country in which they live. These are only a few factors that may each singly or in combination influence subjects' responses.

In addition to the age, gender, or ethnicity of subjects that might influence responses, characteristics of the assessor can often influence the subjects' responses as well. Human assessors differ from each other in gender, age, birth cohort, ethnic background, socioeconomic class, and all the other variables that produce heterogeneity in subjects. When multiple assessors evaluate the same subject, interassessor variability frequently reflects heterogeneity among human assessors.

The combination of heterogeneity of human subjects with heterogeneity of human assessors makes it a safe bet that in any research study of a sample of subjects from a human population—no matter how restrictive the inclusion and exclusion criteria, no matter how well trained the assessors—one may expect heterogeneity of response.

This situation is disquieting, perhaps even frightening, to scientists who wish to study human populations. In hard science, scientists "control" sources of heterogeneity: temperature, time, size, and other factors that might produce heterogeneity in the results or in the replications of an experiment. They achieve control by standardizing or systematically varying sources of heterogeneity. Scientists who do not design and execute their experiments to control such factors are, we are early taught, sloppy. Their results will likely not be reproducible by other scientists and thus not highly regarded as science.

In mathematics, one "assumes" away sources of heterogeneity. One assumes that one leg of the triangle is exactly equal to another, that observations in a population are normally distributed with equal variance, and so on. The results of a mathematical proof are based on these assumptions. When the assumptions do not hold, the mathematical proof does not hold as well. In mathematics, there is no limit on what one can and cannot assume. What is important is that assumptions are explicit and that the inductive or deductive process leading from assumptions to conclusions (the proof) is done properly.

When a mathematical theorem is applied in hard science, what is assumed in the mathematics must correspond to what is controlled in the laboratory in order that the deductive or inductive process of the mathematics can then produce valid and reproducible conclusions.

In the following section, we discuss the ways that scientists studying human populations often try to mimic these approaches.

Control the Sources of Heterogeneity by Very Restrictive Inclusion and Exclusion Criteria

A study of coronary artery disease might sample only men between 40 and 50 years of age who are white and are receiving health care from a certain tertiary care facility. Such a strategy, however, cannot succeed in removing all the sources of heterogeneity. Even men so selected might differ in terms of fitness, diet, and family history, all of which may influence coronary artery disease. Nevertheless, such a strategy does succeed in limiting the generalizability of any results. Whether the results of such a study apply to women, to men at other ages, to men of other ethnic or socioeconomic groups, to men from other geographical areas, or to men receiving health care from primary health care facilities cannot be assured.

Until quite recently, FDA trials of efficacy and safety of drugs tended to exclude females, ostensibly for safety reasons. As a result, it is not clear whether many drugs currently widely prescribed for females have ever been adequately evaluated for efficacy and safety for women.

Similarly, studies of efficacy, effectiveness, and safety of drug treatments often include subjects with only one disorder, the "pure" group with no comorbidity. In many situations, particularly with older subjects or with other high-risk populations, comorbidity is the rule, not the exception. In such cases, the most convincing demonstration of efficacy and safety for the pure diagnostic group gives no assurance of efficacy and safety for the very subjects for whom the results might be of greatest clinical importance—who may constitute the majority of people with the disorder of interest.

Assume the Heterogeneity Away or Create Mathematical Models That "Remove" It

As noted above, in stating and proving a mathematical theorem, the mathematician can make any assumptions she or he chooses as long as those assumptions are stated clearly. But when applying such a theorem in a research study of a population, the biobehavioral scientist must check the appropriateness of the assumptions in the context in which that scientist proposes to use it. For example, many mathematical models assume equal variance in subgroups (e.g., a t-test) or a linear relationship (e.g., product–moment correlation or linear regression).

When the researchers make mathematical assumptions that may or may not be true and that they cannot or do not check, the risk is that the inductive and deductive procedure, however precise and elegant in mathematical terms, will produce results that misrepresent the population. The results may be no more true than are the assumptions. It is not unusual to see publication of data from two groups to which a t-test is applied, where the sample sizes in the two groups are very unequal, and the standard deviation in the smaller sized group may be many fold larger than that in the larger sized group, a situation that exaggerates the statistical significance level. In such a case, the researchers are either unaware of the underlying assumption of equality of variance in the two-sample t-test and what influence this assumption has on correct comput-ation of significance level, or are simply ignoring their own data, which would tend to cast doubt on the validity of the test they chose to apply.

Use of problematic mathematical models is frequently justified, not in terms of demonstration that the assumptions are reasonable in the con-text of use, but by examining the goodness of fit of the model. Thus, for example, many standard statistical tests are based on assumptions of linear relationships (simple and linear regression, product–moment cor-relation, and most standard multivariate analyses). In some cases, re-searchers run a preliminary test to test the linearity. However, sample sizes are often too small and measures are not of high enough quality to detect deviations from complex mathematical models. The more complex the model, the more problematic the situation. As a result, a statistically significant lack of the fit of the model indeed demonstrates that the model is a poor one and should be rejected, for the assumptions of the model empirically do not hold. However a nonsignificant test does not prove that the model is adequate, only that its inadequacy cannot be demonstrated given the sample available. The validity of any conclusions based on the assumptions of the model must remain in doubt.

Even more problematic is the situation in which researchers compare two groups (let us say two intervention groups) that differ from each other in terms of age, sex, socioeconomic class, etc., using values adjusted for or controlling for such differences. In such cases, a linear model govern-ing the relationships between variables is proposed. Researchers assume that the same relationship exists in both the groups and use this model to remove the heterogeneity of the groups before using a t-test to compare the adjusted or controlled values. Mathematical models are thus created that may or may not be true, where power typically is not sufficient to check their adequacy, and then used to remove sources of variance.

Ignore the Heterogeneity; Pretend It's Not There

Ultimately every researcher must focus on certain sources of hetero-geneity and ignore others. In summary, biobehavioral researchers face situations in which there is always heterogeneity. Much (perhaps most) of this heterogeneity cannot be controlled in the research design and imple-mentation. Either to pretend to control it or to assume that there is no heterogeneity or to assume that the heterogeneity is controlled by mathe-matical modeling is likely to produce invalid and misleading results.

I suggest a view of heterogeneity contrary to that implied in seeking such control, one that might succinctly be stated as follows: The scientific study of human populations is in essence the study of heterogeneity within those populations. Thus, far from controlling away or assuming away or ignoring heterogeneity, the focus of all human research should be on detecting sources of heterogeneity.

In the next two sections I provide two examples of how pretending to control heterogeneity, or assuming that one has control of heterogeneity when one probably does not, and pretending there is no heterogeneity when there is can produce statistical artifacts. The first section is an example of certain statistical artifacts that have been studied in the methodological literature under the names Simpson's paradox, the ecological fallacy, and pseudocorrelation. The second section is an example of artifacts that casual and uninformed use of linear models might produce.

SIMPSON'S PARADOX AND ASSOCIATED STATISTICAL ARTIFACTS

In 1975, Bickel, Hammel, and O'Connell published a paper entitled "Sex Bias in Graduate Admissions: Data from Berkeley." The problem they discuss is variously referred to as or related to Simpson's paradox, the ecological fallacy, or psuedocorrelation (Bickel et al.).

Bickel and colleagues (1975) were interested in the issue of possible gender bias in graduate school admission to the University of California at Berkeley (hereafter Cal) in 1973. They examined all decisions on applications to the entering class for the fall 1973 quarter. There were 12,763 applicants in all. Most (67%) of the applicants were male. Of the male applicants, 44% were admitted, and 35% of the female applicants were admitted. One must conclude that there is a gender bias somewhere in the system.

To understand how important this issue was at that time, recall that Title VII of the Civil Rights Act in 1964 made such discrimination on the basis of gender illegal and that in 1972 this act was explicitly extended to apply to universities receiving federal funds, of which Cal was a prime example. The consequences of such a proof of discrimination could include withdrawal of all federal funding and preclusion from any further participation as a federal contractor. Thus any finding of a gender bias in admission in 1973 on the part of Cal graduate programs, many of which were supported by federal funds, was not a trivial matter.

Applicants to Cal were heterogeneous, not only in terms of gender, age, ethnic group, socioeconomic class, etc. but also in terms of the department or unit to which they applied and by which they were evaluated. A man or woman who applied to the modern language department would be disconcerted indeed if he or she were admitted to the physics department, and vice versa. Similarly, an application might be read and an applicant evaluated very differently by a member of the admissions committee of the modern language department than it would by a member of the physics department. While there are many other sources of heterogeneity, certainly the department to which application was made and by which it was processed must be a source of heterogeneity in this population that cannot be ignored.

The issue of gender bias could be evaluated for only 85 of the 101 graduate departments because 16 of the departments either had no female applicants or admitted all applicants, male or female. Of the 85 remaining departments, the admission rates of males and female applicants did not statistically differ for 75 departments (some admittedly too small to provide convincing evidence either way), 4 significantly favored males over females, and 6 favored females over males. Since most of the departments demonstrated no gender bias, and of those that did more showed bias favoring females than favoring males, where did the gender bias seen in the total population come from? In this case the apparent gender bias resulted from a statistical artifact called Simpson's paradox (Blyth, 1972; Simpson, 1951; Wagner, 1982).

A careful examination of the sources of heterogeneity indicated that there was major heterogeneity between departments in the percentage of female applicants, ranging approximately from 0% to 80%. At the same time there was major heterogeneity between departments in the percentage of applicants admitted: Some departments admitted as few as 5%, and others admitted 100%. Finally, a positive correlation appears between the percentage of female applicants and the admission rates across the departments. Such a correlation that exists between characterstics (percent female applicants versus admission rate) of departments is called an *ecological correlation*, where the ecological units are the departments. In contrast, a correlation that exists between gender and admission within each department is the *individual correlation*. In this case, there appears to be no substantial or consistent individual correlation, but there is a substantial and positive ecological correlation.

Among the relatively large departments, two clusters appear: (Cluster 1) those with fewer than 25% female applicants, with a median admission rate of approximately 60% (for both male and female applicants), and (Cluster 2) those with more than 25% female applicants with a median admission rate of approximately 25% (again for both male and female applicants). Cluster 1 departments appear to be those with a strong prerequisite in mathematics (the hard sciences and mathematical fields); Cluster 2 departments are those with weak or no prerequisites in mathematics (the humanities and the social sciences).

Of course there is a gender bias. It is shown, first of all, in the choice to go to graduate school. That bias is evidenced by the fact that there were about twice as many male applicants as female. The gender bias also lies in the choice of fields female and male applicants elect to pursue. Males were more likely to apply to high-math (Cluster 1) departments than were females. However, neither the decision to apply to graduate school nor the choice of department to which to apply is under the control of the graduate divisions of Cal. Thus these data, while they do indicate bias somewhere in the system, do not indicate a gender bias in graduate school admission process per se.

Does that mean that there was no gender bias in the admission process at UC Berkeley? That we cannot tell, for there is probably still substantial, unaccounted for heterogeneity. For example, there is undoubtedly heterogeneity in entry qualifications among the applicants to any department. A department that admitted 50% of its 100 male applicants and 50% of its 20 female applicants to fill its 60 positions might well appear to be "gender blind." However, if the 20 female applicants were uniformly better prepared and were more competent than the 100 male applicants, a truly gender-blind admission policy should have admitted 100% of the females and only 40% of the males to make up its class of 60. And if 60 of the male applicants were better prepared and qualified than all 20 female applicants, a truly gender-blind admission policy should have admitted 60% of its male applicants and 0% of its female applicants. Considering the sources of heterogeneity they focused on (department characteristics), Bickel et al. (1975) could not document any gender bias. Whether that conclusion would stand or fall, were other sources of heterogeneity considered, remains unanswered.

The Bickel et al. (1975) study illustrates several vital principles in the study of human populations. First, every human population is made up of what I will, for historical reasons, call "ecological units." Such units can be defined in many ways. They may be administrative units: departments, schools, classes, cities, counties, states, clinics, practices, hospitals, or catchment areas. They may be social units: families, neighborhoods, or clubs. They may be units defined by gender, age, birth cohort, ethnic or racial identification, or ability level. They may have an identity as units only within the context of a particular research study: recruitment or referral source, therapy group, or exercise group.

Within a population, patterns that are true of one ecological unit may not be true of another. Thus one cannot generalize either from a study done on one ecological unit to another or from one ecological unit to its parent population. Thus the results from the Bickel et al. (1975) study, for example, cannot be generalized to years other than 1973 or to Stanford University in 1973, and certainly not to universities in general.

Furthermore, patterns that are true across ecological units (i.e., ecological correlation) may or may not describe patterns that are true across subjects within any ecological unit (i.e., individual correlation). Thus one cannot infer individual correlation from ecological correlation or vice versa (the "ecological fallacy"); Goodman, 1959; Kraemer, 1978; Robinson, 1950). More generally, the Bickel et al. (1975) study illustrates the principle that a pattern that is seen for a total population is a composite of the corresponding patterns seen within each of its ecological units and the pattern seen across its ecological units (Kraemer, 1978) (where a pattern might be described by a mean, a variance, a correlation coefficient, etc.). How much each source influences the total pattern depends on the homogeneity or heterogeneity within each ecological unit and the homogeneity or heterogeneity across ecological units. Thus, just as one cannot generalize from one population to another or from one population to a more general one, one can never particularize from a total population to any one of its ecological units.

In the Bickel et al. (1975) study, the total correlation between being female and admission was negative and of moderate size. The ecological correlation (i.e., between departmental admission rates and department percentage of female applicants) was negative and large. The individual departmental correlations (i.e., the correlation between being female and admission within each department) ranged from large and positive to large and negative, with most either nonsignificant and near zero. Which is the right answer? We would suggest that they are all "right" answers but to different questions. Each answer shed further light on the sources of heterogeneity: heterogeneity between applicants within departments, between departments, and between groups of departments (Cluster 1 vs. Cluster 2). Having a better grasp of sources of heterogeneity, we understand the issues of gender and admission better than we did before, but we also know that additional questions exist, and we can develop some ideas as to where we should direct those questions.

COLLINEARITY, INTERACTIONS, MODELS, AND THE STATISTICAL ARTIFACTS THEY INDUCE

One idea generated from the Bickel et al. (1975) study is that to understand gender biases in admission, one needs minimally to take into account the heterogeneity between "high math" departments (Cluster 1) versus "low math" departments (Cluster 2). Let us pursue how we might address the issues related to this type of heterogeneity and some questionable approaches to such issues that have been used.

Suppose we are studying Hypothetical University (hereafter HU). In order to investigate the issues of heterogeneity in admissions at HU, we propose a study where gender (male vs. female) and field (high math vs. low math) are the independent variables and admission the dependent variable. The actual population figures (usually unknown at the planning stage) appear in Tables 1 and 2.

In Table 1, we see that according to the records at HU, as was also true in 1973 at Cal, most of the total applicants are male (66%). More males

TABLE 1. The Distribution of Applications by Gender and Field at Hypothetical University

	High math	Low math	Total
Males	60%	6%	66%
Females	10%	24%	34%
Total	70%	30%	100%

apply to high-math fields than do females (91% vs. 29%), and more applicants to high-math fields are male than applicants to low-math fields (86% vs. 20%). However looked at, there is a strong correlation between gender (male, female) and field (high math, low math). When such a correlation exists between variables defined as the independent variables in a study, this is called *collinearity* or *multicollinearity*. Collinearity is different from an interaction effect as the following example shows.

In Table 2, we see the admission rates for each of these four subgroups defined by gender and field. The admission rate is the *dependent* (or outcome) variable. We see that the overall admission rate is higher for males than for females (79% vs. 41%). Once again we see a gender bias like that seen in the Bickel et al. (1975) study. We also see that the overall admission rate is higher for high-math fields than for low-math fields (81% vs. 31%). In addition, in the high-math fields, the admission rates for females is higher than that for males (90% vs. 80%), and in the low-math fields, the admission rates for females is much lower than that for males (20% vs. 90%). This type of pattern, where the relationship between one independent variable (gender) and the outcome (admission) changes depending on the value of other independent variables (field), is called an *interaction effect*.

Collinearity and interactions are concepts that are often confused. It is possible to have collinearity between the independent variables either with or without interaction effects on the dependent variable. It is possible to have noncollinear independent variables that either have or do not have an interaction effect on the dependent variables. Two independent

TABLE 2. The Admission Rates by Gender and Field at Hypothetical University

	High math	Low math	Total
Males	80%	90%	79%
Females	90%	20%	41%
Total	81%	31%	100%

variables either are or are not collinear in a population or sample, regardless of what the dependent variable is. However, two independent variables (collinear or not) might have a strong interactive effect on one dependent variable but not on another in the same population. In this case, the dependent variable is admission to graduate school, and there appears to be an interactive effect of sex and field on that dependent variable. If we proposed to study not the admission of applicants, but the Graduate Record Exam scores of applicants, there might be no interactive effect of sex and field. Both collinearity and interactions affect heterogeneity in a population, and how researchers deal with them in analysis influences how well or badly heterogeneity is dealt with.

The most common approach to analyzing the data from the population described in Tables 1 and 2 is based on a linear mathematical model. In this process, one hypothesizes that some scaling f(.) of the outcome measure is a linear function of the following type:

$$f(y) = \beta_0 + \beta_1 G + \beta_2 F + \beta_3 GF$$

where y is the admission rate in a particular cell, G represents a coding of gender (here males are coded 0 and females 1), F a coding of field (here high math is coded 0 and low math 1).

We could choose to model the raw admission rates ($f(y) = y$) or to model a rescaling such as its logit, its logarithm, its arcsine transformation, etc. The statistical reasons for choosing one scaling or another of these rescalings in applications are not relevant to the present discussion. For simplicity, we will use the raw admission rates, for the principles here apply to whatever scaling one chooses.

Also, we have chosen to code the independent variables as indicated ($G = 0$ for males and $G = 1$ for females; $F = 0$ for high math and $F = 1$ for low math), but it must be remembered that the coding is arbitrary. Again, the principles here will apply to whatever coding one chooses.

With the scaling and coding used, the intercept ($\beta_0 = .8$) is the admission rate for males in high math ($G = 0$ and $F = 0$ in the model above). The "main effect of gender" ($\beta_1 = 0.1$) is the difference between the admission rate for females and males in high-math fields ($G = 1$ and $F = 0$ vs. $G = 0$ and $F = 0$). The "main effect of field" ($\beta_2 = .1$) is the difference between the admission rates for low math versus high math for males ($G = 0$ and $F = 1$ vs. $G = 0$ and $F = 0$). The "interaction effect" ($\beta_3 = 0.8$) is the difference between the admission rate for females in low math ($G = 1$ and $F = 1$) and the sum of the intercept plus the main effects.

It should be noted that if we had chosen to use, not the raw admission rate, but its logit, its logarithm, its arcsine, etc., the entries in each cell would change and thus the value of the parameters would also change. Furthermore, if we had chosen to code males as $G = 0.5$ and females as $G = 0.5$ or some other such coding or to code field (F) differently, the parameters would also change. To understand the sources of heterogeneity correctly, how one codes the dependent and independent variables must be understood and correctly interpreted. Yet many researchers use programs in standard statistical packages and interpet the results generated from those programs without knowing how the program codes the independent variables.

With these parameters I have perfect fit between what would be predicted from the effects and the true cell admission rates. If I had chosen a different scaling of response, or a different coding of the independent variables, the intercept, both main effects and the interaction effects might be different. Yet whatever scaling or coding I might choose, the fit would remain perfect. The message is very simple: *A model is a model is a model.* There are always an infinity of mathematical models that one could choose, each of which could produce perfect fit but different parameter estimates and thus different insights as to the sources of heterogeneity. No model is the "real thing."

Use of a mathematical model allows us to study and develop hypotheses about the functioning of complex systems that we cannot otherwise directly study. Think about using a model of a human (a dummy) in automobile crash tests. One can gain insights into how much protection various types of seatbelts or airbags afford in crashes at various speeds. These are the kinds of insights that could not possibly be gained by using real humans in such tests. Yet the dummy is not a human. There are certain reactions to crashes one could not possibly learn from studying the reaction of dummies in crash tests (e.g., the emotional responses, pain and suffering, costs of subsequent medical care). Nevertheless, we can learn a great deal of real value. In much the same way, no mathematical model reproduces the system it is meant to represent. Yet if one is careful in the structuring and interpreting a mathematical model of a system, one can gain valuable insights into how that system might work.

Back to HU: We do not actually know what the population at HU looks like (i.e., the contents of Tables 1 and 2 are not known to us). To estimate the parameters (i.e., the intercept, the main effects and interactions) that underlie Tables 1 and 2, we propose to sample that population, mathematically fit the model we have chosen, estimate the parameters, and test the null hypothesis that each (the main effect of gender, the main effect of field, and the interactive effect of gender and field) is zero. We discuss three of many research strategies that could be proposed to do this task.

Strategy 1. We propose to draw a random sample of N subjects from the pool of applicants to HU and to fit all the parameters of the above model, using the estimation procedure previously explained.

In this case, the estimates we derive will be unbiased estimates of the population counterparts. The lack of bias can be mathematically proved. The precision of these estimates, of course, will depend on the size of N, as will the power of the tests for these parameters. In addition the sample size in each of the cells also influences the precision of estimates and power of tests. If, for example, $N = 100$, one would expect to see only 6 male applicants to the low-math fields, which would result in a very unstable estimate of the admission rate in that cell and thus instability in any parameter estimate that involved that estimated admission rate. In this case, $N = 100$ would be considered a very small sample size. In other situations, $N = 100$ might be an adequate sample size indeed (for example, using Strategy 3 to be described below).

The estimators obtained in this strategy, no matter how inaccurate or unstable they might be, will produce perfect fit to the sample data, just as the model perfectly fits the population. However, it must be remembered that whatever the choice of scaling of the dependent variable or the choice of coding of the independent variables, the estimators would be different, but the fit remains perfect. Another simple message: Poor fit of a model to data indicates a poor model. Good, even perfect, fit of a model to data does not mean the model is the "right" one.

Strategy 2.   Once again we propose to draw a random sample of N subjects from the applicant pool to HU. However, now we decide that the interaction effect is of no research interest, since our primary question concerns the main effect of gender. Even the main effect of field is only a "nuisance" effect that must be dealt with. Why should we waste the time, effort, and sample size to fit an uninteresting interaction effect? So we propose to ignore interaction in fitting the model.

When we choose not to fit interaction effects, we assume that those effects are zero. When we then use some algorithm to fit the selected model to data, that algorithm will struggle to get the very best fit it can get with the materials offered (here with the intercept and the two main effects). If there really is a population interaction effect, as in Table 1, that we have elected to ignore, the algorithm will do the very best it can to absorb that interaction effect into the estimated main effects. As a result, the estimators of the main effects will now be biased estimators of the true main effects unless one of two situations pertains: Either the real interaction effect is zero (and thus our assumption is correct) or there is no collinearity between the two independent variables.

If neither of these protections hold, as in Table 1, the estimated main effect of gender will be biased in a direction and with a degree of bias that will be influenced by the direction and magnitude of the interactive effect we chose to ignore and by the direction and magnitude of the collinearity between the independent variables. It is quite possible that a main effect of gender that is truly zero may be estimated as high positive or negative, and even be found statistically significant, or that a main effect of gender that is truly large may be estimated as zero. The upshot is that the effects we have ignored because we claim they are "uninteresting" compromise the validity of what we learn about the effects that were important to us. In short what matters are the true sources of heterogeneity, not which sources of heterogeneity are of interest to the researcher. Ignoring true sources of heterogeneity may compromise the validity of the inferences about the sources of heterogeneity of interest to the researchers.

With Strategy 2, of course, one would not typically get a perfect fit between what would be predicted on the basis of the estimated parameters and the observed data. One might then argue that the protection against being misled lies in doing some type of goodness-of-fit test, often included in standard statistical packages. However, whether or not one would reject the null hypothesis of such a test depends on the sample size, the quality of measurement, the size of the omitted interaction effect, and the collinearity between the independent variables. Thus a nonstatistically significant goodness-of-fit test does not guarantee that the estimates of the interesting parameters are unbiased.

It is easy to be statistically righteous and warn against omission of interaction effects that may or may not be important when there are only two independent variables and thus only one interaction effect. The difficulty, of course, is that users of linear models frequently have not merely two, but many, independent variables. With m independent variables, there are 2^m possible effects, including the intercept and m main effects. To estimate all these effects well, one should have a sample size at least 10 times as large as the number of effects to be estimated. Thus with merely 5 independent variables, one has 32 effects, made up of the intercept, 5 main effects, and 26 interaction effects. To estimate 32 parameters well in a linear model, one might require a minimum of 320 subjects. Moreover, if there are collinearities among those 5 independent variables, because collinearities "eat up" power, one may need even more subjects to obtain stable estimates and powerful tests.

Whatever the righteous statistician might recommend, it is not surprising that many researchers simply choose to ignore all the interactions (i.e., to assume that all of these are zero), or to ignore all but the first order interactions, in order to achieve a promising ratio of sample size to number of effects. Indeed there is nothing wrong with that approach, as long as one remembers that the limitations of mathematical modeling are now compounded by the assumptions that certain, perhaps important, interactions are arbitrarily assumed to be zero. If that assumption is wrong, any conclusions about the effects that are included will be biased accordingly.

The message here: Whether or not a researcher is interested in a particular parameter in a model is not the deciding factor in whether that effect should be included in the model. Nor is the inadequacy of the sample size a good basis on which to decide to exclude effects. What is crucial is whether that effect is zero or not in the population to which the model is to be applied, that is, what the true (usually unknown) sources of heterogeneity are in the population. Thus one should always take the results of mathematical modeling as suggestive, worthy of further consideration but not conclusive until independently confirmed in further studies that do not reproduce the same biases.

Strategy 3.   Instead of taking a random sample from the application pool of HU, we propose to take a random sample of $N/4$ subjects from each of the four cells of Table 1: a stratified sample. Thus, although only 6% of the application pool are males applying to low-math fields and 60% are males applying to high-math fields, 25% of our sample will be in each of those cells.

By sampling this way, we remove any collinearity between the independent variables in the sample. Now 50% of the females and 50% of the males are in the low-math subsample, and 50% of both the low-math and high-math fields subsamples are females. Now it does not matter whether we fit the full model or omit the interaction. The results will come out the same, whether or not the interaction is truly there in the population. All estimators will be unbiased. Indeed the precision of estimation and power of tests will, in general, increase over what it would be from a random sample of N subjects in the same population.

There is a price, however. In a random sample, one can estimate the admission rates of males, females, or applicants to high-math fields, or of applicants to low-math fields. With the stratified sample described, the expected proportion of males in the sample admitted is 85% (the average of 80% and 90%), not 79% as it is in the total population. The expected proportion of females in the sample admitted is 55% (the average of 90% and 20%), not 41%, etc. In order to obtain unbiased admission rates from a stratified sample, one needs additional information (corresponding to that in Table 1) in order to know how to weight the admission rates from each cell. A mistake researchers frequently make is that, having stratified a sample for good and valid reasons, they generate statistical artifacts by using estimation and testing methods appropriate for random samples. That would, of course, once again misrepresent the sources of heterogeneity in the population. Fundamentally, there are not absolutely right and wrong ways to analyze. The analytic procedure must be consistent with the sampling, design, and measurement decisions and thus may be right under one circumstance and wrong in another.

Statistical Significance.   One final comment that applies to all strategies concerns the term *statistical significance*. If Table 2 represents the population, all the true effects of the model we have chosen are nonzero. Consequently, a large enough sample size with any of the strategies will produce statistically significant effects. It is important to realize that statistical significance does not mean an effect is large or important. It means that the sample size, the quality of measurement, and the design were all sufficient to prove "beyond reasonable doubt" ($p < .05$ or $p < .01$) that the observed result was not consistent with the null hypothesis.

Thus a statement of statistical significance is largely a statement about the quality of the study, not specifically about the size or importance of the effect.

Nonstatistically significant effects may or may not be important, for a "nonstatistically significant result" indicates that the study is not adequate to settle the question. Statistically significant effects, on the other hand, should be closely examined to determine whether their size indicates that they are important or trivial. In short, to describe an effect in terms of whether it was or was not statistically significant, or with its p-level, is remarkably uninformative about the results of any study.

Studies like the Bickel et al. (1975) study clarify that there is always heterogeneity of response that one ignores only at peril of statistically artifactual results. To begin to understand heterogeneity of response, mathematical modeling is essential, and linear models are most commonly used (multiple linear or logistic regression, structural equation models, Cox proportional hazards model, etc.). To use such models to develop insights into complex biobehavioral processes is necessary and important, but to check those insights in the real world, not viewed through the faulty filter of a mathematical model, is essential.

Thus for a reasonably chosen model that fits reasonably well—however we sampled, whatever the scaling of the dependent variables, whatever independent variables we selected, whatever the coding of those independent variables, whatever interactions we included in or excluded from the fitting of the model—we should show any statistically significant effects as they appear in the data. Thus whichever strategy we elected to use to study HU shows us the entries of Table 2 as estimated in the sample, that is, as descriptive statistics absent any model that shows the size of effects found. If then we were to report that we assumed certain interaction effects to be zero, and thus found highly statistically significant gender effects, readers could examine Table 2 and begin, quite properly, to question our conclusions. It is astounding how many times statistically significant results cannot be seen in the data that generated them because of faults in the choice or fitting or interpretation of the mathematical model or the statistical results.

CONCLUSIONS AND DISCUSSION

Whatever population of human subjects one elects to sample and study, that population is likely to be heterogeneous. Moreover, the population one elects to sample and study is usually part of a more heterogeneous parent population and simultaneously the parent of multiple more homogeneous subpopulations. Under the best of circumstances, one cannot generalize from the population of study to its parent population, nor can one too readily particularize from the population of study to each of its offspring populations. Within that study population, one cannot identify, successfully control, or "model away" all the sources of heterogeneity. If one chooses to ignore them or pretend to control them, perhaps by unjustified use of mathematical models, statistical artifacts may result.

That realization can lead to despair. One could say that since one cannot control heterogeneity and its effect on conclusions, one should either not study human populations at all or should find it acceptable to do such studies badly. Instead I suggest that heterogeneity and its effect on conclusions are the proper focus of good biobehavioral research.

In practice, each study should have a very particular goal, a certain limited set of research hypotheses or questions, and a specific population of interest. Then the study should be optimally designed to answer those research questions for that population. One study, I would suggest, cannot possible be optimally designed to answer many different research questions for many different populations of interest. The direction of much current biobehavioral research is toward massive collections of data with no a priori specific questions, in the hopes that once one has the data, true answers will emerge. We suggest such serendipity is very unlikely.

When we have the answer to those few specific research questions for the population of interest, that is the time to consider possible sources of heterogeneity within that population. Can one, on an exploratory level, find subpopulations in which the answers might appear to differ from that of the parent population? If so, this forms the basis for proposals of next generation studies.

That is also the time to consider any parent populations that might be of interest. Such consideration is facilitated if multiple researchers ask the same research questions for several different populations of interest. Are the conclusions the same? If not, is there any indication of what characteristics heterogeneous between the populations studied might explain the heterogeneity of results? As hypotheses emerge, they also become the focus for proposals of next-generation studies.

And so, study by study, an understanding of the biobehavioral phenomenon addressed in the research study would begin to emerge. The difficulty lies in a reluctance to see each of our research studies as only one small piece in a very large puzzle, a small piece that has no meaning unless supplemented by other small pieces from the research efforts of others and by pieces from next-generation research studies. Each of us wants our study to be the definitive study, but given the heterogeneity of human populations, that will never be.

REFERENCES

Bickel, P. J., Hammel, E. A., O'Connell, J. W. (1975). Sex bias in graduate admissions: Data from Berkeley. *Science, 187,* 398–404.

Blyth, C. R. (1972). On Simpson's paradox and the sure-thing principle. *Journal of the American Statistical Association, 68*, 746.

Goodman, L. A. (1959). Some alternatives to ecological correlation. *American Journal of Sociology, 64*, 610–625.

Kraemer, H. C. (1978). Individual and ecological correlation in a general context: The investigation of testosterone and orgasmic frequency in the human male. *Behavior Science, 23*, 67–72.

Robinson, W. S. (1950). Ecological correlations and the behavior of individuals. *American Sociological Review, 15*, 351–357.

Simpson, E. H. (1951). The interpretation of interaction in contingency tables. *Journal of the Royal Statistical Society, Series B., 13*, 238–241.

Wagner, C. H. (1982). Simpson's paradox in real life. *The American Statistician, 36*, 46–48.

PART II

LIFE-SPAN ISSUES IN HEALTH PSYCHOLOGY

CHAPTER 3

Issues of Age and Health

MONISHA PASUPATHI

INTRODUCTION

Knowing the age of people tells us something about their physical health. It also tells us something about their cognitive abilities, accumulated knowledge, coping strategies, and environment. Age tells us what kinds of historical events people have lived through, what their daily activities and concerns might be, and how others might perceive their abilities. Not surprisingly, age is an important variable for health psychology.

When we say *age*, we are typically referring to the number of years since birth, known as chronological age. Chronological age, however, does not cause anything—it is simply a measure of time in which events happen (Wohlwill, 1970). Age differences are not caused by age per se but by the actions of other mechanisms that covary with passing time. Identifying those mechanisms should be one of the primary objectives in research on age and health outcomes. The multiple correlates of age, however, do not make this a simple task. Broadly, age differences can be caused by biological factors, psychological factors, social and contextual factors, or by some interaction of these factors.

In this chapter, I briefly outline some important concerns for developmental research in health psychology. I first give a short review of relationships between age and other variables, such as biological and psychological functioning. Then I discuss the influence of age on a person's

MONISHA PASUPATHI • Department of Psychology, Stanford University, Stanford, California 94305.

Handbook of Diversity Issues in Health Psychology, edited by Pamela M. Kato and Traci Mann. Plenum Press, New York, 1996.

environment, and conclude with a discussion of interpreting age differences.

AGE-RELATED PHENOMENA

Biology and Age: Normal Development

Chronological age is related to physiological functioning in systematic ways. Physical maturation from childhood into early adulthood is associated with increasing mastery of physical abilities, as strength, motor coordination, and stamina all improve over the childhood and adolescent years. Many of the major organ systems attain an adult level of function. While increasing physical prowess may seem a unitary move toward good health, new abilities and new independence expose children to more health risks (Maddux, Roberts, Sledden, & Wright, 1986).

Development from early adulthood through old age is associated with mild to moderate decline in physical ability and in the functioning of the major organ systems. The actual onset and rapidity of decline may vary substantially from system to system within one person, and across people as well. In particular, declines in homeostatic functioning (Zarit & Zarit, 1987) make it more difficult for the elderly person to recover from day-to-day stresses as well as disease. Most of the time, however, age-related declines do not alter daily functioning. The largest age-related declines occur in vision and hearing; both can be reduced or eliminated by corrective measures.

In addition to basic biological function, age is also associated with changes in disease prevalence, symptomatology, prognoses, and treatments—all discussed below.

Age and Disease Processes

People of different ages have different illnesses (Aldwin, 1991), and different illnesses can mean different outcomes—from prognosis to coping and treatment compliance. Even when people of different ages have the same underlying illness, differences in symptoms, prognosis, and treatment may exist.

Age can be related to symptomatology within one disorder. For example, the diagnostic criteria for depression are slightly different for children than they are for adults (APA, 1994). Symptomatology may be related to prognosis even within a disorder and may influence the choice of particular treatments.

Age also affects prognosis and treatment independently of symptoms. For example, chicken pox is more serious when contracted by adults than when contracted by children. Not only does the general prognosis of some disorders and injuries vary with age, but treatments may be more or less effective at different ages. For example, children and elderly people sometimes respond differently to drugs than do young and middle-aged adults. The elderly, and elderly women in particular, are more sensitive to drug effects and may need lower than typical doses (Gatz, Harris, & Turk-Charles, in press). Differential treatment response may or may not account for age differences in prognosis.

Age and Psychology

Age may be related to changes in conceptions of illness, coping processes, and treatment compliance, although there is less evidence for these relationships than there is for age–biology relationships.

Illness conceptions may have much to do with health outcomes. Understanding illness and treatment is important for treatment seeking, compliance with treatment, and with preventative behaviors, all of which predict health outcomes (Maddux et al., 1986). For example, children who think of their illness as a punishment for having been "bad" are, understandably, less likely to report symptoms. This delays treatment and possibly worsens the course of an illness (Burbach & Peterson, 1986).

Conceptions of illness do change as children develop increasingly sophisticated cognitive capacities, and older children have more complex and accurate concepts about diseases (Perrin & Gerrity, 1981; Bibace & Walsh, 1980; Burbach & Peterson, 1986). In fact, what child psychologists refer to as "mental age," or the quality of a child's intellectual functioning, is highly correlated with disease conceptions. There is far less research on adult developmental changes in disease conceptions. Elderly adults may accumulate increasing knowledge about illnesses or be more sophisticated consumers of health care. They might also be motivated to change or distort their conceptions of illness and disease to maintain a view of themselves as healthy.

Coping has also been proposed to influence health outcomes. Theories of coping typically emphasize two aspects of coping processes. Problem-focused coping encompasses strategies that are directed at the illness (seeking treatment, seeking information). Emotion-focused coping encompasses strategies that are aimed at managing the stress and arousal associated with the illness—in short, emotion-regulation strategies (Lazarus, 1993). Emotion-regulation capacities emerge early in life, but may improve continuously over the life span (Lawton, Kleban, Rajagopal, & Dean, 1992). Such capacities include controlling the expression and experience of emotions in various ways. Children may use problem-focused coping earlier than they use emotion-focused coping (see Compas, Banez, Malcarne, & Worsham, 1991 for a review), suggesting that younger children may require particular support in dealing with the emotional aspects of illness.

Adults in later life appear to cope better with illness-related stress than do younger adults (Aldwin, 1991). The improvement may be due to a change in the relationship between perceived controllability of an illness and a patient's perception of their coping abilities for that illness. Elderly adults think they can cope well with illness regardless of the controllability of the illness, while younger adults tend to perceive uncontrollable illnesses as much more difficult to cope with (Aldwin, 1991).

Health outcomes are also related to compliance with treatment regimens—better compliance typically leads to better recovery from illnesses. Some researchers report that compliance has a curvilinear relationship with age, decreasing from early childhood to adolescence and then rising again in old age (Bond, Aiken, & Somerville, 1992; Smith & Yawn, 1994). Very old adults may show declines in adherence once again (Park & Kidder, in press). Children have higher treatment compliance when they are younger, probably because their parents help ensure compliance, and nondemented elderly are also highly likely to comply, perhaps because of the importance placed on health by elderly people. However, elderly adults with cognitive impairment, and very old adults, do show difficulties with medication adherence (Park, Willis, Morrow, Diehl, & Gaines, 1994), suggesting that declines in basic psychological capacities produce changes in health-related processes.

In sum, age is related to illness understanding, coping strategies, and compliance with treatment, and age differences in health outcomes may reflect the operation of these variables.

Age, Mind, and Body

Of course, illness understanding, coping strategies, and treatment compliance are all related to biological variables as well, further complicating discussions of age and health. Both coping and compliance will vary according to whether the disease is acute or chronic and whether it is terminal. For example, compliance with a short-term regimen of penicillin is far different from compliance with daily insulin shots for many years. Coping with a terminal illness is quite different from managing a brief bout with the flu. Similarly, the relationship between mental and physical disease, roughly speaking, may also be important. As Zeiss, Lewinsohn, and Rohde (this volume) note, illness and depression are highly interrelated, at least in elderly populations.

In fact, the interplay between psychological factors and physiological effects may be stronger at some ages than at others. For example, some findings suggest that the relationship between psychosocial characteristics and physical outcomes is stronger in old age. Berkman and Syme (1979) showed that social embeddedness—having intimate and satisfying relationships with others—is related to mortality at all ages. However, the relationship gets stronger in older cohorts. Rowe and Kahn (1987) review a number of studies that reach similar conclusions. Both the higher mortality rates of older cohorts and the age-associated declines in homeostatic regulation of physiological processes (Zarit & Zarit, 1987) may explain this effect.

Children, who are not finished growing, may also be more vulnerable to the effects of psychological variables on biological outcomes. Gardner (1972) suggested that a lack of affection and stimulation for children could lower the production of pituitary hormones and lead to what she termed "deprivation dwarfism" in the most severe cases. The long-standing literature on failure to thrive similarly implies that children require affection as well as food and shelter in order for normal physical development to occur (Ward, Kessler, & Altman, 1993).

In sum, both biological and psychological aspects of the person vary with age, and all of these factors can interact. In the next section, I consider the influence of age on a person's environment across the life span.

AGE AND THE ENVIRONMENT

Until now, I have treated age as an individual difference variable— that is, a characteristic of a person. Age also has implications for a person's environment over time, and these implications are important for health outcomes. I'll talk about three ways in which age relates to environment: age as cohort, age as determining current life tasks, and age-related prejudices.

Cohort

An *age cohort* is a group of people who share a similar birth period— for example, everyone born in 1942 or everyone born in the 1960s. A *cohort effect* means that a difference between groups is due to variables associated with their birth period. For example, Elder and Meguro (1987) show that birth year is a critical factor in men's wartime experience, which not only exposes them to the risks of combat but also alters the timing with which they marry and start families.

More generally, age cohorts can differ in their exposure to prenatal care; public health and safety measures; knowledge of illnesses; and exposure to natural disasters, war, or major political upheavals. Health differences between people who are currently children and people who are currently young adults can be due to these kinds of cohort-related differences rather than age per se.

Current Life Tasks

Current life tasks are also age graded—we assign normative ages for events like marriage and childbirth and normative age periods for schooling, child rearing, and grandparenthood, just to mention a few examples (Neugarten & Neugarten, 1987). The result is that individuals of different ages face very different day-to-day stressors and have very different day-to-day exposure to the potential for illness and injury. For example, manual labor may be free from managerial stressors like responsibility for hiring and firing decisions. On the other hand, manual work may expose people to job-related illness and injury. As Leffert and Petersen (this volume) note, adolescents experience a number of normative changes—decreasing supervision and increasing opportunity to experiment with new behaviors—changes that increase their exposure to health risks.

Life circumstances can also be related to treatment and compliance. For example, working-class adults may be unable to take time from work in order to seek care. When adults in their working years do seek care, compliance may be difficult (particularly when treatment involves rest) because of their other responsibilities. Adolescents, who are experiencing decreased adult supervision, may also be less likely to comply with treatments.

Age-Related Prejudice

Stereotypes of old age include many negative qualities, particularly cognitive incompetence (Kite & Johnson, 1988).[1] Not surprisingly, doctors treat elderly patients with less engagement, patience, and respect than they treat young adult patients. Further, they give elderly patients less information and support (Greene, Adelman, Charon, & Hoffman, 1986). These differences exist despite the absence of differences in patient behavior and jeopardize the quality of health care that elderly individuals receive. Physicians also seem to implicitly endorse the stereotype that old dogs cannot learn new tricks. Young and Kahana (1989) showed that physicians did not recommend lifestyle changes for cardiac patients who were over 60 years of age, but did recommend such changes for patients under 60 years of age. This bias occurred despite the fact that patient compliance for the two age groups studied was the same and behavioral interventions have been shown to work with equal treatment effectiveness in young and elderly adult groups. In this volume, Levy and Langer discuss the ways in which an antiaging social context can influence the cognitive performance of elderly people.

---

[1]Although mild cognitive deficits are a part of normal aging, only 5% of elderly people are demented (Crook, 1987).

Just as interactions between older adults and physicians can be harmful, the interactions between physicians and young children can also create problems. Physicians may use terms that are above the child's level of understanding, focusing their attention entirely on the parents when dispensing information about the illness and possible treatments. Children can develop serious misunderstandings about their illness and the proposed treatment based on what they overhear physicians say to their parents, as in the famous example where "edema in your belly" becomes "a demon in my belly" (Perrin & Gerrity, 1981). These misunderstandings can lead to guilt, excessive fear, and may make it difficult for children to report symptoms when future episodes of illness occur. Adults' misconceptions about children can have serious implications. For example, Kasson, Sentivany, and Kato (this volume) discuss conflicting myths held by health professionals and parents about children's experience of pain and the resulting problems with pain mismanagement.

Age affects physical and psychological development and also determines a person's environment, although it is important to remember that in many cases (e.g., pain), age does not make a great deal of difference (Kasson et al., this volume). Because age does predict health, particularly in late adulthood, it is important to consider age in research on health. Because of the many possible mechanisms by which age groups can come to differ in health, namely, biological, psychological, and environmental health, examining these mechanisms is a critical issue in understanding age differences in health.

WHAT DO AGE EFFECTS MEAN?

Interpreting age effects is a difficult business. In this section, I will consider a study on the prognosis of patients with osteosarcomas (bone-related cancers; Bentzen et al., 1988). Bentzen and colleagues find that for adults over 25, age is a good predictor of health outcomes. Further, adults between 25 and 30 years of age have the best prognosis. Increasingly older patients have increasingly poorer prognoses.

The association between age and survival could be due to biological factors, psychological factors, or even social and contextual factors. Why might adults between 25 and 30 years of age have the best prognosis? Many adults are in peak physical condition between 25 and 30 years of age, and perhaps they are more resilient than patients of other ages. Alternatively, perhaps 25 to 30 year olds have a greater ability to handle the stresses of cancer treatment than do older age groups, who have multiple other stressors in addition to cancer. Even environmental factors may play a role—for example, perhaps treatment regimens and surgery techniques have been disproportionately tested on 25- to 30-year-old adults, resulting in better treatment efficacy for those age groups.

Based on this particular study, we know that age is related to prognosis, but not why.

Beyond explaining age differences, two other concerns warrant mention. First, within-age-group variability is important even when researchers are focusing on differences between age groups. Because variability on almost every measureable characteristic increases in old age (Dannefer & Perlmutter, 1990), even statistically significant age effects may be small relative to the variation within an age group. So, despite the fact that, on average, elderly adults cope more effectively with illnesses than young adults (Aldwin, 1991), there may still be substantial and important variability in how elderly adults cope with illnesses.

A second concern revolves around the plasticity of age effects, particularly when causal mechanisms are not well understood. Consider that deteriorating cardiovascular health is typically assumed to be a biological process associated with old age.[1] When Bortz (1982) looked at young adults who were undergoing bedrest, however, he found that they exhibited many of the cardiovascular effects previously associated with later life. He concluded that much of the age-related biological decline that researchers observe might be attributed to disuse rather than to inevitable, genetically programmed decline.

CONCLUSION

Because age is related to almost everything of interest to health psychologists, from physical condition to social context, it is critical that age be addressed by researchers. However, a focus on age should be tempered by attempts to address explanatory variables and by attention to within-age-group variability and plasticity.

This chapter has not addressed the relationship between age and other social categories like gender, race, sexual orientation, or class. Age does interact with these other variables in the few domains where data exits; for example, as Jackson and Sellars (this volume) discuss, the health disadvantage of African-Americans reverses in late life so that very elderly African-Americans are actually healthier than same-aged European Americans. In general, however, there is no literature on the health psychology of those in "double" or "triple" jeopardy, even though variables like race, class, gender, and sexual orientation influence health over the entire life span by impacting access to and utilization of health care services throughout life. In fact, perhaps the most telling point for health psychologists from a life-span perspective is that health in old age is the outcome of thousands of choices and circumstances from before birth to the end of a person's life.

---

[1]It is important to note that no satisfactory biological model of aging has yet been proposed, although progress has been made recently (Johnson, 1994).

REFERENCES

Aldwin, C. M. (1991). Does age affect the stress and coping response? Implications of age differences in perceived control. *Journal of Gerontology, 46,* 131–136.

American Psychiatric Association. (1994). *Diagnostic and statistical manual of mental disorders (4th ed.).* Washington, DC: American Psychiatric Association.

Bentzen, S. M., Poulsen, H. S., Kaae, S., Jensen, O. M., Johansen, H., Mouridsen, H. T., Daugaard, S., & Arnoldi, C. (1988). Prognostic factors in osteosarcomas: A regression analysis. *Cancer, 62(1),* 194–202.

Berkman, L. F., & Syme, S. L. (1979). Social networks, host resistance, and mortality: A nine-year follow-up study of Alameda County residents. *American Journal of Epidemiology, 109,* 186–204.

Bibace, R., & Walsh, M. E. (1980). Development of children's concepts of illness. *Pediatrics, 66,* 912–917.

Bond, G. G., Aiken, L. S., & Somerville, S. C. (1992). The health belief model and adolescents with insulin-dependent diabetes mellitus. *Health Psychology, 11,* 190–198.

Bortz, W. M. (1982). Disuse and aging. *Journal of the American Medical Association, 248,* 1203–1207.

Burbach, D. J., & Peterson, L. (1986). Children's concepts of physical illness: A review and critique of the cognitive-developmental literature. *Health Psychology, 5,* 307–325.

Compas, B. E., Banez, G. A., Malcarne, V., & Worsham, N. (1991). Perceived control and coping with stress: A developmental perspective. *Journal of Social Issues, 47,* 23–34.

Crook, T. (1987). Dementia. In L. L. Carstensen & B. A. Edelstein (Eds.), *Handbook of clinical gerontology* (pp. 96–111). New York: Pergamon.

Dannefer, D., & Perlmutter, M. (1990). Development as a multidimensional process: Individual and social constraints. *Human Development, 33,* 108–137.

Elder, G. H., & Meguro, Y. (1987). Wartime in men's lives: A comparative study of American and Japanese cohorts. *International Journal of Behavioral Development, 10,* 439–466.

Gardner, L. I. (1972). Deprivation dwarfism. *Scientific American, 227,* 76–82.

Gatz, M., Harris, J. R., & Turk-Charles, S. (in press). Older women and health. In A. L. Stanton & S. J. Gallant (Eds.), *Women's psychological and physical health: A scholarly and social agenda.* Washington, DC: American Psychological Association.

Greene, M., Adelman, R., Charon, R., & Hoffman, S. (1986). Ageism in the medical encounter: An exploratory study of the doctor–elderly patient relationship. *Language and Communication, 6,* 113–124.

Johnson, T. E. (1994). *Testing biological theories of aging: Facts versus theory.* Paper presented at the 1994 convention of the Gerontological Society of America, Atlanta, GA.

Kite, M. E., & Johnson, B. T. (1988). Attitudes towards older and younger adults: A meta-analysis. *Psychology and Aging, 3,* 233–244.

Lawton, M. P., Kleban, M. H., Rajagopal, D., & Dean, J. (1992). Dimensions of affective experience in three age groups. *Psychology and Aging, 7,* 171–184.

Lazarus, R. (1993). Coping theory and research: Past, present, and future. *Psychosomatic Medicine, 55,* 234–247.

Maddux, J. E., Roberts, M. C., Sledden, E. A., & Wright, L. (1986). Developmental issues in child health psychology. *American Psychologist, 41,* 25–34.

Neugarten, B. L., & Neugarten, D. A. (1987). The changing meanings of age. *Psychology Today, May,* 29–33.

Park, D. C., & Kidder, D. P. (in press). Prospective memory and medication adherence. In M. Brandimonte, G. Einstein, & M. McDaniel (Eds.), *Prospective memory: Theory and applications.* Hillsdale, NJ: Lawrence Erlbaum Associates.

Park, D. C., Willis, S. W., Morrow, D., Diehl, M., & Gaines, C. L. (1994). Cognitive function and medication usage in older adults. *Journal of Applied Gerontology, 13,* 39–57.

Perrin, E. C., & Gerrity, P. S. (1981). There's a demon in your belly: Children's understanding of illness. *Pediatrics, 67,* 841–849.

Rowe, J. W., & Kahn, R. L. (1987). Human aging: Usual and successful. *Science, 237,* 143–149.

Smith, C. M., & Yawn, B. (1994). Factors associated with appointment keeping in a family practice residency clinic. *Journal of Family Practice, 38,* 25–29.

Ward, M. J., Kessler, D. B., & Altman, S. C. (1993). Infant–mother attachment in children with failure to thrive. *Infant Mental Health Journal, 14,* 208–220.

Wohlwill, J. F. (1970). The age variable in psychological research. *Psychological Review, 77,* 49–64.

Young, R. F., & Kahana, E. (1989). Age, medical advice about cardiac risk reduction, and patient compliance. *Journal of Aging and Health, 1,* 121–134.

Zarit, J. M., & Zarit, S. H. (1987). Molar aging: The physiology and psychology of normal aging. In L. L. Carstensen & B. A. Edelstein (Eds.), *Handbook of clinical gerontology* (pp. 18–32). New York: Pergamon.

CHAPTER 4

Touch Therapies across the Life Span

TIFFANY M. FIELD

The *Ayur-Veda*, the earliest known medical text from India (around 1800 B.C.), lists touch therapy (massage therapy), diet, and exercise as primary healing practices of that time. As Jules Older notes, even the English word *shampoo* comes from the word *champna*, which is an ancient Indian word meaning *to press* (Older, 1982). From early times, massage has been effectively used for many medical and psychiatric conditions, including dropsy; mental illness; torpor; spasm; stomach pain; heart disease; labor pain; delivery; postpartum bleeding; infertility; dysmenorrhea; stimulating the breast for milk; postsurgery to speed healing; as an adjunct to plastic surgery; discomforts and disorders of the joints; to restore movement in strained, fractured, or wounded limbs; lumbago; rheumatic diseases; and aging.

Anecdotally massage therapy has been noted to improve circulation, help eliminate waste, dissolve soft adhesions, reduce swelling, and soothe the peripheral and central nervous system. Other uses include treating pressure sores in bedridden patients, relieving edema and varicose ulcers, gum massage for gum disease, and prostate massage for the treatment of prostatitis. The only conditions that have been listed as potential contraindications to massage are arthritis, inflammation due to infection,

TIFFANY M. FIELD • Touch Research Institute, University of Miami School of Medicine, Miami, Florida 33101.

Handbook of Diversity Issues in Health Psychology, edited by Pamela M. Kato and Traci Mann. Plenum Press, New York, 1996.

phlebitis for varicose veins, cellulitis, and bursitis. However, these contraindications are not based on research data.

Exotic uses of massage have been described for various cultures (Older, 1982). Older noted that in New Zealand, the pre-European Maori mothers massaged their children's noses to improve the shape, and they massaged their children's legs to lengthen and straighten them. In Cuba garlic and oil massages are prepared and applied to the stomach following "a meal lodged in the stomach where it caused pain and fever" (Older, 1982). In Samoa, massage is used for every disorder from diarrhea to migraine headache, using a mixture of coconut milk, flowers from trees and plants, and roots of grasses (Older, 1982).

Massage therapy is one of the most popular touch therapies because it lends itself to so many conditions. In addition, people without illness often use it as a preventive measure to reduce stress, and it is one of the oldest touch therapies. Of the massage therapies, Swedish massage is the most popularly used. Swedish massage is generally divided into six types in order of increasing pressure applied: (1) *effleurage or stroking*; (2) *friction or movement* of the hands over the body with more force than effleurage; (3) *pressure without movement*; (4) *petrissage* or kneading in which the hands are stationary, but the fingers work their way into sore muscles; (5) *vibration* for which a machine, as opposed to human touch, is typically used for vibration; and (6) *percussion*, or slapping, pounding, and tapping.

Most of the reports on massage therapy in the literature unfortunately are anecdotal case studies. The effects they report could merely be placebo effects because the subjects are receiving additional attention and have certain expectations about being treated that then translate into positive effects. Studies, of course, need to include control groups (those who receive some attention but no massage therapy) or treatment comparison groups (those who receive, for example, relaxation therapy vs. massage therapy). In this chapter only studies that have used control or comparison groups will be reviewed, although some of those studies are still in progress, limiting those discussions to preliminary results. The studies are briefly summarized in abstract form and in alphabetic order of condition.

AGE DIFFERENCES IN MASSAGE THERAPY APPROACHES

The studies are also ordered by age group because touch therapies differ by age group on several dimensions, including the type of touch (simple for children, more complex for adults), type of touch therapist (parents for children, professionals for adults), indications for touch therapy, (typically for pain in young children, for stress in adults), and measures of effects (nonverbal or observational measures for children, self-report measures for adults). The simplest massage is performed with newborns to reduce pain associated with medical procedures and to enhance weight gain. Simple stroking is performed because newborns (in contrast to adults) prefer simple, familiar stimulation. Like adults, however, newborns prefer some pressure, and also like adults, they prefer being massaged with oil.

As infants grow older they come to prefer novel stimulation and more variety so at this age stroking is combined with twisting (milking) motions and circular stroking. Rubbing can now occur all over the body including the chest (where most newborns do not like being rubbed). At the infancy stage, massage is generally used to calm and quiet, for example, to reduce crying associated with colic and to enhance sleep. Typically, parents are taught the massage by infant-massage instructors so that the parents can provide this treatment on a daily basis.

Older children become somewhat shy about being massaged in most places except their backs and heads, so the massage becomes more like a back rub during this period. Again, bedtime massage is a good ritual for alleviating stress in the child and enhancing the parent–child interaction. Also during this stage of development, parents are taught massage to enhance the other treatments children may be receiving for chronic diseases such as asthma, cancer, and diabetes, reducing the parent's sense of helplessness and the child's awareness of pain during painful medical procedures.

Adults prefer very complex massage techniques that can be learned from a professional therapist or videotapes. At this time, a significant other is needed for daily massages to be affordable, and typically they are used to reduce stress and thereby enhance job performance, immune function, and many other functions in the body.

MASSAGE THERAPY WITH CHILDREN

Preterm Infants

Most of the data on the positive effects of infant massage come from studies on preterm (premature) infants. During the last two decades, a number of studies were conducted, most of them labeled tactile/kinesthetic stimulation because of the negative connotations of the word *massage* (Barnard & Bee, 1983; Rausch, 1981; Rice, 1977; Solkff & Matuszak, 1975; White & LaBarba, 1976). The results published by these investigators were generally positive. A recent global analysis of data from 19 of these studies revealed that 72% of the massaged infants were positively affected (Ottenbacher et al., 1987). Most of them experienced greater weight gain and better performance on developmental tasks. Those studies that did not report significant weight gain used the wrong kind of touch, a light-stroking procedure. Babies do not like light touch, probably because it feels like tickling. The babies who gained weight had been given deeper pressure massage, thus stimulating both tactile and pressure receptors.

One of the studies used in this global analysis was conducted in our lab (Field et al., 1986). In that study we gave massage therapy to premature newborns for 45 minutes a day (in doses of 3 15-minute periods) for 10 days. The infants were 9 weeks premature, weighed about 2 pounds, and were treated in intensive care for about 3 weeks before the study. The study was started when they had graduated from the "grower nursery." At this time their main agenda was to gain weight. The massage therapy sessions were divided into 3 5-minute phases. During the first and third phases the infants were stroked. The newborns were placed on their stomachs and given moderate pressure stroking of the head and face region, neck and shoulders, back, legs, and arms for 5 1-minute segments. The Swedish-like massage was given because, as already noted, infants prefer some degree of pressure. During the middle phase, the infants' arms and legs were moved back and forth in bicycling-like motions while the infants were lying on their backs.

The massaged infants in this study gained 47% more weight (even though the groups had the same amount of formula; see Figure 1). Compared to the control infants they were awake and active more of the time even though we expected that they would sleep more, and they were more alert and responsive to social stimulation (like a person's face). The massaged infants also showed better performance on a newborn test, including more organized limb movements and more attentiveness to stimulation. Finally, they were discharged from the hospital 6 days sooner, saving approximately $3,000 per infant in hospital costs.

In another study on the use of massage with premature infants, 33 mother–infant pairs were randomly assigned to one of three groups:

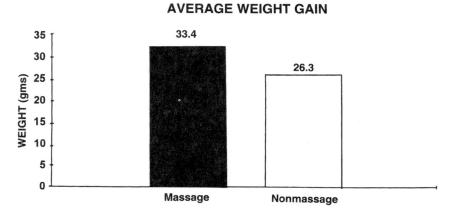

FIGURE 1. Average weight gain of infants with and without massage.

control, talking, or interactive groups (White-Traut & Nelson, 1988). The interactive group received massage, talking, eye contact, and rocking. The treatments were given at specific times 24 hours after delivery. Before being discharged, the mothers and infants were observed during a feeding. The interactive group who received the massage had better feeding interactions.

In still another study, preterms' biochemical and clinical responses to massage were assessed (Acolet et al., 1993). The 11 infants in the study were born 11 weeks prematurely, weighed approximately 2 pounds, and were hospitalized for 3 days. Blood samples were obtained for stress hormone (cortisol) levels 45 minutes before the start of massage and approximately 1 hour after the end of the massage. Cortisol levels decreased consistently after massage. There was also a slight decrease in skin temperature.

Around the time we were conducting our preemie studies, our colleagues at Duke University Medical School were conducting similar studies but on rat pups (Schanberg & Field, 1988). Schanberg and his colleagues were removing rat pups from their mother to explore touch deprivation. As mentioned earlier, the researchers stroked the depressed rat pups with a paint brush much as the mother rat would tongue lick them so the rat pups would grow normally. In several studies the Duke team noted that growth hormone decreased when the pups were removed from their mother. This decrease was noted in all body organs including heart, liver, and brain, and these values returned to normal once the pups were stroked with the paint brush. Their more recent discovery of a growth gene that responds to touch, suggests a strong genetic influence on the relationship between touching and growth (Schanberg, 1995).

This observation plus the results of a study in Sweden led us to some ideas about mechanisms that might explain the touch–weight gain relationship (Uvnas-Moberg, Widstrom, Marchine, & Windberg, 1987). The Swedish study reported that stimulating the mouth of the newborn (and the breast of the breast-feeding mother) led to an increase in food absorption hormones such as gastrin and insulin. Massage therapy on different body parts might also lead to an increase in food absorption hormones. The increase in these hormones could explain the weight gain. We began measuring these hormones (glucose and insulin), and we are finding that the massaged infants have higher glucose and insulin levels. Unfortunately, breast-feeding mothers (who do not want to gain weight) might gain weight for the same reason.

Abused and Neglected Children

Massage therapy has been successfully used with sexually and physically abused and neglected children living in a shelter (Field, 1995). Staff members and volunteers gave the children a 15-minute massage every day for a 1-month period. After 1 month of massage therapy, the children's sleep increased and they became more alert. The children's caregivers also reported that the children became more active and sociable.

Asthmatic Children

Massage therapy has also been used with asthmatic children to reduce anxiety levels and asthma symptoms (Field, Henteleff, & Mavunda, 1994). Twenty-minute daily bedtime massages were given to the children for a 1-month period by their mothers. The data show that immediately after the first and last day massage sessions the children's self-reported anxiety levels decreased and their mood improved. By the end of the study, the children had fewer asthma attacks, and peak air flow readings were higher, suggesting more efficient respiration (see Table 1).

Autistic Children

In this study we wanted to determine whether massage therapy improved the classroom behavior of preschool autistic children (Field et al., 1994b). After 1 month of massage therapy, the autistic children had less touch aversion, they were less distracted by sounds, they were more attentive in class, and they related socially to their teachers more (see

TABLE 1. Means for Asthma Massage Therapy Group

	First day		Last day	
	Pre	Post	Pre	Post
Pre/post measures				
Self-report				
Parent anxiety (STAI)	30.1	27.9[1]	30.4	27.1[1]
Child anxiety (STAIC)*	31.7	28.6[2]	28.7	27.1[1]
Child depressed mood* (POMS)	15.9	10.8[3]	8.6	4.4[3]
Child behavior				
Affect	2.3	2.5	2.3	2.8[3]
Anxiety*	2.0	1.9	2.4	2.6[1]
Fidgetiness	2.3	2.6[3]	2.5	2.7
Child physiology				
Saliva cortisol (ng/ml)	1.3	.9[2]	1.1	.9
First day/last day measures				
Self-report	First day		Last day	
Parent depression (CESD)	16.2		13.3[1]	
Parent asthma attitude	6.2		7.0[1]	
Child asthma attitude	5.2		6.9[4]	
Peak air flow	279.2		308.6[1]	

Note. Asterisks indicate significantly different presession values on first day versus last day. Superscripts indicate significance of adjacent numbers: [1]$p < .05$, [2]$p < .01$, [3]$p < .005$, [4]$p < .001$.

TABLE 2. Mean Change Scores for Touch Autism Therapy
and Attention Control Group

Variables	Touch therapy	Touch control	Optimal direction
Classroom observations			
Touch aversion	-2.6_a*	-3.0_a*	neg.
Off-task behavior	-12.8_a*	-12.3_a*	neg.
Orienting to irrelevant sounds	-2.1_a*	$-.7_b$*	neg.
Stereotypical behaviors	-8.2_a*	$-.3_b$*	neg.
Autism behavior checklist			
Sensory	-2.4_a*	$-.4_b$*	neg.
Relating	-3.2_a*	1.3_b	neg.
Object use	-2.3_a	-2.4_a	neg.
Language	-1.1_a	$-.4_a$	neg.
Social skills	-2.4_a	-1.7_a	neg.
Total	-10.6_a*	-5.0_b	neg.
Early social communication scales			
Joint attention	2.3_a*	-2.5_b	pos.
Behavior regulation	6.3_a*	$-.5_b$	pos.
Social	5.0_a*	1.8_b	pos.
Initiating	2.3_a*	-1.3_b	pos.

*Significant changes (@ $p < .05$) from beginning to end of therapy. When one group changes significantly more than the other (@ $p < .05$), the groups have different subscripts.

Table 2). These were surprising findings because we had expected that autistic children would find touch aversive. Touching during massage may be less aversive than other touch for autistic children because it is predictable. Autistic children typically find unpredictable stimulation too arousing.

Developmental Delays

In this pilot study, massage therapy was given to 13 developmentally delayed preschool children (Linkous & Stutts, 1990). The massage therapy increased muscle activation and thus increased muscle tone in 13 hypotonic developmentally delayed children. The authors of this paper were also reluctant to call their treatment massage therapy and instead called it "passive tactile stimulation."

Diabetes

Parents' typical involvement in the treatment of this condition is negative, for example, monitoring dietary compliance, and taking blood samples, and giving insulin shots. The purpose of this study was to give parents a more positive role in their children's treatment by massaging their children daily before bedtime (Field, Delamater, Shaw, & LaGreca, 1996). A preliminary data analysis of pilot data on a sample of 13 children revealed the following significant effects: (1) immediately after the massage therapy sessions, parents' anxiety and depressed mood levels were lower and their children's anxiety levels and depressed mood levels were lower; and (2) at the end of the 1-month period, the parents' insulin and food regulation scores improved, and the children's blood glucose levels decreased from 158 to the normal range (118).

Posttraumatic Stress Disorder

This study was conducted with children who were traumatized by Hurricane Andrew (Field, Seligman, Scafidi, & Schanberg, 1996). Massage therapy was expected to reduce their depression, anxiety, and behavior problems associated with posttraumatic stress disorder. The children were massaged three times weekly for 1 month, and the control group children watched relaxing videotapes during their sessions. After 1 month the massaged children had lower depression and anxiety levels than the control group, they had lower cortisol levels (stress hormone), and their drawings were happier (see Figure 2).

TABLE 3. Means for Diabetes Pre–Post Massage/
Relaxation (in Parentheses) Measures for First and Last
Day Treatment

Measure	First day		Last day	
	Pre	Post	Pre	Post
Parent anxiety (STAI)	33.6_a	$27.10_b{}^2$	30.0_a	28.1_a
	(37.1)	(32.2)	(37.1)	(37.4)
Child anxiety (STAIC)	27.9_a	$25.7_b{}^1$	31.0_a	29.3_a
	(26.5)	(27.6)	$(27.5)_a$	$(24.4)_b$
Child pulse	108.0_a	$74.0_b{}^1$	97.6_a	85.6_a
	(99.3)	(89.4)	(99.9)	(87.8)

	First day	Last day
Family cohesion	7.4_a	$8.4_b{}^1$
	(7.0)	(7.3)
Parent sense competence	44.9_a	$47.3_b{}^1$
	(49.7)	(48.6)
Parent coping	49.2_a	$52.9_b{}^1$
	(41.4)	(45.8)
Food regulation	4.4_a	$4.6_b{}^1$
	(4.3)	(4.4)
Glucose level	166.0_a	$124.9_b{}^1$
	(159.3)	(139.0)

Note. Subscripts indicate values that significantly differ from adjacent values. Superscripts indicate significance of adjacent numbers: [1]$p < .05$, [2]$p < .01$.

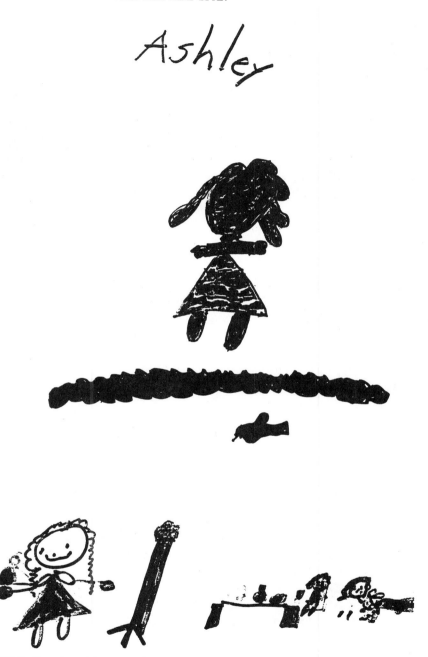

FIGURE 2. Drawing at top completed by 6-year-old girl at beginning of massage therapy study on Posttraumatic Stress Disorder following Hurricane Andrew. Drawing at bottom completed by same 6-year-old girl at end of massage therapy study.

MASSAGE THERAPY WITH ADOLESCENTS

Depression following Childbirth

Depression after childbirth has negative effects on infants' growth and development if the mothers' depression continues for several months. In this study, depressed adolescent mothers received a 25-minute massage twice a week for a 5-week period. The adolescent mothers reported less anxiety and more positive mood immediately after the massage, and their fidgeting decreased, their talking increased, and their facial expressions were more positive after massage over the 5-week period. Their stress hormone levels (cortisol) and their depression decreased.

Eating Disorders

Adolescents with eating disorders such as bulimia (overeating and vomiting) or anorexia (undereating) are often depressed. This study was focused on decreasing depression and anxiety and improving body image in adolescents with eating disorders (Mueller et al., 1996). The adolescent girls were massaged twice weekly for a 5-week period. At the end of the study, the massaged adolescents had fewer depressive symptoms than the control group, a less distorted body image, increased satisfaction with overall appearance, and improved self-esteem.

Psychiatric Problems

In this study 52 hospitalized depressed and conduct-disorder (behavior problem) adolescents received a 30-minute back massage for a 5-day period every day (Field et al., 1992). Compared to a control group who watched relaxing videotapes, the massaged subjects were less depressed and anxious and had lower stress hormone (saliva cortisol) levels after the massage (see Table 4). In addition, nurses rated the massage recipients as less anxious and more cooperative on the last day of the study, nighttime sleep increased over this period (the adolescents were videotaped during their sleep for this measure), and urinary cortisol and norepinephrine levels (stress hormones) decreased.

MASSAGE THERAPY WITH ADULTS

Alcohol and Drug Addiction

In a study by another research group, massage therapy was given to clients and counselors in chemical dependency treatment programs and

TABLE 4. Depressed Subjects Who Received Massage Therapy

	First day			Last day		
	Pre	Post	p level	Pre	Post	p level
Self-report						
State anxiety	34.7	27.3	.001	319	27.6	.01
Depressed mood (POMS)	20.4	16.4	.005	14.7	14.7	NS
Behavior observation						
State	2.4	1.5	.001	2.5	1.7	.001
Affect	2.0	2.3	.005	2.0	2.3	.01
Vocalizations	1.8	1.1	.005	1.8	1.2	.001
Activity	1.7	1.2	.001	1.7	1.4	.001
Anxeity	1.7	1.2	.005	1.4	1.2	.05
Fidgeting	1.5	1.2	.01	1.4	1.1	.05
Nurses' ratings						
Affect	1.9			2.3		.05
Anxiety	2.1			1.8		.05
Fidgeting	1.8			1.5		.05
Cooperation	2.1			2.3		.05
Sleep behaviors						
Deep sleep	79.7			91.3		.01
Awakenings	15.2			4.0		.05
Physiological measures						
Activity watch	5.0	1.5	.001	3.4	1.7	.01
Pulse	88.0	79.0	.001	87.0	82.0	.001
Biocemical						
Saliva cortisol	1.8	1.4	.05	2.2	1.4	.001
Urine cortisol	99.0			64.0		.01
Urine norepinephrine	39.0			29.0		.05

to recovering patients after treatment (Adcock, 1987). The primary benefits were deeper relaxation, greater self-acceptance, and quicker detoxification.

Breast Surgery

Common procedures after breast surgery for cancer include augmentation or reduction mammoplasty and breast reconstruction. Postoperative complications include infection, poor wound healing, and pain. In this study, scar formation (which may disrupt the normal breast contour) was reduced by frequent massaging of the scar (Field & Miller, 1992). Unfortunately, following breast surgery, many women do not enjoy massaging themselves or having significant others massage them, so these factors combined make it very difficult to assess the effects of massage on breast-scar reduction.

Burns

Burn patients were randomly assigned to massage therapy or a standard treatment control group at the beginning of the scar formation stage. The massage therapy group received 30 minutes of massage with cocoa butter two times a week for 5 weeks. The massage therapy group patients had more optimal self-reports on anxiety, depression, pain, and itching immediately after the first and last therapy sessions than the standard treatment group, and their ratings on these measures improved over the 5-week period.

Cancer

In this study we examined the effects of gentle back massage on the well-being of female patients who were receiving radiotherapy for breast cancer, using subjects as their own controls (Sims, 1986). Patients reported less distress, greater tranquility and vitality, and less tension and tiredness following the back massage therapy versus before the therapy.

Chronic Fatigue Syndrome

Twenty chronic fatigue syndrome subjects were randomly assigned to a massage therapy or a SHAM TENS (transcutaneous electrical stimulation) control group. Immediately following the massage therapy versus SHAM TENS on the first and last days of the study, the massage therapy group had lower depression and anxiety scores and lower cortisol levels. Longer term effects (last day versus first day) suggested that the massage therapy versus SHAM TENS group had lower depression, emotional distress, and somatic symptom scores; more hours of sleep, and lower epinephrine and cortisol levels.

Headaches

Twenty-one female patients suffering from chronic tension headache received 10 sessions of upper-body massage (not including the head), consisting of deep-pressure techniques in addition to softer massage used in the beginning (Puustjarvi, Airaksinen, & Pontinen, 1990). Trigger points (knots in the muscles) were carefully but forcefully massaged. At the end of the study, the range of neck movement had increased, and the number of days with headaches had decreased. Lower Beck Depression Inventory scores also suggested less depression at the end of the treatment period than at the beginning.

HIV

In this study we examined massage therapy effects on anxiety and depression levels and on immune function in adult gay men with HIV

(Ironson, 1996). The subjects received a 45-minute massage five times a week for a 1-month period. At the end of the treatment period, anxiety and distress levels were reduced, and serotonin levels were increased. Natural killer cells (the front line of the immune system) and natural killer cell cytotoxicity also increased. The increase in natural killer cell number suggests that massage therapy helped the immune system by reducing the probability that these men would experience opportunistic infections such as pneumonia.

Immune Function

In another immune study, 50 healthy college students were assigned to one of several relaxation methods—progressive muscle relaxation (tightening and relaxing muscles sequentially throughout the body), visual imagery, massage, lying quietly with eyes closed, or a control group (Green & Green, 1987). Immunoglobulin A (immune response) and cortisol levels (stress hormone) were measured from saliva samples taken before and after the 20-minute sessions. The massage group subjects showed the largest increase in salivary immunoglobulin concentrations.

Job Stress

Our job stress study was designed to reduce job stress and anxiety, as well as increase productivity and job satisfaction (Field, Ironson, Pickens, Nawrocki, Fox, Scafidi, Burman, & Schanberg, 1986). A 15-minute chair massage was given during the lunch period in the subject's office twice a week for 5 weeks. After the massage sessions, the participants reported feeling less anxiety and fatigue and being able to think more clearly. Their brain waves (EEG alpha, beta, and theta waves) changed in ways that are consistent with increased relaxation (i.e., increased theta) alertness (i.e., decreased alpha and beta). In addition, they were able to complete math computations in half the time with half the errors.

Cancer Pain Relief

This study, by another group, compared different procedures for coping with cancer pain (Weinrich & Weinrich, 1990). Pain management, perceived ability to decrease pain, and pain intensity ratings were measured before and after distraction, relaxation, and massage. Results suggested that these methods were effective.

In another cancer study, 28 patients were randomly assigned to a massage or control group. The patients in the massage group were given a 10-minute back massage while the patients in the control group were simply visited for 10 minutes. Pain levels decreased after the massage, but curiously only for males.

Fibromyalgia

Thirty adult fibromyalgia syndrome subjects were randomly assigned to a massage therapy, a transcutaneous electrical stimulation (TENS), or a transcutaneous electrical stimulation no-current group (SHAM TENS) for 30-minute treatment sessions two times per week for 5 weeks. The massage therapy subjects reported lower anxiety and depression, and their cortisol levels were lower immediately after the therapy sessions on the first and last days of the study (see Table 5). The TENS group showed similar changes but only after therapy on the last day of the study. The massage therapy group improved on the dolorimeter measure of pain. They also reported less pain last week, less stiffness and fatigue, and fewer nights of difficult sleeping. Thus massage therapy was the most effective therapy with these fibromyalgia patients.

General Pain

Massage therapy is usually given by someone else, but in this study a nonelectrical touch device, called the Dermapoints Massageroller, was used (Naliboff & Tachiki, 1991). This is a steel hand-held rod that has wheels of small, pointed, steel triangles that move across the skin as you roll it, much like a miniature rolling pin for dough but with points. In this

TABLE 5. Means for Fibromyalgia Massage Therapy Group

	First day		Last day	
	Pre	Post	Pre	Post
Variables*				
Pre/post therapy				
Anxiety (STAI)	45.4	35.0[d]	38.6	34.1[a]
Depression (POMS)	17.3	12.9[a]	21.3	12.0[a]
Stress hormone (ng cortisol)	1.9	1.2[a]	1.8	1.0[a]
First day–last day physician's assessment	First day		Last day	
Rating of clinical condition (0–10)	4.3		1.8[a]	
Dolorimeter value (kg)	3.4		4.5[b]	
Self-report				
Pain and sleep symptoms				
Pain	8.6		5.3[d]	
Pain last week	7.8		6.0[b]	
Stiffness	8.6		6.8[b]	
Fatigue	7.4		4.5[b]	
# nights difficult sleeping	6.1		3.4[c]	
Depression scale (CESD)	31.9		26.8	

*All variables are ratings except where otherwise specified.
[a] = 0.05; [b] = 0.01 ;[c] = 0.005; [d] = 0.001 for adjacent values.
PRE = pretherapy; POST = posttherapy.

study stimulation by the massageroller led to increased skin temperature and decreased muscle tension.

In another study connective tissue massage was given by a therapist to relieve pain (Kaada & Torsteinbo, 1989). Beta-endorphins were measured in the blood of the 12 volunteers before and after a 30–minute session of connective tissue massage. There was a moderate increase in beta-endorphin levels lasting for about 1 hour. The release of beta-endorphins was linked with pain relief and feeling of well-being after the treatment.

Postoperative Pain

Researchers studied postoperative pain in 116 patients who underwent a thoracotomy (Lepresle, Mechet, & Debesse, 1991). Pain was assessed using a visual analog scale (a ruler with pain measured from 1 to 10). Those who received massage reported significantly lower pain as measured by the visual analog scale.

MASSAGE THERAPY FOR OLDER ADULTS

Slow-Stroke Back Massage

This study examined the effects of slow-stroke back massage on systolic and diastolic blood pressure, heart rate, and skin temperature of 30 middle-aged-adult hospice patients (Meek, 1993). Systolic BP, diastolic BP, and heart rate decreased, and skin temperature increased following back massage.

Pain Management

One pain-management paper presents techniques that can be used with middle-aged adults in the home or a hospice setting and are relatively low risk, simple, and inexpensive (McCaffery & Wolff, 1992). The techniques include massage, superficial heat and cold, menthol application to the skin (such as Bengay), transcutaneous electrical nerve stimulation (TENS—transmitting a very weak electrical current through the body), positioning, and movement.

Grandparent Volunteers Giving versus Receiving Massage

Hospital volunteers (typically of grandparent age, namely, 60 to 80 years old) were taught to massage babies at our hospital so that the therapy could be cost effective. The volunteers reported feeling better themselves after massaging the infants. Thus in this study we compared the effects of grandparent volunteers giving infants massage versus receiving massages themselves (Field et al., 1996). After the massage sessions the volunteers reported lower anxiety and improved mood, and after a month-long study they reported increased self-esteem and a better lifestyle (e.g., fewer doctor visits and more social contacts). These effects were stronger for the volunteer grandparents after a month of massaging the infants than after receiving massage therapy themselves.

SUMMARY

In summary, massage therapy has been effective in our studies (and studies by other groups) regardless of age or condition. Generally, the massage therapy results in lower anxiety levels (both self-reported and observed), lower stress hormones (cortisol), and better mood (less depression). Other findings that were unique to specific studies would probably generalize to all ages and conditions if these measures were used in all studies. The measures include enhanced alertness and math performance (along with the EEG pattern of heightened alertness), improved sleep, and enhanced immune function. These changes may be related to increased vagal activity (resulting from tactile and pressure stimulation). Increasing vagal activity typically slows the nervous system to a more

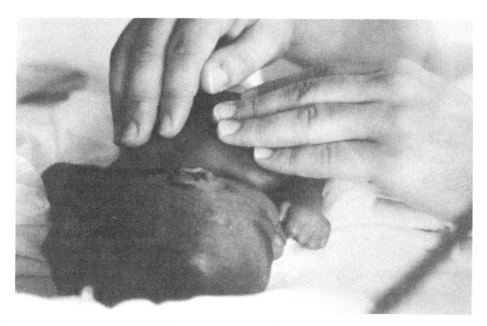

FIGURE 3. Premature infant being massaged.

alert, relaxed (parasympathetic) state during which stress hormones (cortisol) are decreased. Since increased cortisol is associated with compromised immune function, it is not surprising that the immune system would also benefit from massage therapy.

Other results may be specific to the condition and probably would not generalize to other conditions. For example, the preemie needs to gain weight (see Figure 3), but a full-term newborn does not, and a postpartum mother would certainly not want to gain weight from massage. For another example, the asthmatic needs to breathe better, and a side effect of the massage therapy is better breathing, probably again because of increased vagal activity and parasympathetic activation. The degree to which massage therapy alters or prevents these conditions is not clear at this time, but inasmuch as most diseases are exacerbated by stress and massage therapy alleviates stress, massage should probably be high on the health priority list, along with diet and exercise, as it was around 1800 B.C. in India. Everyone loves a little touch therapy.

ACKNOWLEDGMENTS

This research was supported by an NIMH Research Scientist Award (#MH00331) and an NIMH Research Grant (#MH46586) to Tiffany Field.

REFERENCES

Acolet, D., Giannakoulopoulos, X., Bond, C., Weg, W., Clow, A., & Glover, V. (1993). Changes in plasma cortisol and catecholamine concentrations in response to massage in preterm infants. *Archives of Disease in Childhood, 68,* 29–31.

Adcock, C. L. (1987). Massage therapy in alcohol/drug treatment. *Alcoholism Treatment Quarterly, 1,* 87–101.

Field, D. A., & Miller S. (1992). Cosmetic breast surgery. *American Family Physician, 45,* 711–719.

Field, T. (1995). Massage therapy for infants and children. *Developmental and Behavioral Pediatrics, 16,* 105–111.

Field, T., Delamater, A., Shaw, K., & LaGreca, A. (1996). Diabetic children's adherence and glucose levels improve after touch therapy. In review.

Field, T., Grizzle, N., & Scafidi, F. (1996). Massage and relaxation therapies' effects on depressed adolescent mothers. *Adolescence* (in press).

Field, T., Henteleff, T., & Mavunda, K. (1994a). Asthmatic children have less anxiety and respiratory problems after touch therapy. In review.

Field, T., Ironson, G., Pickens, J., Nawrocki, T., Fox, N., Scafidi, F., Burman, I., & Schanberg, S. (1996). Massage effects on job stress, EEG and math computations. *International Journal of Neuroscience* (in press).

Field, T., Lasko, D., Mundy, P., Henteleff, T., Talpins, S., & Dowling, M. (1994b). Autistic children's attentiveness and responsivity improved after touch therapy. *Journal of Autism and Developmental Disabilities* (in press).

Field, T., Morrow, C., Valdeon, C., Larson, S., Kuhn, C., & Schanberg, S. (1992). Massage therapy reduces anxiety in child and adolescent psychiatric patients. *Journal of the American Academy of Child and Adolescent Psychiatry, 31*, 125–131.

Field, T., Schanberg, S., Scafidi, F., Bower, C., Vega-Lahr, N., Garcia, R., Nystrom, J., & Kuhn, C. M. (1986). Tactile/kinesthetic stimulation effects on preterm neonates. *Pediatrics, 77(5)*, 654–658.

Field, T., Seligman, S., Scafidi, F., & Schanberg, S. (1996). Alleviating posttraumatic stress in children following Hurricane Andrew. *Journal of Applied Developmental Psychology* (in press).

Field, T., Wheeden, A., Burman, I., Schanberg, S., & Kuhn, C. (1996). Grandparent volunteers benefit from massaging infants. In review.

Green, R. G., & Green, M. L. (1987). Relaxation increases salivary immunoglobulin A. *Psychological Reports, 61*, 623–629.

Ironson, G., Field, T., Scafidi, F., Hashimoto, M., Kumar, M., Kumar, A., et al. (1996). Massage is associated with enhancement of the immune system's cytotoxic capacity levels. *International Journal of Neuroscience, 84*, 205–217.

Kaada, B., & Torsteinbo, O. (1989). Increase of plasma beta-endorphins in connective tissue. *General Pharmacology, 20*, 487–490.

Lepresle, M. I., Mechet, C., & Debesse, B. (1991). Postoperative pain after thoracotomy. A study of 116 patients. *Revue des Maladies Respiratoires, 8*, 213–218.

Linkous, L. W., & Stutts, R. M. (1990). Passive tactile stimulation effects on the muscle tone of hypotonic, developmentally delayed children. *Perceptual and Motor Skills, 71*, 951–954.

McCaffery, M., & Wolff, M. (1992). Pain relief using cutaneous modalities, positioning, and movement. *Hospice Journal, 8*, 121–153.

Meek, S. S. (1993). Effects of slow stroke back massage on relaxation in hospice clients. *Image—The Journal of Nursing Scholarship, 25*, 17–21.

Mueller, C., Field, T., Yando, R., Harding, J., Gonzalez, K. P., Lasko, D., & Bendell, D. (1995). Under-eating and over-eating concerns among adolescents. *Journal of Child Psychology and Psychiatry*. In review.

Naliboff, B. D., & Tachiki, K. H. (1991). Autonomic and skeletal muscle responses to non-electrical cutaneous stimulation. *Perceptual and Motor Skills, 72*, 575–584.

Older, J. (1982). *Touching is healing*. New York: Stein and Day.

Ottenbacher, K. J., Muller, L., Brandt, D., Heintzelman, A., Hojem, P., & Sharpe, P. (1987). The effectiveness of tactile stimulation as a form of early intervention: A quantitive evaluation. *Journal of Developmental and Behavioral Pediatrics, 8*, 68–76.

Puustjarvi, K., Airaksinen, O., & Pontinen, P. J. (1990). The effects of massage in patients with chronic tension headache. *Acupuncture and Electro-Therapeutic Research, 15*, 159–162.

Rausch, P. B. (1981). Neurophysiological development in premature infants following stimulation. *Developmental Psychology, 13*, 69–76.

Rice, R. D. (1977). Neurophysiological development in premature infants following stimulation. *Developmental Psychology, 13*, 69–76.

Schanberg, S. (1995). The genetic basis for touch effects. In T. Field (Ed.), *Touch in early development*. Hillsdale, NJ: Erlbaum.

Schanberg, S., & Field, T. (1988). Maternal deprivation and supplemental stimulation. In T. Field, P. McCabe, & N. Schneiderman (Eds.), *Stress and coping across development*. Hillsdale, NJ: Erlbaum.

Sims, S. (1986). Slow stroke back massage for cancer patients. *Nursing Times, 82*, 47–50.

Solkoff, N., & Matuszak, D. (1975). Tactile stimulation and behavioral development among low-birthweight infants. *Child Psychiatry and Human Development, 6*, 33–37.

Uvnas-Moberg, K., Widstrom, A. M., Marchine, G., & Windberg, J. (1987). Release of GI hormone in mothers and infants by sensory stimulation. *Acta Paediatrica Scandinavia, 76*, 851–860.

Weinrich, S. P., & Weinrich, M. C. (1990). The effect of massage on pain in cancer patients. *Applied Nursing Research, 3,* 140–145.

Wheeden, A., Scafidi, F. A., Field, T., Ironson, G., & Valdeon, C. Massage effects on cocaine-exposed preterm neonates. In press.

White, J. L., & LaBarba, R. C. (1976). The effects of tactile and kinesthetic stimulation on neonatal development in the premature infant. *Developmental Psychobiology, 6,* 569–577.

White-Traut, R. C., & Nelson, M. N. (1988). Maternally administered tactile, auditory, visual, and vestibular stimulation: Relationship to later interactions between mothers and premature infants. *Research in Nursing & Health, 11,* 31–39.

CHAPTER 5

The Context of Development for Young Children from Cocaine-Abusing Families

LINDA C. MAYES AND MARC H. BORNSTEIN

INTRODUCTION

Prolonged cocaine addiction by its very intractable nature defines a way of life, and popular notions about the lifestyle of cocaine abuse have always abounded in stereotypes (Courtwright, 1982; Musto, 1973). One view persisting from the late 19th century portrays the innocent or eccentric but wildly imaginative individual jump-starting his creative slumps with an occasional, absolutely controlled, if not misguided, use of cocaine. Poets, painters, successful businessmen, professors, and physicians may have fallen prey to the temptation from time to time, but at their core they were still contributing members of society. The other, currently more popular, stereotypic extreme is the sinister, dangerous derelict, a thief at the least and murderer at the worst, whose life has been self-destructed by irresponsible cocaine abuse. These are the individuals whom communities abhor, enact laws against, and pursue—they are nameless and isolated outcasts, the criminals, prostitutes, and misfits. Similar negative stereotypes about cocaine use are seen in images of parents who abuse

LINDA C. MAYES • Child Study Center, Yale University, New Haven, Connecticut 06510.   MARC H. BORNSTEIN • National Institute of Child Health and Human Development, 9000 Rockville Pike, Bethesda, Maryland 20892.

Handbook of Diversity Issues in Health Psychology, edited by Pamela M. Kato and Traci Mann. Plenum Press, New York, 1996.

cocaine and in portrayals of children who were exposed to cocaine prenatally. That is, no one abusing cocaine can care for children, and children exposed to cocaine prenatally are universally and irrevocably damaged.

Effect of Stereotypes about Substance Abuse

As in most instances of widely diverging stereotypes, such images leave out more than they reveal and are rarely rooted in empirical study (Fitzpatrick & Gerard, 1993; Mayes, Granger, Bornstein, & Zuckerman, 1992; Mayes, in press-a). But they do permit society to distance itself from a problem that is fundamentally about losing and regaining control over personal deficiencies and impairments, setbacks, fears, and despair and has always involved addicted individuals, their families, and children in inescapable tragedies and loss. So certain and pervasive are the stereotypes about cocaine abuse that they have often influenced and clouded efforts to understand the range of individual variation and patterns among adults who are cocaine abusing (Cohen & Harrison, 1986; Gossop, Griffiths, Powis, & Strang, 1994) and the cumulative effects of cocaine abuse on an individual adult's psychological and physical development and functioning.

Rarely too do these popular views allow a closer appreciation of all those people, including children, who may be caught up in the world of cocaine abuse but are not themselves addicts. The effect of stereotypes and attitudes about substance abuse on the care of addicts has not been systematically studied. However, models of other stereotypes regarding, for example, race, gender, or AIDS suggest that attitudes do shape assessments of need as well as the expectations of peers, teachers, physicians, or other service providers (DeJong, Van den Brink, & Jansen, 1993; Garretson, 1993; Snell, Finney, & Godwin, 1991). The influence of any given set of stereotypes may lead service providers to expect less of a given group of individuals or to be pessimistic about an individual's capacity to change or use services. Thus biases regarding substance abusers may also implicitly shape the composition and distribution of drug-abuse intervention and rehabilitation services, and they may have explicit effects on the availability of overall health care services for all substance abusers and most dramatically for women substance abusers (and their children).

Epidemiology of Substance Abuse

Viewed at close range, the world of cocaine abuse is multidimensional in its origins and outcomes. It cuts across socioeconomic class and gender (and did so in the late 19th as it does in the late 20th century; Musto, 1973). It involves individuals who come to cocaine abuse after a series of extraordinarily traumatic life events: those who began their use as a way of being with peers, those who started their abuse in early adolescence and have known little else since, and those who use cocaine as a means of medicating what they perceive as their own personal deficits. The cocaine abusing adult may be a productive, regular member of the work force or professional community, or the abuser may be a high school dropout, unemployed, single mother of five. He or she may have sustained years of heavy use with little visible effect or be seriously physically and psychologically ill after only a few years of use (Khalsa, Anglin, Paredes, Potepan, & Potter, 1993). The addicted adult may have tried repeatedly to stop his or her use or adamantly refused to acknowledge his or her degree of dependence or accept any intervention. In short, there is no single pattern of cocaine abuse, but in the last decade, two trends have raised concern.

The first is the increasing use of cocaine and other substances of abuse among women living in impoverished inner city neighborhoods (Amaro, Zuckerman, & Cabral, 1989; Zuckerman, Frank, Hingson, & Amaro, 1989). Some major cities in the United States report 50% of women receiving prenatal care at inner-city hospital clinics have used cocaine regularly during their pregnancy and for several years before (Amaro, Fried, Cabral, & Zuckerman, 1990; Osterloh & Lee, 1989); in addition, the majority of urban areas across the Untied States report a persistently high (10%–20%) incidence of cocaine abuse among women of childbearing age (Chasnoff, Landress, & Barrett, 1990; Frank et al., 1988). The second related trend is the increasing number of children born to cocaine-using women, growing up with substance abusing parents, or both (Scherling, 1994). No one estimate is certain, but currently perhaps more than 350,000 infants are born per year to mothers who have used cocaine with or without other substances (such as alcohol) throughout their pregnancy (Besharov, 1990; Gomby & Shiono, 1991). These trends have, in turn, led to two expanding areas of research, the first being a focus on the effects of prenatal cocaine exposure on infants' and children's development and the second on studies of the characteristics of women who abuse substances and the effects of that substance abuse on their ability to parent.

Health Care Policy for Substance-Abusing Parents and Their Children

This chapter reviews the accumulated data in both of these research areas, summarizes the principal research themes, and concludes with an overview of the health and developmental needs of substance-abusing women and their children. A focus on young children from cocaine-abusing families represents a significant area for health psychology. As will be outlined, children from cocaine-abusing families have multiple unmet developmental and health care needs, and their parents often have great difficulty meeting those needs or accessing care for themselves. Furthermore, very few health care programs combine substance-abuse treatment, basic pediatric care, and psychosocial developmental interventions for the children. In short, few programs addressing an adult's addiction address how that addiction affects the children and the family and that adult's role as a parent. Understanding the developmental and physical needs of children from substance-abusing families along with the needs of their parents will inform the development of more integrated health care services for children from substance-abusing families.

Moreover, policies regarding the health care of multiply disadvantaged children from multiply disadvantaged families are better informed by specific data about the developmental and health needs of this population. Particularly in regards to substance abuse, health and legal policies made apart from existing data have tended to be punitive toward substance abusing parents and not always in the best interests of their children (Garrity-Roukas, 1994). For example, mandatory reporting to child protective agencies of positive urine screens during pregnancy presumes the pregnant woman will be unable to care for her newborn but does not take into account the possibility that such regulations may dissuade substance abusing mothers from seeking either prenatal care or well-child care. In this way, the policy regarding mandatory reporting may work against mothers and children receiving adequate health care and is not informed by data about either the neurodevelopmental status of cocaine-exposed newborns or about the parenting capacities of cocaine-using adults.

When we look beyond the stereotypes and popular opinions, the problem of prenatal cocaine exposure is marked by multiple levels of interaction between prenatal and postnatal factors and between biologic vulnerabilities and disordered environments. Investigators seeking to understand further the effects of prenatal cocaine exposure on children's psychological development face the dilemma that cocaine affects development through multiple pathways and that rarely, if ever, is it possible to speak of a "pure" cocaine effect or a singular and identifiable effect on one aspect of brain development or, for that matter, on parental function (Mayes & Bornstein, 1995b). Because cocaine is a potentially teratogenic agent with profound effects on the child's immediate parental and more global social environment, as well as the child's pre- and postnatal development, studies of the outcome of prenatally cocaine-exposed infants necessarily involve biologic–environment interaction models (Bergeman & Plomin, 1989). For the child and parent, the multiple pathways of effect of prenatal cocaine exposure and ongoing cocaine use also represent risks for numbers of other problems, such as homelessness, involvement in violence and crime, poor school performance and early school dropout, and multigenerational drug abuse, problems that trap both parent and child in poverty and despair. We begin with a summary of the pathways through which prenatal cocaine exposure and ongoing parental cocaine use can affect both child and family.

PATHWAYS OF COCAINE EFFECTS ON CHILDREN'S DEVELOPMENT

Effects on Fetal Brain Development

Guiding much of the research focused on the consequences of prenatal cocaine exposure is the hypothesis that cocaine has a direct effect on developing fetal brain such that either structure, function, or both, are altered adversely. Sufficient data are now available from animal models to indicate that prenatal cocaine exposure does alter monoaminergic neurotransmitter function particularly in those areas of the brain involved in the regulation of attention and states of arousal (Mayes, in press-a; Mayes & Bornstein, 1995b). Because of a cocaine-related vasoconstrictive effect on placental blood flow and on developing fetal vasculature, prenatal cocaine exposure also affects fetal brain growth as well as overall fetal growth (Coles, Platzman, Smith, James, & Falek, 1992; Singer, Farkas, & Kliegman, 1992; Woods, Plessinger, & Clark, 1987). In addition to these direct effects of prenatal cocaine exposure on fetal brain development, cocaine affects development via at least four other possible pathways.

Postnatal Exposure

One pathway for the effect of cocaine on child development is through continued postnatal cocaine exposure for the infant via passive absorption of crack smoke (Kjarasch, Glotzer, Vinci, Wietzman, & Sargent, 1991). Brain development continues through at least the first 12 months after birth with extensive synaptic remodeling, pruning, and actual structural refinement, and monoaminergic neurotransmitter systems are involved in the regulation of these areas of postnatal brain growth (Goldman-Rakic, 1987). Because of the effect of cocaine on monoaminergic neurotransmitter function, passive exposure postnatally to cocaine may affect these processes of synaptic remodeling, loss, and genesis.

Adult Psychopathology

The second pathway relates to issues that bring adults to abuse cocaine initially. For many substance-abusing adults, psychiatric disorders, such as depression or even attention deficit disorder, appear to predate substance abuse per se and, at least for some, may represent a significant factor in initial experimentation with cocaine or other substances (Khantzian, 1985; Khantzian & Khantzian, 1984; Woods, Eyler, Behnke, & Conlon, 1991). This circumstance has two consequences: (1) Drug-abusing parents may suffer other psychiatric symptoms and associated psychological and social disorders, and (2) drug-abusing parents may pass to their offspring an increased genetic risk for these psychiatric conditions.

Several investigators have noted the association between active substance abuse and major psychopathology. Among substance-abusing adults, the incidence of major depression, recurrent and early psychiatric hospitalizations, and, for men, conduct problems often resulting in criminal prosecution is higher than that of the general population (Mirin, Weiss, Griffin, & Michael, 1991; Rounsaville et al., 1991). Among substance abusers' parents and siblings, there is also an increased rate of psychiatric disorders such as depression and antisocial personality disorder, which are comorbid with substance abuse (Mirin et al.; Rounsaville et al.). The comorbidity appears not to be an aggregation of specific disorders, that is, a concordance for depression or antisocial personality, but rather a general conveyance of risk and an elevation in the incidence of several disorders (Luthar, Anton, Merikangas, & Rounsaville, 1992; Merikangas, Rounsaville, & Prusoff, 1992).

Parental death or desertion, marital discord, divorce, substance abuse, and high rates of physical and sexual abuse have also been identified as characteristics of the families of origin of substance abusers (Chambers, Hinesby, & Moldestad, 1970; Raynes, Clement, Patch, & Ervin, 1974). Rounsaville, Weissman, Wilber, and Kleber (1982) reported that disruptive events such as family violence, hospitalizations, or unexpected separations were common historical incidents in the early experiences of substance abusers. Early traumatic experiences such as these are also associated with later impairments in parenting and dysfunctional parenting styles regardless of whether or not the adult also becomes a substance abuser.

This comorbidity of substance abuse with other psychiatric conditions will have implications as well for the genetic transmission of disorders in the second-generation offspring of these families (Pauls, 1991). In particular, both affective disorders and impairments in attention regulation may be at least partially genetically transmitted from the substance-abusing adult to child. Thus, while not directly related to the cocaine exposure itself, maternal cocaine addiction may serve as a marker for genetic loading for affective disorders in the child.

Parenting among Substance-Abusing Adults

The third pathway of effect of cocaine on developmental outcome relates to the effects of these comorbid psychiatric disorders on the substance-abusing adult's actual parenting behaviors. Impairments in parenting by a cocaine-abusing adult may reflect preexisting psychological and psychiatric conditions, which contributed to the individual's addiction. An extensive literature describes the detrimental effects of maternal postpartum depression on maternal responsivity and sensitivity to the infant and, in turn, on the infant's active engagement and affective range (Field, 1995). The substance-abusing adult's depression may be worsened by poor social supports, the repeated stress of poverty and violence, and the often poor physical health associated with their addiction (Zuckerman, Amaro, Banchner, & Cabral, 1989). Severe depression may also make it more difficult for an adult to decrease or stop using cocaine. Thus the adult becomes a more dysfunctional parent because of both depression and worsening drug abuse.

Similar impairments in the substance-abusing adult's capacity to respond to his or her child may also reflect the effects of chronic cocaine use on specific neuropsychological domains that are crucial for certain aspects of parenting (Bauman & Dougherty, 1983; Mayes, 1995). All substances of abuse alter the individual's state of consciousness, memory, affect regulation, and impulse control in varying degree and may become so addictive that the adult's primary goal is to supply his or her addiction to the exclusion of other activities and other people in her or his life. These types of alterations will markedly influence the adult's capacity, for example, to sustain important responsive interactions with an infant or young child at any given moment (Bornstein, 1995).

No studies have specifically examined how the duration of an adult's cocaine abuse impacts on the degree of parenting dysfunction. However, prolonged cocaine abuse that results in neuropsychological impairments in memory, verbal fluency, attention, persistence, and task orientation might be expected to influence parenting behaviors such as the capacity to sustain an interaction (Ardila, Rosselli, & Strumwasser, 1991; Beery, Van, Herzberg, & Hinkin, 1993; Manschreck et al., 1990; O'Malley, Adamse, Heaton, & Gawin, 1992). Similarly, the neuropsychological effects of prolonged addiction on memory, persistence, and concentration may also impede an adult's response to drug-treatment interventions and contribute to an intractable addiction involving multiple drugs in addition to cocaine including alcohol, marijuana, and tobacco, factors that also influence parenting.

Substance-Abusing Environment

The fourth potential pathway of cocaine-related effects on infant and child relates to the global amount of family discord, virtual homelessness, poverty, and on a more basic level, chronic uncertainty, despair, and fear in both adults and children that characterize the cocaine-using world. Abuse of cocaine often involves the user directly or indirectly in criminal activities such as prostitution, theft, or actual drug dealing (Boyd & Mieczkowski, 1990) and exposes the user as well as her or his children to personal and property violence. Because of these activities, cocaine- abusing adults are more likely to be arrested and incarcerated repeatedly, exposing their children to multiple episodes of parental separation and placements usually with a series of foster families or with other (often substance-abusing) neighbors or relatives (Lawson & Wilson, 1980). The levels and types of violence that the children of cocaine-abusing mothers are exposed to range from verbal abuse between adults to physical fights with deadly weapons. Children 5 to 6 years of age living in this world see and participate in scenes well beyond their psychological capacities either to understand or cope.

Acute and chronic trauma affect children's brain development and psychological functioning. We might readily surmise that children developing amidst drug-associated violence, poverty, discord, neglect, and uncertainty experience a level of acute and ongoing stress and trauma of potentially sufficient intensity and chronicity to alter the development of centrally regulated, basic psychophysiological functions. Moreover, many of these children may have impairments in the capacity to regulate states of arousal in response to novel or highly stimulating situations and are thus exposed to conditions that further stress dysfunctional regulatory systems. In the central nervous system, stress-related neurotransmitters potentially contribute to increased sensitivity and altered arousal regulatory mechanisms in the face of overwhelming, stressful events (Pittman, 1988). Compromise in arousal regulation secondary to traumatic events and response to stimulation may further impede the child's already compromised ability to respond to ongoing discord and chaos in the world around him.

Relation of Levels of Effect to Attention

Each of these pathways along with a potentially direct effect of cocaine on prenatal brain development is bidirectional and interacts with the others. For example, a direct effect of prenatal exposure may be expressed as dysfunction in attentional regulation. Attentional dyfunction also shapes the infant's response to his or her environment both in terms of the parent's activities and the more distal factors cited such as severe neglect or recurrent violence. In turn, infants with attentional problems may require their parents to adjust their responses and methods of caring but such a level of sensitivity to the individual infant's needs is potentially compromised by the adult's addiction.

PRENATAL COCAINE EXPOSURE AND
DEVELOPMENTAL OUTCOME

General Developmental Outcome

In this section, we review what is currently known about the long-term developmental outcome of prenatally cocaine-exposed children. The pathway of effect implicit in most of these studies is a direct effect on prenatal brain development. However, each of the pathways specified above is operative in every available study to date, although rarely examined explicitly. Studies of the developmental effects on children of prenatal cocaine exposure have for the most part utilized general measures of developmental integrity or competency (Mayes, in press-a), such as the Bayley Scales of Infant Development (BSID; Bayley, 1969, 1993). In early reports of infants exposed to cocaine as well as combinations of heroin, methadone, and marijuana, cocaine exposure was predictively linked to moderate to severe developmental delays across diverse developmental domains (see Mayes, 1992).

Subsequent studies have reported mild to no impairments in overall developmental functioning in cocaine-exposed children compared to non-cocaine-exposed groups (Anisfeld et al., 1991; Arendt, Singer, & Minnes, 1993; Chasnoff, Griffith, Freier, and Murray, 1992; Griffith, Azuma, & Chasnoff, 1994; Mayes, in press-a; Scherling, 1994; Zuckerman & Frank, 1992). Chasnoff and colleagues reported on the developmental profiles of a group of cocaine/alcohol exposed 24-month-olds followed from birth compared to the performance of non-cocaine-exposed but marijuana-exposed, and/or alcohol-exposed children (Chasnoff et al., 1992). Mothers of infants in the non-cocaine-using comparison groups were similar to the cocaine-using mothers on socioeconomic status, age, marital status, and tobacco use during pregnancy. On repeated developmental assessments using the BSID at 3, 6, 12, 18, and 24 months, albeit with a high rate of attrition from the original cohort, there were no mean differences across groups in either the mental or motor domains. The investigators cautioned, however, that a higher percentage of cocaine-exposed infants scored 2 standard deviations below the mean (Chasnoff et al., 1992). Cocaine-exposed children from this cohort followed through age 3 years continued to show no differences on overall performance on the Stanford-Binet form the non-cocaine-exposed controls (Griffith et al., 1994; although the cocaine-exposed group scored significantly lower on verbal reasoning).

Findings such as these have resulted in the reevaluation of early concerns about global developmental delay in prenatally cocaine-exposed children. However, studies of more specific developmental functions suggest that cocaine-exposed infants and young children may have impairments in attention and state or arousal regulation (Mayes & Bornstein, 1995b). For example, it has been reported that, despite no apparent differences on either motor or mental indexes on the BSID, cocaine-exposed 24-month-old children appear to have more difficulty attending to several objects at the same time, and they fail more often in structuring an approach to a nonfamiliar task in the context of developmental assessment (Hawley & Disney, 1992).

Arousal and Attention

A few studies have examined attention, novel responsivity, and state regulation in cocaine-exposed infants in the first year of life. Differences between cocaine-exposed and non-cocaine-exposed infants have been reported in startle responsivity, neonatal orientation, motor and state regulatory capacities, habituation, recognition memory, and reactivity to novelty. Anday, Cohen, Kelley, and Leitner (1989) observed the cocaine-exposed newborns were more reactive to reflex-eliciting stimuli as well as to specific auditory stimuli. In the neonatal period, findings of neurobehavioral impairments as measured by the Neonatal Behavioral Assessment Scales (NBAS; Brazelton, 1984) have been reported but are inconsistent (Chasnoff, Griffith, MacGregor, Dirkes, & Burns, 1989; Coles et al., 1992; Eisen et al., 1990; Mayes, Granger, Frank, Bornstein, & Schottenfeld, 1993). Two studies (Eisen et al., 1990; Mayes et al., 1993) found significant deficits in cocaine-exposed newborns in habituation performance on the NBAS.

Habituation and the complementary processes of novelty responsiveness and recognition memory provide information about the organization of looking behavior and attention in the first years of life, and the habituation process represents an early form of some type of information processing and encoding by the infant and child (Bornstein, 1985a; Bornstein & Mayes, 1992; Colombo & Mitchell, 1990; Lewis, Goldberg, & Campbell, 1969; Lewis & Brooks-Gunn, 1981). Habituation measures discriminate among samples of infants differing in risk status (reviewed in Bornstein, 1985a; Mayes & Bornstein, 1995a). Attention indexed by habituation also involves arousal and arousal regulation (Mayes & Bornstein, 1995a, b). Sustained attention to a novel stimulus entails not only the active intake of information but also more tonic alteration in state or arousal. A deficit in the modulation of arousal or in the activation of states of arousal will influence attentional processes and habituation performance (Pribram & McGuiness, 1975; Ruff, 1988). Links between the monoaminergic neurotransmitter system, through which most of the central effects of cocaine are mediated, and arousal regulation, as well as attentional mechanisms that are indexed by the habituation process (Coles & Robbins, 1989), make it plausible to hypothesize that prenatal cocaine exposure could affect the infant's early habituation performance, the processes related to habituation such as recognition memory or novelty responsiveness, and the infant's reactivity or regulation of arousal to novel stimulation. Studies examining habituation and its related processes in cocaine-exposed infants have suggested specific impairments in recognition memory, novelty responsiveness, and in arousal and reactivity to novel stimuli in infants 3 to 12 months of age (Alessandri, Sullivan, Imaizumi, & Lewis, 1993; Mayes, Bornstein, Chawarska, & Granger, 1995; Struthers & Hansen, 1992).

In summary, available findings suggest that the neurodevelopmental effects of cocaine exposure before birth may be expressed primarily in the general area of arousal regulation in novel or stimulating, potentially stressful situations. Impaired arousal regulation in turn influences the child's attention, reactivity, and response to both nonsocial and social situations. However, the biologically or genetically based developmental trajectory of capacities for the regulation of states of arousal and of attention is also sensitive to environmental influences. Infants exposed prenatally to cocaine are exposed to a number of environmental risk factors that may impair the development of attention and arousal regulatory mechanisms (Mayes, 1992, in press-a; Mayes et al., 1992) as outlined in the previous section. Any one of these pathways may compound possible direct cocaine effects on the development of early attentional and arousal regulatory functions in infants. Thus, the dilemma for understanding the relation of prenatal cocaine exposure to impairments in such basic functions as arousal or state regulation is that the cocaine-related effect may be mediated simultaneously through effects on brain development and through effects on the child's postnatal environment including parenting.

THE EFFECTS OF SUBSTANCE ABUSE ON PARENTING

How the abuse of cocaine as well as alcohol and other agents affects an adult's ability to parent has received less attention than the possible developmental sequelae of actual prenatal exposure (Mayes, 1995; Mayes & Bornstein, 1995b). A central methodologic issue is: Do cocaine-abusing parents have impaired relationships with their children that are different from impairments found in other dysfunctional or disadvantaged families not affected by substance abuse? If so, are the patterns of parenting impairment uniquely related to the effects of cocaine on adult psychological functioning or to other conditions that are also associated with substance abuse (e.g., depression, history of early abuse, and neglect)?

Indirect Measures of Parenting

Parenting functions among substance-abuse human adults have been examined primarily with indirect and global measures such as surveys of the incidence of child abuse and of the home environment to assess the adequacy of the child's physical care. That parents who are actively abusing cocaine and other substances have problems caring for their children is indicated in part by the increased incidence of physical abuse and neglect in such families and by the proportionately higher than national average numbers of children from substance-abusing families who are in foster care or other types of placements (Lawson & Wilson, 1980; Rogosch, Cicchetti, Shields, & Toth, 1995). In a case-control study of all consecutive emergency room or hospital evaluations of injuries thought to be secondary to abuse, children who were physically abused were significantly more likely to come from households with cocaine-abusing adults as parents (Wasserman & Leventhal, 1993). Black and

Mayer (1980) reported on a sample of 200 addicted parents, 92 of whom were alcoholics and 108 opiate addicts. In approximately 20% of the families, a child was physically or sexually abused, and in over 40%, children had been physically neglected.

Other commonly used measures of parental functioning among substance-abusing adults include questionnaires that assess the adult's own experience of being parented (e.g., Bernardi, Jones, & Tennant, 1989) or the parent's perception of his or her role, use of social supports, and techniques of parental control (Wellisch & Steinberg, 1980). On measures such as these, substance-abusing mothers report a broad range of parenting difficulties, including reliance on a more disciplinarian, threatening style of parenting and negative reinforcement (Bauman & Dougherty, 1983). However, such measures do not usually examine how mothers perceive the effects of their substance abuse on their parenting. For example, maternal attitudes toward the child are influenced in part by worries and guilt over potentially damaging her child through cocaine use. Such worries may be sufficient to adversely affect mothers' participation in treatment programs for themselves or for their children, for fear that others will remind them of the harm they believe they have done through their addiction. Moreover, because of the associated depression and impairments in attention and concentration associated with active substance abuse, self-report instruments are often inaccurate when completed by substance-abusing adults and do not address the question of whether or not active cocaine abuse limits or disrupts a mother's immediate interactions with her children.

Observations of Parenting Skills of Substance-Abusing Adults

Direct observations of interactions between substance abusing parents and their children have utilized observations of children's and mothers' responses to brief separations and of play interactions between mothers and infants. Studies of separation paradigms and attachment patterns among the children of substance-abusing adults suggest an increased incidence of disrupted or disturbed relationships between parents and children and higher rates of disorganized attachment behaviors (Main & Solomon, 1986; Rodning, Beckwith, & Howard, 1989, 1991). Drug-exposed children reared in foster care may be less likely to be insecurely attached than those living with their biological mothers (Rodning et al., 1989) although these differences in attachment patterns by rearing conditions have not been found consistently (Rodning et al., 1991). However, failure to find a difference between prenatally exposed infants in foster care and those in the care of their biological mothers does not provide sufficient evidence for a relation between prenatal cocaine exposure and infant attachment behaviors inasmuch as children in foster care have often been in their biological parents' care for months to years and may have experienced more than one foster placement. Indeed, defining the primary caregiver is a difficult problem in studies of substance-abusing parents and reflects a difficult dilemma in all studies of parenting of cocaine-exposed children, since in many substance-abusing families, a child may be in the care of many different adults in the course of a week or months. Moreover, disordered attachment patterns are reported increased among families with overall increased disorganization, stress, abuse, and exposure to violence with or without substance abuse (Carlson, Cicchetti, Barnett, & Braunwald, 1989; O'Connor, Sigman, & Brill, 1987).

Direct observational measures of child and parent together have been employed less often with substance-abusing families and have mainly included measures of parental involvement and intrusiveness (e.g., for heroin/methadone-using families, Bernstein, Jeremy, Hans, & Marcus, 1984, and Bernstein, Jeremy, & Marcus, 1986; for cocaine-using adults, Burns, Chethik, Burns, & Clark, 1991). Bernstein and colleagues (1984) reported that mothers participating in a methadone-maintenance program in comparison to a non-opiate-addicted group reacted less often and less contingently to their 4-month-old infants' communicative bids and tried less often to elicit or encourage communicative play with their infants. Similar impairments in maternal responsiveness and reciprocity were reported by Burns and colleagues (1991) in a group of 5 polydrug-using mothers, two of whom used cocaine primarily, with no comparison group. Polydrug (including cocaine) abusing mothers showed a reduction in reciprocal behaviors with their infants and infrequently structured and mediated the environment, findings suggestive of problems with attention-directing, structuring activities. Far more work is needed using direct observational measures of interactions between cocaine-using parents and their children.

Importantly, although substance-abusing mothers generally engage in more impaired interactions with their children than comparison groups, not all substance-abusing parents interact poorly with their children. A number of associated factors in addition to, or instead of, substance abuse may predict dysfunctional parenting behaviors. For example, Bernstein and colleagues (1984) reported that 47% of a group of methadone-maintained women received adequate scores for interaction and communication with their infants. Women with poor interaction scores showed lower IQs, lower socioeconomic status (based on a combination of maternal education and family income), and had fewer contacts with their child's father (methods described in Marcus, Hans, Patterson, & Morris, 1984).

Effect of Infant Behavior on Parenting

Infant behavior also affects parenting behaviors (Lewis & Rosenblum, 1974). Diverse infant characteristics, and thus infant behaviors, related to the effects of prenatal drug exposure, as with fetal-alcohol effects, narcotic withdrawal, or the more general contributions of prenatal drug exposure to prematurity and intrauterine growth retardation (Zucker-man et al., 1989), may make the infant more difficult to care for. Only recently have investigators of parenting by substance-abusing mothers begun to employ interactive models that examine how variations in infant characteristics influence maternal behaviors (Griffith & Freier, 1992). For example, in a study of maternal alcohol use, maternal–infant interaction, and infant cognitive development, O'Connor, Sigman, and Kasari (1992, 1993) reported that the direction of strongest association was between maternal prenatal alcohol use and the effects on infant affective regula-tion, which in turn influenced mother–infant interaction and subsequent infant cognitive outcome. Postnatal maternal alcohol consumption did not relate to maternal interactive characteristics.

More detailed studies of the specific alterations in parenting associ-ated with substance abuse are needed not only to guide the design of more effective interventions for substance-abusing parents but also because developmental trajectories for domains such as attention and arousal regulation in infants are influenced by parental interactions (Bornstein, 1985b; Bornstein & Lamb, 1992; Bornstein & Tamis-LeMonda, 1990; Tamis-LeMonda & Bornstein, 1989). Infant attention, exploration, and use of language are influenced by maternal activity. Although attention and reactivity reflect neuropsychological functions that are biologically based, these functions are sensitive to the level of environmental organi-zation, responsivity, and adaptability. The degree of sensitivity is individ-ually variable among infants, but those with problems in reactivity to novelty or in the regulation of states of arousal overall may be more sensitive to parental disorganization and inconsistency. Problems in the regulation of arousal in infants may also contribute to an infant's being more difficult to care for, which further influences the potentially compro-mised cocaine-abusing adult's ability to respond to and support that particular infant's needs. Finally, because of the debilitating effects of chronic cocaine abuse on overall adult psychological and physical health, parental responsiveness and adaptation may deteriorate over time or vary depending on the severity of the cocaine abuse and intoxication.

THE INTERVENTION NEEDS OF COCAINE-EXPOSED CHILDREN AND THEIR COCAINE-USING PARENTS

The increased prevalence of drug abuse in women has also raised special issues regarding their drug-abuse treatment and special health care needs (Mendelson, Weiss, Griffin, Mirin, et al., 1991) and the needs of their children. Developing new drug-abuse-treatment programs or revis-ing existing interventions specifically tailored to meet the needs of women substance abusers and their children is a very recent concern, and very little intervention research has been done in this area. The relevant questions are (1) Are there differences between men and women in their patterns of drug use that may alter their response to drug treatment interventions? (2) Are there different patterns of associated or comorbid disorders for men and women substance abusers that may also influence their response to drug treatment interventions? (3) What are the additional needs of women that affect their participation in drug treatment programs (e.g., when the woman is also a mother and needs to find care for her children while she participates in treatment)? (4) Are the intervention needs of children from substance-abusing families different from children from similar high-risk but non-drug-using environments, and what are those needs? For each of these questions, some current data can inform program development, but far more systematic research is needed.

Gender Differences in Patterns of Substance Abuse

Patterns of drug use do vary between men and women substance abusers. For cocaine users, Griffin, Weiss, Mirin, and Lange (1989) found that women tended to begin their drug use at earlier ages than men did and, concomitantly, to seek drug treatment at an earlier age. (Opposite patterns pertain for opiate abuse in which women addicts are older, tend to begin using later, and have longer histories of addiction before they seek treatment; Moise, Reed, & Ryan, 1982). When compared to women with primary alcohol dependence, women who abused cocaine with alcohol were significantly more likely to have dropped out of school before attaining a high school degree, had been drinking at a much younger age, and had also been sexually active much earlier in adolescence than those women who abused only alcohol (Mendelson et al., 1991). Women more often use drugs at home or alone (Lester, 1982). Women also more often cite emotional or life-event reasons for beginning substance abuse (depression, feeling unsociable, worry over health, or family pressures), whereas men are more likely to cite no specific reason for initiating substance use (Griffin et al., 1989). These same types of emotional or interpersonal factors are also more predictive of relapse in women participating in substance-abuse-treatment programs: that is, women are more likely to return to drug use when faced with social or interpersonal stressors such as social isolation. How being a parent moderates these patterns of drug use between men and women has not been systematically studied. Indeed, many studies regarding differences between male and female addicts do not report whether or not either were also caring for children.

Gender Differences in Psychiatric Comorbidity

There are also marked differences in psychological and psychiatric conditions associated with substance abuse between men and women.

Female addicts tend to have fewer financial resources, less job or employment experience, more instability in their relationships and more partners with substance-abuse problems, and overall more disturbances
among members of their families (Moise et al., 1982). Female addicts are
also more likely to have experienced sexual or physical abuse prior to
their substance abuse (Harrison, 1989) and more often attribute their
drug abuse to critical life events such as abuse, divorce, or death
(Chatham, 1990). Multiple studies have now shown the markedly increased incidence in major depression in women substance abusers compared to male addicts, a finding that is consistent across alcohol, opiates,
and cocaine (Blume, 1986; Griffin et al., 1989; McClellan et al., 1983).
Conversely, male cocaine and opiate addicts are more often involved in
criminal activities with antisocial personality characteristics (Rounsaville
et al., 1982; Hesselbrock, Meyer, & Keener, 1985). Women substance
abusers report more social isolation and, if they report a social group
while they are addicted, tend more often to have a network of substance-
abusing friends or to be living with a substance-abusing partner. They
also consistently report lower self-esteem than do drug-dependent men
(Colten, 1980; Reed, 1985). The depressive symptoms in women substance abusers remit significantly more slowly with treatment than in
men, although there is a suggestion that persistent depression after a
month of cocaine abstinence is a prognostically good indicator for sustained abstinence (Carroll, 1989). (Similar findings have been reported for
women alcoholics; Rounsaville, Dolinsky, Babor, & Meyer, 1987.) Again,
how pregnancy and parenting moderate these experiences has not been
examined empirically, although substance-abusing women may be more
available to intervention and treatment during pregnancy (Smith, Dent,
Coles, & Falek, 1992).

Intervention Needs of Women Substance Abusers

These differences in patterns of drug use and in associated psychiatric and psychological conditions point to special intervention needs for
female substance abusers. In addition, women substance abusers are
more likely to be responsible for children. In a day-treatment program for
alcoholics, 75% of women had children (Shulte & Blume, 1979), and
similar percentages are reported from treatment programs for heroin
addicts (Hanke & Faupel, 1993; Marsh & Miller, 1985). Moreover,
substance-abusing women are much less likely to seek professional services of any kind for their children or, for that matter, for themselves (Reed
& Leibson, 1981).

Several programs have documented that women tend to need more
ancillary interventions during participation in the intervention (Marsh &
Miller, 1985). These include housing services, since women substance
abusers are more often homeless or in housing that is inadequate for

children. Women substance abusers quite frequently require obstetric and gynecologic care because of frequent pregnancies and high-risk sexual behaviors (multiple partners, increased incidence of sexually transmitted diseases, failure to use or have available adequate contraception). They may need on-site child care services in order to facilitate their remaining in treatment, since women substance abusers very often have inadequate social and family networks to help them care for their children. Legal services are needed to address custody as well as civil and criminal charges, and vocational training with employment counseling may be critical to helping substance-abusing women maintain their abstinence when they are discharged from treatment programs. Substance-abuse-treatment programs and their ancillary services may need to have more female counselors and health care providers, since female addicts may have serious difficulties relating to men and thus be reluctant to enter treatment with them (Hanke & Faupel, 1993; Stevens, Arbiter, & Glider, 1989).

Female cocaine-abusers receiving treatment for their addiction face a number of obstacles, including most prominently a shortage of treatment programs for women. Many health care clinics are reluctant to treat pregnant cocaine addicts because of their higher risk for obstetric complications and also because of their poor compliance. Additionally, pregnant cocaine-using women are often excluded from treatment programs because of concerns about the safety of detoxication while the mother is pregnant or lack of facilities to care for a newborn so that the mother may continue to participate in treatment. Chavkin (1989) found that 54% of drug treatment programs in New York City excluded pregnant women and an additional 13% rejected pregnant women on Medicaid. Only 13% of programs accepted pregnant women on Medicaid who were cocaine or crack addicted. The marked shortage of programs for pregnant cocaine-using women is reflected also in a survey of major hospitals in large American cities in which approximately 60% reported having no referral resources for pregnant addicts.

Intervention Needs of Children of Substance-Abusing Parents

The lifestyle imposed by cocaine abuse often compromises the health care of the children involved. Cocaine-abusing adults on average comply poorly not only with substance-abuse-treatment interventions but also with health care interventions centered around basic child needs such as prenatal care and well-child care (Chan, Wingert, Wachsman, Schuetz, & Rogers, 1986; Funkhouser, Butz, Feng, McCaul, & Rosenstein, 1993). Although not well documented or well studied to date, the children of substance-abusing women are much more likely to receive little preventative or well-child care, to have inadequate or no immunizations, and to be seen for minor illnesses in emergency rooms where their more basic primary care needs cannot be addressed. As the special needs of women substance abusers are more adequately defined, it has recently been advocated that substance-abuse-treatment programs for women also include on-site pediatric care for their children (Brown, 1992).

Integrating health care services for children with on-going substance abuse treatment programs for their mothers will also facilitate providing psychosocial and developmental interventions in these same programs. Indeed, because substance-abusing families often find it difficult to access intervention services delivered in multiple sites, providing developmental and psychosocial interventions for children in the same setting as substance-abuse treatment and health care for adults and children may reach more children at psychosocial risk than separate referrals to outside agencies. Several substance-abuse-treatment programs specifically for women have integrated on-site day care and nursery programs into their daily milieu and have made available developmental evaluations and individual child-oriented educational and therapeutic interventions (Harvey & Comfort, 1992; Pawl, 1992; Saunders, 1992). These services are particularly critical for preschool children who are not in school during the time their mothers need to participate in treatment programs and who, precisely because they are not in any intervention program, are often exposed throughout the entire day to the chaos and disorganization of their parent's substance-abusing lifestyle.

Programs for preschool children in the same site as the substance-abuse-treatment program also remove one additional barrier to an adult's move toward acknowledging his or her addiction and seeking help for it; that is, child care is removed as a reason for not participating. Until recently, few programs acknowledged the need for child care as an obstacle to parents' beginning treatment and rarely did a program accommodate children. For example, Magjaryi (1990) found that only 4% of publicly funded California drug-treatment programs treated women with their children. When services are provided for children, adults appear to remain in treatment longer and participate more consistently (Coletti & Hamilton, 1991). In addition to improving acceptance of treatment, when children are in the same program as their mothers, multiple opportunities arise for child development and adult professionals to work together on how the mother's substance abuse affects the family and her role as a parent. Parent-education programs gain an immediacy and relevance when the mother's child is next door in the nursery or when she helps other mothers care for the children in the day care center under the support and guidance of early-childhood professionals. Finally, though as yet not studied, interventions directed toward helping adults reflect on the effect of their substance abuse on their children may provide another therapeutic technique for helping substance-abusing adults, who are also parents, achieve abstinence. The point of therapeutic intervention becomes not just the effect of the addiction on the mother herself but on how her addiction potentially harms her children.

It is not clear whether or not the children of cocaine-abusing families will require special developmental and psychosocial services that differ from those appropriate to children from generally disadvantaged circumstances (Mayes et al., 1992). In other words, it is quite likely true that cocaine-exposed children living with cocaine-using parents will have special intervention needs, but it is unclear if those needs will be different because of their prenatal and postnatal cocaine exposure. It may be that the problems with attention and arousal regulation described earlier will contribute to special educational needs by early preschool and first grade—a hypothesis for which there is as yet no systematic data. However, there are some risks to presuming and labeling cocaine-exposed children as uniquely different in their needs from other children from disadvantaged circumstances. Labels often become self-fulfilling in that expectations for the children are lowered (Rosenthal & Jacobson, 1968). Attributing to cocaine-exposed children dysfunctions beyond the capacity of existing systems to remediate makes it very difficult to find services for the children (including foster or adoptive homes). Also, as suggested in the beginning of this chapter, labels and stereotypes may bias clinical decisions. For example, given equivalent extent of illegal drug use by pregnant women, physicians and clinics are more likely to report to law-enforcement agencies black women or women on welfare than white or middle-class women (Chasnoff et al., 1990). While not studied, it may be that given equivalent developmental needs, teachers are more likely to focus more on the child from a presumed non-drug-using background than on a cocaine-exposed child if the presumption of irremediable difficulty and unique needs prevails. Such presumptions then lead us to overlook what can be done and what has long been known about the effects of early intervention and remediation (Meisels & Shonkoff, 1990).

From the other side, cocaine-exposed children do represent a special population of children with special needs that are different in degree, if not content, from those children who are non-drug-exposed but living in psychosocial adversity. The effect of parental substance abuse on the children's environment likely exposes children of substance-abusing families to greater chaos and inconsistency, higher levels of stress and violence, and greater risks for abuse and abandonment. These events are not different from those that may happen for a non-drug-exposed child, but they occur more frequently and are of greater severity among substance-abusing families. Also, because of their prenatal biologic exposure and associated developmental dysfunctions or impairments, cocaine-exposed children may be more susceptible to the detrimental effects of environmental stress. Similar to other groups of infants born with biologic risks (e.g., premature infants), their biologic risks may be ameliorated or worsened by environmental conditions. Thus, cocaine-exposed children represent a special population at both biologic and environmental risk for developmental impairments. These children require interventions that address both the biologic and environmental contributions, and the interactions between these conditions, to their developmental trajectories.

With these caveats in mind, the infants and children of substance-abusing families should receive comprehensive services, provided in the same site as their mothers' substance-abuse treatment, that include adequate nutrition, health care, immunizations, and developmental and psychosocial interventions. Very few published reports evaluate what types of developmental and psychosocial interventions work most effectively. However, accumulated experience of working with children from disadvantaged backgrounds does inform the basic components of these types of interventions (Meisels & Shonkoff, 1990). At the very least, children from substance-abusing households will likely need special language services, not necessarily because of a specific effect of cocaine on language development, but because of the generally understood delays in language and communication seen in children from disruptive, sometimes neglectful circumstances. They will also need smaller programs that offer more opportunities for intensive individualized attention from an adult and more supervision of group interactions with smaller groups of children. Within these small programs, the level of stimulation will need to be closely monitored and altered to suit the individual child. Such attention to the level of stimulation and environmental novelty is not because cocaine-exposed children may be more easily overstimulated but more generally because children from neglectful or disadvantaged environments are often more sensitive and easily overwhelmed by too much novelty (Cohen & Taharally, 1992). Finally, programs that work with parents and permit some parent participation in caring for the children will provide preschool children the opportunity to be with their mothers in a supportive, developmentally nurturing setting and to be with adults behaving consistently toward them.

CONCLUSIONS

Cocaine abuse defines not only a medical and psychiatric condition but also a lifestyle and a social or community context. The latter set of circumstances contributes to the varying outcome of infants and young children prenatally exposed to cocaine and also to the special health care needs of substance-abusing women and their children. Children developing within an environment of violence, poverty, and discord that is increasingly common in inner city neighborhoods are at risk for dysfunctional development on a number of accounts—in addition to their prenatal exposure to cocaine. Even if controversy and conflicting findings surround the long-term effects of cocaine on cognitive and intellectual development, suggestive findings point to impairments in more basic neurodevelopmental domains of arousal and attentional regulation, functions that underlay learning and information processing. The postnatal cocaine-abusing environment, both in its more general factors of poverty, homelessness, and violence and in the specific dysfunctions of parenting that accompany cocaine abuse, almost certainly exacerbate the effects of prenatal substance exposure whatever they may be. Additionally, female cocaine abusers have special psychological and medical care needs that transcend treatment of their addiction and reflect on their role as parents and the chronic psychologic, physical, and economic morbidities that contribute to the context of development under the influence of cocaine abuse. In summary, cocaine-abusing parents and their children represent a special population that has, until recently, been understudied. Interventions that address the medical and psychological needs of cocaine-abusing parents and their children together is a critically needed area of service development.

ACKNOWLEDGMENTS

This chapter summarizes selected aspects of our collaborative research, and portions of the text have appeared in our previous scientific publications cited in the references. We thank D. Cohen, R. Granger, and R. Schottenfeld as well as O.M. Haynes for support of our studies of prenatal cocaine exposure.

REFERENCES

Alessandri, S. M., Sullivan, M. W., Imaizumi, S., & Lewis, M. (1993). Learning and emotional responsivity in cocaine-exposed infants. *Developmental Psychology, 29*, 989–997.

Amaro, H., Fried, L. E., Cabral H., & Zuckerman B. (1990). Violence during pregnancy and substance use. *American Journal of Public Health, 80*, 575–579.

Amaro H., Zuckerman B., & Cabral H. (1989). Drug use among adolescent mothers: Profile of risk. *Pediatrics, 84*, 144–151.

Anday, E. K., Cohen, M. E., Kelley, N. E., & Leitner, D. S. (1989). Effect of in utero cocaine exposure on startle and its modification. *Developmental Pharmacology and Therapeutics, 12*, 137–145.

Anisfeld, E., Cunningham, N., Ferrari, L., Melendez, M., Ruesch, N., Soto, L., & Wagnon, D. (1991). Infant development after prenatal cocaine exposure. *Society for Research in Child Development* [abstract].

Ardila, A., Rosselli, M., & Strumwasser, S. (1991). Neuropsychological deficits in chronic cocaine abusers. *International Journal of Neuroscience, 57*, 73–79.

Arendt, R., Singer, L., & Minnes, S. (1993). Development of cocaine exposed infants. *Society for Research in Child Development* [abstract].

Bauman, P. S., & Dougherty, F. E. (1983). Drug-addicted mothers' parenting and their children's development. *International Journal of the Addictions, 18*, 291–302.

Bayley, N. (1969). *Manual for the Bayley scales of infant development.* New York: Psychological Corporation.

Bayley, N. (1993). *Bayley scales of infant development* (Rev. ed.). New York: Psychological Corporation.

Beery, J., Van, G. W. G., Herzberg, D. S., & Hinkin, C. E. (1993). Neuropsychological deficits in abstinent cocaine abusers: Preliminary findings after two weeks of abstinence. *Drug and Alcohol Dependence, 32,* 231–237.

Bergeman, C. S., & Plomin, R. (1989). Genotype-environment interaction. In M. H. Bornstein & J. S. Bruner (Eds.), *Interaction in human development* (pp. 157–171). Hillsdale, NJ: Lawrence Erlbaum Associates.

Bernardi, E., Jones, M., & Tennant, C. (1989). Quality of parenting in alcoholics and narcotic addicts. *British Journal of Psychiatry, 154,* 677–682.

Bernstein, V., Jeremy, R. J., Hans, S., & Marcus, J. (1984). A longitudinal study of offspring born to methadone-maintained women: II. Dyadic interaction and infant behavior at four months. *American Journal of Drug and Alcohol Abuse, 10,* 161–193.

Bernstein, V., Jeremy, R. J., & Marcus, J. (1986). Mother-infant interaction in multiproblem families: Finding those at risk. *Journal of the American Academy of Child Psychiatry, 25,* 631–640.

Besharov, D. J. (1990). Crack children in foster care. *Children Today, 19,* 21–25.

Black, R., & Mayer, J. (1980). Parents with special problems: Alcoholism and opiate addiction. *Child Abuse and Neglect, 4,* 45–54.

Blume, S. B. (1986). Women and alcohol. *Journal of the American Medical Association, 256,* 1467–1470.

Bornstein, M. (1985a). Habituation as a measure of visual information processing in human infants: Summary, systemization, and synthesis. In G. Gottlieb & N. Krasnegor, (Eds.), *Development of audition and vision during the first year of postnatal life: A methodological overview* (pp. 253–295). Norwood, NJ: Ablex.

Bornstein, M. H. (1985b). How infant and mother jointly contribute to developing cognitive competence in the child. *Proceedings of the National Academy of Science* (U.S.A.), *85,* 7470–7473.

Bornstein, M. H. (1995). Parenting infants. In M. H. Bornstein (Ed.), *Handbook of parenting* (Vol. 1). Hillsdale, NJ: Erlbaum.

Bornstein, M. H., & Lamb, M. E. (1992). *Development in infancy: An introduction* (3rd ed.). New York: McGraw-Hill.

Bornstein, M. H., & Tamis-LeMonda, C. S. (1990). Activities and interactions of mothers and their firstborn infants in the first six months of life: Covariation, stability, continuity, correspondence, and prediction. *Child Development, 61,* 1206–1217.

Bornstein, M. H., & Mayes, L. C. (1992). Taking a measure of the infant mind. In F. Kessell, M. H. Bornstein, & A. Sameroff (Eds.), *Contemporary constructions of the child: Essays in honor of William Kessen* (pp. 45–56). Hillsdale, NJ: Erlbaum.

Boyd, C. J., & Mieczkowski, T. (1990). Drug use, health, family, and social support in "crack" cocaine users. *Addictive Behaviors, 15,* 481–485.

Brazelton, T. B. (1984). *Neonatal behavior assessment scale.* (Clinics in Developmental Medicine, No. 88, 2nd ed.). Philadelphia, PA: Lippincott.

Brown, E. (1992). Program and staff characteristics in successful treatment. In M. M. Kilbey & K. Asghar (Eds.), *Methodological issues in epidemiological, prevention, and treatment research on drug-exposed women and their children* (NIDA Research Monograph No. 117 305–313). Washington, DC: U.S. Government Printing Office.

Burns, K., Chethik, L., Burns, W. J., & Clark, R. (1991). Dyadic disturbances in cocaine-abusing mothers and their infants. *Journal of Clinical Psychology, 47,* 316–319.

Carlson, V., Cicchetti, D., Barnett, D., & Braunwald, K. (1989). Disorganized/disoriented attachment relationships in maltreated infants. *Developmental Psychology, 25,* 525–531.

Carroll, K. M. (1989). Psychiatric diagnosis and cocaine treatment response. Paper presented at the 142nd annual meeting of the *American Psychiatric Association,* San Francisco, CA.

Chambers, C. D., Hinesby, R. K., & Moldestad, M. (1970). Narcotic addiction in females: A race comparison. *International Journal of the Addictions, 5,* 257–278.

Chan, L. S., Wingert, W. A., Wachsman, L., Schuetz, S., & Rogers, C. (1986). Differences between dropouts and active participants in a pediatric clinic for substance abuse mothers. *American Journal of Drug and Alcohol Abuse, 12*, 89–99.

Chasnoff, I., Griffith, D. R., MacGregor, S., Dirkes, K., & Burns, K. (1989). Temporal patterns of cocaine use in pregnancy. *Journal of the American Medical Association, 261*, 1741–1744.

Chasnoff, I. J., Landress, H. J., & Barrett, M. E. (1990). Prevalence of illicit drugs or alcohol abuse during pregnancy and discrepancies in mandatory reporting in Pinellas County, Florida. *New England Journal of Medicine, 322*, 102–106.

Chasnoff, I. J., Griffith, D. R., Freier, C., & Murray, J. (1992). Cocaine/ polydrug use in pregnancy: Two-year follow-up. *Pediatrics, 89*, 284–289.

Chatham, L. R. (1990). Understanding the issues: An overview. In R. C. Engs (Ed.), *Women: Alcohol and other drugs.* Dubuque, IA: Kendall/Hunt.

Chavkin, W. (1989, July 18). Help, don't jail addicted women. *New York Times*, A21.

Cohen, A., & Harrison, M. D. (1986). The "urge to classify" the drug user: A review of classifications by patterns of abuse. *International Journal of the Addictions, 21*, 1249–1260.

Cohen, S., & Taharally, C. (1992). Getting ready for young children with prenatal drug exposure. *Childhood Education, 69*, 5–9.

Coles, B. J., & Robbins, T. W. (1989). Effects of 6-hydroxy-dopamine lesions of the nucleus accumbens septi on performance of a 5-choice serial reaction time task in rats: Implications for theories of selective attention and arousal. *Behavioral Brain Research, 33*, 165–179.

Coles, C. D., Platzman, K. A., Smith, I., James, M. E., & Falek, A. (1992). Effects of cocaine and alcohol use in pregnancy on neonatal growth and neurobehavioral status. *Neurotoxicology and Teratology, 14*, 23–33.

Coletti, S., & Hamilton, N. L. (1991). Treatment for pregnant women and postpartum women and their infants. *National conference on drug abuse research and practice, conference highlights* (DHHS Publication No. ADM91–1818). Washington, DC: U.S. Government Printing Office.

Colombo, J., & Mitchell, D. W. (1990). Individual differences in early visual attention. In J. Colombo & J. Fagen (Eds.), *Individual differences in infancy: Reliability, stability, and prediction* pp. 193–227). Hillsdale, NJ: Erlbaum.

Colten, M. E. (1980). A description and comparative analysis of self-perceptions and attitudes of heroin addicted women. In *Addicted women: Family dynamics, self-perceptions, and support systems.* National Institute on Drug Abuse, Washington, DC: U.S. Government Printing Office.

Courtwright, D. T. (1982). *Dark paradise.* Cambridge, MA: Harvard University Press.

DeJong, C. A., Van den Brink, W., & Jansen, J. A. (1993). Sex role stereotypes and clinical judgement: How therapists view their alcoholic patients. *Journal of Substance Abuse Treatment, 10*, 383–389.

Eisen, L. N., Field, T. M., Bandstra, E. S., Roberts, J. P., Morrow, C., et al. (1990). Perinatal cocaine effects on neonatal stress behavior and performance on the Brazelton scale. *Pediatrics, 88*, 477–480.

Field, T. M. (1995). Psychologically depressed parents. In M. H. Bornstein (Ed.), *Handbook of parenting: Status and social conditions of parenting* (Vol. 3), Hillsdale, NJ: Erlbaum Associates.

Fitzpatrick, J. L., & Gerard, K. (1993). Community attitudes toward drug use: The need to assess community norms. *International Journal of the Addictions, 28*, 947–957.

Frank, D. A., Zuckerman, B. S., Amaro, H., Aboagye, K., Bauchner, H., et al. (1988). Cocaine use during pregnancy: Prevalence and correlates. *Pediatrics, 82*, 888–895.

Funkhouser, A. W., Butz, A. M., Feng, T. L., McCaul, M. E., & Rosenstein, B. J. (1993). Prenatal care and drug use in pregnant women. *Drug and Alcohol Dependence, 33*, 1–9.

Garretson, D. J. (1993). Psychological misdiagnosis of African-Americans. *Journal of Multicultural Counseling and Development, 21*, 119–126.

Garrity-Roukas, F. E. (1994). Punitive legal approaches to the problem of prenatal drug abuse. *Infant Mental Health, 15,* 218–237.

Goldman-Rakic, P. S. (1987). Development of cortical circuitry and cognitive function. *Child Development, 58,* 601–622.

Gomby, D. S., & Shiono, P. H. (1991). Estimating the number of substance-exposed infants. *The Future of Children, 1*(1), 17–25. (Available from Center for the Future of Children, David & Lucile Packard Foundation, Los Altos, CA).

Gossop, M., Griffiths, P., Powis, B., & Strang, J. (1994). Cocaine: Patterns of use, route of administration, and severity of dependence. *British Journal of Psychiatry, 164,* 660–664.

Griffin, M. L., Weiss, R. D., Mirin, S. M., & Lange, U. (1989). A comparison of male and female cocaine abusers. *Archives of General Psychiatry, 46,* 122–126.

Griffith, D., & Freier, C. (1992). Methodological issues in the assessment of the mother-child interactions of substance-abusing women and their children (NIDA Research Monograph No. 117, (pp. 228–247). Washington, DC: U.S. Government Printing Office.

Griffith, D. R., Azuma, S. D., & Chasnoff, I. J. (1994). Three-year outcome of children exposed prenatally to drugs. *Journal American Academy of Child Psychiatry, 33,* 20–27.

Hanke, P. J., & Faupel, C. E. (1993). Women opiate users' perceptions of treatment services in New York City. *Journal of Substance Abuse Treatment, 10,* 513–522.

Harrison, P. A. (1989). Women in treatment: Changing over time. *International Journal of the Addictions, 24,* 655–673.

Harvey, C., & Comfort, M. (1992). Integrating parent support into residential drug and alcohol treatment programs. *Zero to Three, 13,* 11–13.

Hawley, T. L., & Disney, E. R. (1992). Crack's children: The consequences of maternal cocaine abuse. *Social Policy Report of the Society for Research in Child Development, 6,* 1–22.

Hesselbrock, M. N., Meyer, R. E., & Keener, J. J. (1985). Psychopathology in hospitalized alcoholics. *Archives of General Psychiatry, 42,* 1050–1055.

Johnson, H. L., & Rosen, T. S. (1990). Difficult mothers of difficult babies: Mother-infant interaction in a multi-risk population. *American Journal of Orthopsychiatry, 60,* 281–288.

Khalsa, M. E., Anglin, M. D., Paredes, A., Potepan, P., & Potter, C. (1993). Pretreatment natural history of cocaine addiction: Preliminary 1-year follow-up results (NIDA Research Monograph No. 135, 218–235). Washington, DC: U.S. Government Printing Office.

Khantzian, E. J., & Khantzian, N. J. (1984). Cocaine addiction: Is there a psychological predisposition. *Psychiatric Annals, 14,* 753–759.

Khantzian, E. J. (1985). The self-medication hypothesis of addictive disorders: Focus on heroin and cocaine dependence. *American Journal of Psychiatry, 142,* 1259–1264.

Kjarasch, S. J., Glotzer, D., Vinci, R., Wietzman, M., & Sargent, T. (1991). Unsuspected cocaine exposure in children. *American Journal of Diseases of Children, 145,* 204–206.

Lawson, M., & Wilson, G. (1980). Parenting among women addicted to narcotics. *Child Welfare, 59,* 67–79.

Lester, L. (1982). The special needs of the female alcoholic. *Social Casework, 63,* 451–456.

Lewis, M., Goldberg, S., & Campbell, H. (1969). A developmental study of information processing within the first three years of life: Response decrement to a redundant signal. *Monographs of the Society for Research in Child Development, 39,* 9 (Serial No. 133).

Lewis, M., & Rosenblum, L. A. (1974). *The effect of the infant on its caregiver.* New York: Wiley.

Lewis, M., & Brooks-Gunn, J. (1981). Visual attention at three months as a predictor of cognitive functioning at two years of age. *Intelligence, 5,* 131–140.

Luthar, S., Anton, S. F., Merikangas, K. R., & Rounsaville, B. J. (1992). Vulnerability to substance abuse and psychopathology among siblings of opioid abusers. *Journal of Nervous and Mental Disorders, 180,* 153–161.

Magjaryi, T. (1990, September). Prevention of alcohol and drug problems among women of childbearing age: Challenges for the 1990s. Paper presented at the OSAP conference Healthy Women, healthy Pregnancies, healthy Infants, Miami, FL.

Main, M., & Solomon, J. (1986). Discovery of an insecure-disorganized/disoriented attachment pattern. In T. B. Brazelton & M. Yogman (Eds.), *Affective development in infancy* (pp. 95–124). Norwood, NJ: Ablex.

Manschreck, T., Schneyer, M., Weisstein, C., Laughery, J., Rosenthal, J., Celada, T., & Berner, J. (1990). Freebase cocaine and memory. *Comprehensive Psychiatry, 31*, 369–375.

Marcus, J., Hans, S. L., Patterson, C. B., & Morris, A. J. (1984). A longitudinal study of offspring born to methadone-maintained women. I. Design, methodology, and description of women's resources for functioning. *American Journal of Drug and Alcohol Abuse, 10*, 135–160.

Marsh, J. C., & Miller, N. A. (1985). Female clients in substance abuse treatment. *International Journal of the Addictions, 20*, 995–1019.

Mayes, L. C. (1992). The effects of prenatal cocaine exposure on young children's development. *The Annals of the American Academy of Political and Social Science, 521*, 11–27.

Mayes, L. C. (1994). Neurobiology of prenatal cocaine exposure: Effect on developing monoaminergic systems. *Infant Mental Health, 15*, 134–145.

Mayes, L. C. (in press-a). Exposure to cocaine: Behavioral outcomes in preschool aged children. In L. Finnegan (Ed.), *Behaviors of drug-exposed offspring*, NIDA Technical Symposium. Washington, DC: U.S. Government Printing Office.

Mayes, L. C. (1995). Substance abuse and parenting. In M. H. Bornstein (Ed)., *The handbook of parenting*. Hillsdale, NJ: Erlbaum.

Mayes, L. C., & Bornstein, M. (in press). Attention regulation in infants born at risk: Preterm and prenatally cocaine exposed infants. In J. Burak & J. Enns (Eds.), *Development, attention, and psychopathology* New York: Guilford.

Mayes, L. C., & Bornstein, M. (1995b). Developmental dilemmas for cocaine abusing parents and their children. In M. Lewis & M. Bendersky (Eds), *Cocaine mother and cocaine babies: The role of toxins in development* pp. 251–272). Hillsdale, NJ: Erlbaum.

Mayes, L. C., Bornstein, M. H., Chawarska, K., & Granger, R. H. (1995) Information processing and developmental assessments in three month olds exposed prenatally to cocaine. *Pediatrics, 4*, 539–545.

Mayes, L. C., Granger, R. H., Bornstein, M. H., & Zuckerman, B. (1992). The problem of intrauterine cocaine exposure. *Journal of the American Medical Association, 267*, 406–408.

Mayes, L. C., Granger, R. H., Frank, M. A., Bornstein, M., & Schottenfeld, R. (1993). Neurobehavioral profiles of infants exposed to cocaine prenatally. *Pediatrics, 91*, 778–783.

McClellan, A. T., Luborksy, L., Woody, G. E., O'Brien, C. P., & Droler, K. (1983). Predicting response to alcohol and drug abuse treatments: Role of psychiatric severity. *Archives of General Psychiatry, 40*, 620–625.

Meisels, S. J., & Shonkoff, J. P. (1990). *Handbook of early childhood intervention*. New York: Cambridge University Press.

Mendelson, J. H., Weiss, R., Griffin, M., Mirin, S. M., et al. (1991). Some special considerations for treatment of drug abuse and dependence in women (NIDA Research Monograph No. 106, pp. 313–326). Washington, DC: U.S. Government Printing Office.

Merikangas, K. R., Rounsaville, B. J., & Prusoff, B. A. (1992). Familial factors in vulnerability to substance abuse. In M. Glantz & R. Pickens (Eds.), *Vulnerability to drug abuse* (pp. 75–98). Washington, DC: American Psychiatric Association.

Miller, G. (1989, June). Addicted infants and their mothers. *Zero to Three*, pp. 20–23.

Mirin, S. M., Weiss, R. D., Griffin, M. L., & Michael, J. L. (1991). Psychopathology in drug abusers and their families. *Comprehensive Psychiatry, 32*, 36–51.

Moise, R., Reed, B. G., & Ryan, V. (1982). Issues in the treatment of heroin-addicted women: A comparison of men and women entering two types of drug abuse programs. *International Journal of the Addictions, 17*, 109–139.

Musto, D. (1973). *The American disease: Origins of narcotic control.* New Haven: Yale University Press.

O'Connor, M. J., Sigman, N., & Brill, N. (1987). Disorganization of attachment in relation to maternal alcohol consumption. *Journal of Consulting and Clinical Psychology, 55,* 831–836.

O'Connor, M. J., Sigman, M., & Kasari, C. (1992). Attachment behavior of infants exposed prenatally to alcohol: Mediating effects of infant affect and mother-infant interaction. *Development and Psychopathology, 4,* 243–256.

O'Connor, M. J., Sigman, M., & Kasari, C. (1993). Maternal alcohol use and infant cognition. *Infant Behavior and Development, 16,* 177–193.

O'Malley, S., Adamse, M., Heaton, R. K., & Gawin, F. H. (1992). Neuropsychological impairments in chronic cocaine abusers. *American Journal of Drug and Alcohol Abuse, 18,* 131–144.

Osterloh J. D., & Lee, B. L. (1989). Urine drug screening in mothers and newborns. *American Journal of Diseases of Children, 143,* 791–793.

Pauls, D. (1991). Genetic influences on child psychiatric conditions. In M. Lewis (Ed.), *Child and adolescent psychiatry: A comprehensive textbook* (pp. 351–363). Baltimore: Williams and Wilkins.

Pawl, J. (1992). Interventions to strengthen relationships between infants and drug-abusing recovering parents. *Zero to Three, 13,* 6–10.

Pittman, R. K. (1988). Post-traumatic stress disorder, conditioning, and network theory. *Psychiatric Annals, 18,* 182–189.

Pribram, K. H., & McGuiness, D. (1975). Arousal, activation, and effort in the control of attention. *Psychological Review, 82,* 116–149.

Raynes, A. E., Clement, C., Patch, V. D., & Ervin, F. (1974). Factors related to imprisonment in female heroin addicts. *International Journal of the Addictions, 9,* 145–150.

Reed, B. G. (1985). Drug misuse and dependency in women: The meaning and implications of being considered a special population or minority group. *International Journal of the Addictions, 20,* 13–62.

Reed, B. G., & Leibson, E. (1981). Women clients in special women's demonstration drug abuse treatment programs compared with women entering selected co-sex programs. *International Journal of the Addictions, 16,* 1425–1466.

Rodning, C., Beckwith, L., & Howard, J. (1989). Characteristics of attachment organization and play organization in prenatally drug-exposed toddlers. *Development and Psychopathology, 1,* 277–289.

Rodning, C., Beckwith, & Howard, J. (1991). Quality of attachment and home environments in children prenatally exposed to PCP and cocaine. *Development and Psychopathology, 3,* 351–366.

Rogosch, F. A., Cicchetti, D., Shields, A., & Toth, S. L. (1995). Parenting dysfunction in child maltreatment. In M. H. Bornstein (Ed.), *Handbook of parenting* (Vol. 4). Hillsdale, NJ: Erlbaum.

Rosenthal, R., & Jacobson, L. (1968). *Pygmalion in the classroom: Teacher expectation and pupil's intellectual development.* New York: Holt, Rinehart & Winston.

Rounsaville, B. J., Dolinsky, Z. S., Babor, T. F., & Meyer, R. E. (1987). Psychopathology as a predictor of treatment outcome in alcoholics. *Archives of General Psychiatry, 44,* 505–513.

Rounsaville, B. J., Kosten, T. R., Weissman, M. M., Prusoff, B., Pauls, D., Foley, S., & Merikangas, K. (1991). Psychiatric disorders in the relatives of probands with opiate addicts. *Archives of General Psychiatry, 48,* 33–42.

Rounsaville, B. J., Weissman, M. M., Wilber, C. H., & Kleber, H. D. (1982). Pathways of opiate addiction: An evaluation of differing antecedents. *British Journal of Psychiatry, 141,* 437–466.

Ruff, H. A. (1988). The measurement of attention in high-risk infants. In P. M. Vietze & H. G. Vaughan (Eds.), *Early identification of infants with developmental disabilities* (pp. 282–296). New York: Grune and Stratton.

Saunders, E. (1992). Project together: Serving substance-abusing mothers and their chidren in Des Moines. *American Journal of Public Health, 82,* 1166–1167.

Scherling, D. (1994). Prenatal cocaine exposure and childhood psychopathology. *American Journal of Orthopsychiatry, 64,* 9–19.

Shulte, K., & Blume, S. B. (1979). A day treatment center for alcoholic women. *Health Social Work, 4,* 222–231.

Singer, L., Farkas, K., & Kliegman, R. (1992). Childhood medical and behavioral consequence of maternal cocaine use. *Journal of Pediatric Psychology, 17,* 389–406.

Smith, I. E., Dent, D. Z., Coles, C. D., & Falek, A. (1992). A comparison study of treated and untreated pregnant and postpartum cocaine-abusing women. *Journal of Substance Abuse Treatment, 9,* 343–348.

Snell, W. E., Finney, P. D., & Godwin, L. J. (1991). Stereotypes about AIDS. *Contemporary Social Psychology, 15,* 18–38.

Stevens, S., Arbiter, V., & Gilder, P. (1989). Women residents: Expanding their role to increase treatment effectiveness in substance abuse programs. *International Journal of the Addictions, 11,* 19–23.

Struthers, J. M., & Hansen, R. L. (1992) Visual recognition memory in drug-exposed infants. *Journal of Developmental and Behavioral Pediatrics, 13,* 108–111.

Tamis-LeMonda, C. S., & Bornstein, M. H. (1989). Habituation and maternal encouragement of attention in infancy as predictors of toddler language, play, and representational competence. *Child Development, 60,* 738–751.

Wasserman, D. R., & Leventhal, J. M. (1993). Maltreatment of children born to cocaine-abusing mothers. *American Journal of Diseases of Children, 147,* 1324–1328.

Wellisch, D. K., & Steinberg, M. R. (1980). Parenting attitudes of addict mothers. *International Journal of the Addictions, 15,* 809–819.

Woods, N. S., Eyler, F. D., Behnke, M., & Conlon, M. (1991). Cocaine use during pregnancy: Maternal depressive symptoms and neonatal neurobehavior over the first month. Presentation at the Society for Research in Child Development, Seattle, WA.

Woods, J. R., Plessinger, M. A., & Clark, K. E. (1987). Effect of cocaine on uterine blood flow and fetal oxygenation. *Journal of the American Medical Association, 257,* 957–961.

Zuckerman, B., Amaro, J., Bauchner, H., & Cabral, H. (1989). Depressive symptoms during pregnancy: Relationships to poor health behaviors. *American Journal of Obstetrics and Gynecology, 160,* 1107–1111.

Zuckerman, B., & Frank, D. A. (1992). Prenatal cocaine and marijuana exposure: Research and clinical implications. In I. S. Zagon & T. A. Slotkin (Eds.), *Maternal substance abuse and the developing nervous system* (pp. 125–154). Boston: Academic Press.

Zuckerman, B., Frank, D. A., Hingson, R., & Amaro, H. (1989). Effects of maternal marijuana and cocaine use on fetal growth. *New England Journal of Medicine, 320,* 762–768.

CHAPTER 6

The Problem of Pediatric Pain

BETTY R. KASSON, SANDRA K. SENTIVANY,
AND PAMELA M. KATO

INTRODUCTION

The management of pain in children has lagged far behind advances in other areas of medical achievement. In 1968, physicians Swafford and Allen stated, "Pediatric patients seldom need relief of pain after general surgery. They tolerate discomfort well" (p. 133) and reported that during a 4-month period, 96% of the postoperative pediatric patients in their intensive care unit did not receive any analgesics for pain. As recently as the 1980s and 1990s, many infants and children were not receiving any analgesia during and after major surgery (Anand, Brown, Bloom, & Aynsley-Green, 1985). Indeed, postoperative children and those with disease-related pain frequently received no analgesic medication at all (Gauntlet, 1987). When compared with adults undergoing similar surgeries, infants and children received fewer doses and smaller amounts of analgesic medication per kilogram of body weight (Beyer, Ashley, Russell,

BETTY R. KASSON • Departments of Nursing and Pediatric Surgery, Lucile Salter Packard Children's Hospital at Stanford, Palo Alto, California 94304.   SANDRA K. SENTIVANY • Departments of Nursing and Pain Management, Lucile Salter Packard Children's Hospital at Stanford, Palo Alto, California 94304.   PAMELA M. KATO • Department of Psychiatry and Behavioral Sciences, Stanford University School of Medicine, Stanford, California 94305.

Handbook of Diversity Issues in Health Psychology, edited by Pamela M. Kato and Traci Mann. Plenum Press, New York, 1996.

& DeGood, 1983; Eland & Anderson, 1977; Schechter, Allen, & Hansen, 1986). The undertreatment of children's pain is still routine and is striking considering pervasive evidence of children's experience of physiological, behavioral, and emotional effects of pain.

Physiologic Effects of Pain

Children have a significant physiologic stress response to pain, including substantial hormonal–metabolic changes. Infants and children who experience painful procedures without analgesia during the perioperative period demonstrate measurable increases in heart rate, blood pressure, pulmonary vascular resistance, and intracranial pressure, as well as a marked decrease in the transcutaneous partial pressure of oxygen (Anand & Hickey, 1987; Messner, Loux, & Grossman, 1979). Catecholamines and stress hormones (i.e., glucagon, growth hormone, and corticosteroids) are released and insulin production suppressed when children experience pain (Anand, 1986; Anand et al., 1985; Fletcher, 1987; Gauntlett, 1987; Kaplan, 1988; Porter, 1989; Yaster, 1987). These changes result in the breakdown of body tissue (e.g., protein, carbohydrate, and fat stores) leading to hyperglycemia and marked increases in blood lactate, pyruvate, ketones, and nonesterified fatty acids (Anand et al., 1985). In addition, increased metabolic rate, blood clotting, fluid retention, and the triggering of an autonomic "fight or flight" response occur (Acute Pain Management Guideline Panel, 1992; Dinarello, 1984; Egdahl, 1959; Kehlet, 1982).

When children's pain is not treated, their rapid, shallow breathing leads to alkalosis and electrolyte losses; their inadequate ability to cough leads to retention of secretions and to potential pneumonia; and their increased heart rate leads an increased metabolic rate (Eland, 1990b). This hypermetabolic response to pain is associated with cardiac and pulmonary insufficiency and impaired immune response, leading to a higher incidence of morbidity and mortality, especially in critically ill infants and children (Bhatt-Mehta & Rosen, 1991).

Adequate management of pain suppresses these adverse physiologic responses and significantly reduces postoperative morbidity and mortality (Fitzgerald & Anand, 1993). The undertreatment of pediatric pain sets in motion physiologic mechanisms that impede healing and may actually contribute to disability and death.

Behavioral Effects of Pain

Even very young children show behavioral reactions to painful stimuli. As early as 2 to 3 months of age, infants show the ability to attend to or shut out stimuli, to appraise situations, and to prepare themselves before responding (Zeltzer, Anderson, & Schechter, 1990). Even neonates will exhibit rapid limb movements and will turn away from noxious stimuli. When children experience acute uncontrolled or intense pain, they demonstrate negative coping behaviors ranging from active screaming, clawing, and fighting to passive withdrawal and learned helplessness. These reactions require costly energy expenditures in a young organism whose primary work is growth.

The behavioral effects of undertreated pain, compared to physiological effects, are less dramatic in the short term but nevertheless have lasting effects on the young child. Poorly managed childhood pain can establish the basis for a lifetime of maladaptive pain processing behaviors. Uncontrolled pain in children can be manifest as decreased pain threshold whenever pain is encountered throughout life (Gaffney & Dunne, 1987; Ross & Ross, 1984b). Childhood experiences with uncontrolled pain during dental procedures can lead to the development of a fear-avoidance phobia (Tesler, 1994). Adults may consequently avoid dental care based on this attitude formed during childhood. In sum, the behaviors and strategies learned in coping with childhood pain shape the ability of the adult to respond in a mature manner to the challenges of adult pain.

Emotional Effects of Pain

Children experience adverse emotional effects when their pain is undertreated. Severe or unrelieved pain in children can cause emotional problems including feelings of guilt and learned helplessness.

There is evidence that children believe in a "just world," that punishments result from misdeeds (Jose, 1990). Thus children may feel that their pain is punishment for a misdeed. Based on clinical observation, Anna Freud (1952) argued that children in pain believe that their pain is a punishment some transgressions. These children may not be willing to talk about their pain and may actually feel guilty and responsible for causing that pain (Lynn, 1986; McBride, 1977; see Savedra, Gibbons, Tesler, Ward, & Wegner, 1982, for a dissenting view).

If a painful experience has been uncontrollable and impossible to escape for a child, it is likely that he or she will show symptoms of learned helplessness (Seligman, 1975). That is, if the child's pleas for relief of pain are unheard, the child will believe that any efforts to gain pain relief are futile. The child will then give up all attempts to have the pain relieved, even in situations where pleas for pain relief may be effective. The child then adopts many signs and symptoms of depression.

Because infants and children experience adverse physiological, behavioral, and emotional effects from the undertreatment of their pain, it is imperative to make efforts to manage their pain more effectively. Such efforts require, first, an understanding of why children's pain is commonly undertreated. In the following sections, we will examine some of the myths that lie at the foundation of pediatric pain mismanagement. We describe the cognitive developmental abilities of children and implications for the assessment of children's pain. We present some pharmacological and nonpharmacological interventions for pediatric pain. We close with a discussion of possible directions for future research and interventions.

MYTHS ABOUT CHILDHOOD PAIN

Many myths have led health professionals to perceive pediatric pain as difficult and dangerous to manage (Burokas, 1985; Eland, 1990). These inaccurate beliefs comprise the foundation of the mismanagement of pediatric pain. They also underlie mismanagement of adult pain; however, the effects of these beliefs are magnified with children because of their unique coping styles and modes of communication.

Myth 1: Respiratory Depression Is More Common in Children Than in Adults

A potentially serious side effect of opioid administration is respiratory depression. Inappropriate consideration of the fear of respiratory depression is a significant barrier to the proper administration of opioids. Respiratory depression from opioid administration is no more common in children than in adults (with the exception of infants less than one month old who have slower clearance of tissue opioids; Yaster & Deshpande, 1988). Despite this fact, undermedicating pain for fear of respiratory depression is more common among children than among adults (e.g., Beyer & Beyer, 1985).

Health professionals' fear of respiratory depression is often exaggerated. Clinically significant respiratory depression is relatively rare. It occurs in fewer than 1% of hospitalized patients receiving prescribed opioids for pain management (Miller & Jick, 1970). In addition, respiratory depression can usually be treated with naloxone, an agent that reverses the effect of the opioids. Furthermore, over time, patients develop a tolerance to the respiratory depressant effects of opioids while still achieving pain relief. Fear of respiratory depression, then, should not prevent doctors from giving children medication to relieve their pain.

Myth 2: Acute and Chronic Pain Are the Same

Children's pain, especially when chronic, is often mismanaged because acute and chronic pain are thought of interchangeably. These types of pain, however, are different and require different approaches to assessment and treatment. Acute pain in children and adults is a protective mechanism that warns of actual or potential tissue damage. Onset is generally sudden, and the pain usually disappears when the body has healed. A sympathetic nervous system response, including tachycardia, tachypnea, hypertension, dilated pupils, pallor or flushing, muscle tension, nausea, and diaphoresis is associated with acute pain. Acute pain can be objectively assessed as well as subjectively reported.

In contrast, chronic pain persists beyond expected healing time and generally is not related to the effects of a specific injury. When children and adults experience chronic pain, they often do not demonstrate the sympathetic nervous system responses that generally accompany acute pain. The absence of obvious physiological symptoms of pain may cause the inexperienced practitioner to assume a patient is not experiencing pain. As a result, the patient's chronic pain is mismanaged by undermedication. Children may be particularly vulnerable to undermedication because children's subjective reports of pain are believed to be less credible than adults' reports (Zeltzer, Barr, McGrath, & Schechter, 1992).

Myth 3: A Positive Placebo Effect for Pain Indicates That the Pain Is Not Real

A placebo is an agent that has no known pharmacological effect but can cause a therapeutic response. The placebo effect is thought to result from the practitioner–patient relationship, the significance of the therapeutic effort to the patient, and the endorphin response of the patient (Goodwin, Goodwin, & Vogel, 1979). When placebos are given to patients in pain, patients not only report feeling less pain, but objective measurements of outcomes controlled by the autonomic nervous system also indicate alleviation of the pain response.

Some health professionals believe that an analgesic response to a placebo indicates that the pain is not real. As a result, patients in pain who show a positive response to placebo medication are given inadequate analgesia, and in some cases, receive no analgesia at all. This attitude is particularly harmful when directed toward pediatric patients because children are already undermedicated for their pain. In general, placebo effects should never be used as a basis for determining whether or not symptoms are "psychogenic" or "somatic" (Brody, 1982). Multiple assessments of pain should be used, for example, behavioral and self-report assessments.

Myth 4: PRN Means Give as Little as Possible

Pain medications are frequently ordered on a PRN (*pro re nata*), or "as needed" basis. Too often this is interpreted as *give as little as possible*. When medications are ordered PRN, health practitioners often wait until pain is severe before they administer analgesics. In these cases, it often takes more medication to relieve the pain. Patients are caught in a cycle of increasing pain, undermedication, and little relief. Long waits for pain medication may result in preoccupation with pain. Patients may lose faith in the reliability of pain relief and may misreport pain to obtain needed medication (Covelman, Scott, Buchanan, & Rosman, 1990). Since children are more likely than adults to receive inadequate doses of medication ordered, PRN schedules are especially likely to result in insufficient analgesia in children.

Around-the-clock dosing provides more effective pain control because regularly scheduled dosing maintains a constant level of drug in the body and addresses pain before it is out of control (Jacox et al., 1994). Continuous pain requires continuous analgesia in both children and adults (McCaffery & Beebe, 1989).

Myth 5: A Given Event Results in an Expected amount of Pain

Health care professionals often have preconceived ideas of how painful they expect a given event to be and how much medication will be required. These ideas are based on their prior experiences with similar events (Broome & Slack, 1990). However, pain is a complex, individual experience not governed by preset categories of intensity. Each pain experience is different for each individual, and pain responses may be different for the same individual at different times. If the pain intensity of an adult or child falls outside of the experience of the person giving the medication, the sufferer's complaints may not be believed or treated. This may be more likely to occur among children whose experiences and perceptions often differ markedly from the adult who is assessing and treating their pain.

Myth 6: A Child's Pain Is Not as Intense as an Adult's Pain

The incomplete development of the nervous system at birth has led health professionals to believe that children do not feel pain with the same intensity as adults. In the early 20th century, physiological scientists discovered that infants had incomplete myelin sheaths around their nerves. Unmyelinated nerves conduct nerve impulses more slowly. It is therefore a common belief that pain impulses cannot be effectively transmitted over unmyelinated nerves. Consequently, health professionals tend to interpret pain behaviors as indicative of hunger, restlessness, or irritability in infants. Their misinterpretation of pain behaviors leads to inadequate analgesia for these children.

Pain pathways are well developed before birth. While unmyelinated fibers, which in fact are more numerous at birth, may transmit impulses more slowly, the pathways from the site of pain through the spinal cord to the thalamus, limbic system, and cerebral cortex are much shorter in infants than adults. Because the pathways are shorter, impulses reach their destinations quickly. Complete myelinization is, therefore, not necessary for the transmission of nociceptive impulses (Zeltzer et al., 1990).

Myth 7: A Child Behaving Passively or Asleep Is Not in Pain

Health professionals may misinterpret children's passive pain behaviors as evidence of no pain and fail to administer adequate analgesia. Children may appear to be passively responding to painful stimuli because they may interpret the event based on their own limited experience with painful events (Parton, 1976). They do not respond to pain like adults because they lack a comparable context in which to interpret painful events.

Children have many ways of coping with pain. Some children are more active in their coping style, others more passive (Broome, Lillis, McGahee, & Bates, 1992). Some children may attempt to actively distract themselves with activities in order to feel better. Children may sleep, either to escape pain or because they are exhausted from dealing with it. Others may become preoccupied with pain, becoming still and quiet, limiting their interactions with others. (Acute Pain Management Guideline Panel, 1992; Eland, 1990; Rogers, 1989).

As we have discussed in the section on the difficult discrimination of chronic pain, and in the previous section on underreporting pain, behavior alone is only one indicator of pain. Evaluations of pain must include the child's report in addition to other objective measures (Rogers, 1989).

Myth 8: Children Who Take Opioids for Pain Will Become Addicted to Them

Fear of addiction and drug abuse is a concern in both the medical and lay communities (Beyer & Beyer, 1985; Webb, Stergios, & Rodgers, 1989). Although this is a concern with adult patients as well, there is a more intense response to the possibility of addicting an innocent child to drugs. Health care professionals are often reluctant to prescribe or administer opioids to children because of the misguided fear of causing addiction in a child. Children and parents often share this fear of addiction and may refuse opioids prescribed by a physician, despite children's reports of pain. Children are indoctrinated from an early age to "just say no" to drugs, and this leads some children and families to make faulty distinctions between legitimate opioid use for pain and recreational drugs.

Fear of addiction and drug abuse may exist because there is widespread confusion about the concepts of addiction, tolerance, and dependence. Addiction involves a behavioral pattern of compulsive seeking and taking of drugs for psychological reasons, not medical reasons. Children who require opioids for pain relief for known medical or surgical causes cannot, by definition, be characterized as being addicted (Eland, 1990b).

Drug tolerance is a natural physiologic response. It occurs when patients require increasingly larger doses of medication to provide the same analgesic effect as the original dose. Patients in pain require increased amounts of medication for physical reasons.

Physical dependence is also a natural physiologic response. It is an altered physiologic state that results from the repeated administration of an opioid. When someone is physically dependent on a drug, he or she requires the continuing use of the drug to prevent withdrawal symptoms. Children do become dependent on opioids. They must therefore be weaned off opioids in order to prevent withdrawal symptoms.

In sum, opioids can be safely administered to children. Careful attention to their administration and to the cessation of administration can contribute to better pain management for children.

Myth 9: There Is a Very Narrow Range of Safety for Opioid Doses in Children

Many health care professionals assume that it is unsafe and irresponsible to prescribe or administer doses of medication other than those recommended. A fixed milligram per kilogram dose of opioid analgesia is frequently believed to be the only safe dose for a child in pain. Because children are smaller, health professionals fear that even small increases in dosage may have severe physical effects, such as respiratory depression. However, the ranges given in drug formularies are only starting points; the development of physiologic tolerance as discussed above, or individual sensitivities, shows that doses should be adjusted until adequate pain management without oversedation is achieved. There is great variability in the dose of opioids necessary to manage pain in different children; one child may require less than the recommended dose of a medication, and another may require far more of the same medication for comparable analgesia (Tyler, 1992). The use of appropriate assessment tools and sound clinical judgment allows for more objective individualization of pain medication dosing.

ASSESSING PAIN IN CHILDREN

The assessment of pain is a complex, multifaceted task. The definitions of pain itself vary greatly, ranging from "... an unpleasant sensory and emotional experience arising from actual or potential tissue damage or described in terms of such damage" (International Association for the Study of Pain, 1979, p. 249) to "whatever the experiencing person says it is, and arising whenever he/she says it does" (McCaffery, 1979, p. 12). Because the definitions differ, it is often difficult to know for sure exactly what we are assessing when we say we are assessing pain. In children, pain assessment is further complicated by developmental variables.

Children in pain continue to progress through developmental stages that determine how their pain is expressed and impact its successful management. The assessment of childhood pain and the application of effective nonpharmacological strategies depend on an understanding of the developmental capabilities of the child. Adult approaches to pain are not so developmentally determined. Each stage of childhood is characterized by particular ways of responding to noxious stimuli based on the child's development, understanding, and capabilities. In the following sections we discuss stages of childhood development and implications for assessment of pain.

Infancy

Although physiological studies have clearly indicated that infants experience distress, quantification of this response in neonates and premature infants is a challenging task. Infants during the first year pass a series of developmental milestones that gradually enable them to move from a generalized, disorganized response to pain to an ability to localize the pain, to calm themselves, and to respond in a more focused manner. This ability is modified by individual differences in the rate at which infants progress and by temperament. Some infants are able to self-soothe early in life and require less soothing from caregivers; some will continue to demonstrate prolonged distress to painful stimuli despite soothing behaviors (Zeltzer et al., 1990).

Infant pain assessment tools are still the subject of much research. Infants and nonverbal children have no way to clarify the meaning of their behavior (e.g., crying, grimacing, etc.) for observers, and the same behavior can arise from a variety of discomfort states. Gonsalves and Mercer (1993) advocate an assessment of physiological changes, such as increased heart rate in premature infants, as indicative of pain states. Johnson, Stevens, Craig, and Grunau (1993) claim that physiological responses are too variable and argue instead for an assessment of behavioral responses because they are more specific measures of pain states. Current evaluation tools for infants use assessments of physiology, of behavior, or both. They include (1) physiological measures of heart rate, respiration rate, and oxygen saturation; (2) single behavior measures (crying); and (3) multidimensional behavioral scales (crying, facial grimacing, fussiness). Many of these scales have good interrater reliability and promising validity, but not one has emerged as the gold standard for assessing infant pain (Watt-Watson & Donavan, 1992; McGrath, 1987).

Preschool

Preschooler responses include new verbal abilities that may improve or hinder attempts at self-regulation. Immature verbal understanding creates new and frightening ways for children to remember painful experiences. For example, a preschooler told by a nurse that she was going to take his vitals ran down the hall in terror. He wasn't sure what his vitals were, but he wasn't going to let anyone have them! Preschoolers are sensate rather than rational and believe their senses rather than what is told to them. If a needle hurts, it makes no sense that it could make them feel better. Preschool coping behaviors include active behaviors such as verbal protests (e.g., "no, no!"), use of pain words (e.g., "hurt, hurt"), hitting, and fighting to escape (Zeltzer et al., 1990; McGrath & Craig, 1989).

Assessment tools for preschoolers and young schoolaged children require that the children rate their pain by scaling a series of objects or pictures (Beyer & Aradine, 1987; Wong & Whaley, 1986). In order to make these ratings, the children must understand that objects or pictures can be symbolic of their pain, and that in some scales, a larger number of objects represents a greater level of pain, as in the Poker Chip Tool (Hester, 1979). The scale selected for pain ratings must be appropriate for the child's developmental level or the results will not be reflective of the child's pain.

Young children are able to use one to four poker chips to represent increasing amounts of pain (Hester, 1979). Poker Chip Tool information correlates well with observed behavioral information in children 4 to 6 years old. The chips themselves are readily available and easy to disinfect. The Poker Chip Tool has been criticized, however, since it provides no interval information (Aradine, Beyer, & Tompkins, 1988). For example, two poker chips may represent 2 times or 10 times as much pain as one poker chip.

Aradine et al. (1988) demonstrated that children as young as age 3 could sequence the photographs of emotion-laden faces in the Oucher Scale (Beyer & Aradine, 1987) from least amount of pain to greatest amount of pain. Not all young children, however, have mastered seriation. The original Oucher Scale used only Caucasian faces, but Oucher scales using Hispanic, black, and other ethnic faces are now being tested (Villarruel & Denyes, 1991; Denyes, Beyer, Villarruel, & Neuman, 1991). There is also some question as to the specificity of the scale for pain only.

Projective and scaling techniques have been combined for pediatric pain assessment. In this technique, children are asked to choose four colors to represent increasing amounts of pain. They are then asked to use a color indicative of their pain to draw the location of their pain on a body outline (Eland, 1985). This gives quantitative information about multiple pain sites in addition to the qualitative scaling of intensity of the pain. The colors chosen must be carefully validated with the child. There is sketchy support for the validity of children's color choices as indicative of their differing pain levels. This tool is limited to children who are physically comfortable enough to choose crayons and color pictures.

School Age and Adolescence

School-aged children are capable of understanding causal relationships and function well in concrete operational thought, although they may have big gaps in their knowledge. In one study (Alex & Ritchie, 1992), children accurately described what their surgery was for and why they were in the hospital, but they had no concept of how long the postoperative pain was supposed to last, and some thought it might go on forever. School-aged children have learned to inhibit socially unacceptable expressions and are very interested in knowing what the rules are and following them. Some will internalize distress and not ask for medication if they think that is the way to be "good."

Adolescents can understand the physiological and psychological interactions that mediate pain. They have capabilities similar to the adult in evaluating the complex affective, sensory, cognitive, and motivational aspects of pain. However, clinicians tend to overestimate older children's understanding of what is told to them (Perrin & Gerrity, 1981). Children under stress regress to earlier cognitive and behavioral states, and adolescents may regress to concrete operational thought when dealing with pain (Brewster, 1982). In addition, the egocentric, individuating aspects of adolescents tend to focus them inward and this tendency may result in distortions of what is told to them.

Pain assessment among school-aged and adolescent children (ages 6–18) has been studied using verbal reports, interviews, questionnaires, diaries, projective tests, pain drawings, pain maps, pain thermometers, descriptor lists, and self-report scales (McGrath, 1987; Donovan, 1992; see Watt-Watson & Donovan, 1992, for a review of psychometric properties). All of these tools elicit the child's experience of pain, but some are quite lengthy and are limited by the child's attention span, energy level, and willingness to participate.

Common sense and consistency are the most important factors in selecting the tool that will provide the best information on pain. The user must select a tool that will be appropriate to the developmental level and capabilities of the child, choose a tool that has good psychometric properties, and ensure that the tool is used consistently by all personnel.

INTERVENTIONS FOR PAIN IN CHILDREN

Because of the complex nature of pain among children, its treatment must be multidimensional. To address only the physical aspects of pain, while ignoring the emotional and behavioral aspects, is to partially treat the pain problem. As mentioned before, the physiological responses to prolonged or chronic pain return to normal values as the body adjusts to the chronic stress. Consequently, it is the behavioral manifestations which may be most indicative of the patient's actual experience of pain. Affective and behavioral patterns established for coping with pain may persist long after the physical pain is resolved. If the affective and behavioral aspects of pain are addressed along with the physical aspects, patients are better able to return to the developmental tasks of their normal lives.

The multidimensional treatment of pain includes the pharmacological and nonpharmacological management of the physical pain and the psychological management of the cognitive, behavioral, environmental, and affective aspects of the pain. Pharmacological measures use drugs to work directly on the central and peripheral pain receptors, neurotransmitters, and substances that mediate pain. Nonpharmacological techniques also address the central and peripheral nervous systems, but involve a less direct approach to the management of pain. Although nonpharmacological methods may be used alone, especially for short, moderately painful procedures such as venipuncture, they are generally more effective when used in conjunction with pharmacological methods.

Pharmacological Interventions

Drug treatment is generally recognized as the mainstay of acute and some chronic pain control in both adults and children. An understanding of the pharmacodynamics and pharmacokinetics of pain control agents is necessary to prescribe dosages and intervals. Understanding the contributions of tolerance and dependence discussed earlier is critical to adjusting medications for maximum comfort with minimal side effects.

There are 3 classes of analgesic drugs: NSAIDs (nonsteroidal antiinflammatory drugs), which work in the peripheral system; opioids, which work centrally; and adjuvants. These may be used separately or in combination. No one drug is necessarily better than another, but drugs have different actions and may be used for different types of pain. Combinations of centrally and peripherally acting drugs and adjuvants may be more effective than increasing the amount of one type alone. For example, one type of somatic pain results from stimulation of pain-conducting afferent nerves that are found in soft tissues or bones. This type of pain is described as *dull* and *aching* and can usually be well controlled with conventional analgesics such as NSAIDS and opioids. Neuropathic pain, on the other hand, generally develops after an injury to peripheral nerves, rather than stimulation of the nerve endings. Neuropathic pain, described as *sharp, burning,* or *shooting,* usually has a poor response to conventional analgesics and is better managed with adjuvants such as local anesthetics (Galer, 1995; Mercadante et al., 1995).

In both adults and children, the important pain management issue is to recognize the type of pain involved and determine the most effective combination of pharmacological and nonpharmacological strategies. In the following section we review nonpharmacological interventions that are highly effective when used in combination with pharmacological techniques, and even when used alone.

Nonpharmacological Interventions

Numerous nonpharmacological techniques of pain management are available for use with children. Some of these techniques have appeal because they are more interactive than most pharmacological methods of pain management and address some of the affective and behavioral components of pain. They also work well without many of the potential side effects of drugs. As mentioned previously, nonpharmacological strategies offer children a feeling of control during a time when they may have little control over what is happening to them. When a child feels a sense of control over self, the environment, or both, some of the negative responses to pain may be diminished. Perceived control during painful situations has been shown to reduce stress and increase pain tolerance (Weisenberg, 1987). The successful use of some nonpharmacological methods requires training, practice, and time on the part of child, family, and practitioner.

Nonpharmacological peripheral nervous system techniques, involving stimulation of the skin as a means of reducing pain perception, include superficial heat and cold, massage, acupressure/acupuncture, and transcutaneous electric nerve stimulation (TENS; Edgar & Smith-Hanrahan, 1992). Central nervous system interventions, which exert their effects through alterations of affective and sensory factors, include relaxation, imagery and hypnosis, music, distraction, and biofeedback.

Peripheral Nervous System Techniques

Superficial Heat and Cold

Superficial heat is the application of moist or dry heat to the body causing analgesia. Subjectively, heat increases the pain threshold and encourages relaxation of painful muscle spasm. Once the inflammatory response has subsided, heat can reduce pain by means of vasodilation, which improves blood flow, enhancing tissue nutrition and the elimination of noxious cellular metabolites (Mehta, 1986). Pain involving muscles or joints is especially responsive to heat therapy.

The application of superficial cold is not always accepted as readily as heat, but cold is frequently more effective in relieving pain. It decreases edema, inhibits the release of pain-mediating chemicals, and slows the conduction of pain impulses from the periphery. The reduction of muscle spasm causes a decrease in pain sensation.

Most studies on the effectiveness of superficial heat and cold for pain relief have been carried out on adult populations (e.g., Curkovic, Vitulic, Babic-Naglic, & Durrigl, 1993). Although there are no controlled outcome studies on the effectiveness of this technique with children, this treatment is commonly used for pain relief in children.

Massage

Massage has long been used as a treatment for many types of pain. It is thought that the pressure of massage causes a decrease in edema and an improvement in circulation, as well as a sense of relaxation that leads to a decrease in the experience of pain. Research has indicated that massage also causes a release of endorphins (Kaada & Torsteinbo, 1989).

Children are generally amenable to this treatment, and it is often used for their pain relief. Although studies show its effectivness with an adult population (see Goats, 1994, for a review), there are no randomized trials of the effectiveness of massage with children. There are, however, case studies claiming its effectiveness for use with children (e.g., Dietz, Mathews, & Montgomery, 1990).

Acupuncture and Acupressure

Acupuncture and acupressure are therapeutic procedures that originated in China more than 5,000 years ago. They are based on the theory that there is a certain flow of energy (*ch'i*) throughout the body. When this energy flow is obstructed, an imbalance between negative and positive forces (*yin* and *yang*) occurs, resulting in pain or disease. Pain is treated by restoring balance to the system. This balance is achieved by inserting and manipulating fine steel needles at specific acupuncture points or by applying manual pressure to the skin at specific points.

It is not entirely clear, especially to the Western mind, how these techniques work. Perhaps endorphins are released when acupoints are pressed, causing a feeling of well-being and pain relief. Acupoint areas, according to histological studies, are rich with nerves and pressure and stretch receptors, they have lower electrical resistance than surrounding skin. As a result, these points are particularly susceptible to pressure, electrical stimulation, or both.

Acupuncture is more widely used for adults than with children. However, there is some evidence of its use and efficacy among children, and is effective among pediatric patients with migraine headaches (Pothman & Goepel, 1984). Acupressure is used more than acupuncture among children, possibly because it is not an invasive technique.

Transcutaneous Electrical Nerve Stimulation (TENS)

This technique involves the passing of a low-voltage electrical current across skin between two electrodes. TENS exerts its effect by activating large diameter, myelinated A beta fibers, closing the pain gate to painful peripheral impulses. TENS may also initiate the release of endorphins

(Edgar & Smith-Hanrahan, 1992). The use of TENS has proven useful for many types of acute and chronic pain (Eland, 1991; Pothman, 1991), although its efficacy with children has not been tested. It is often used clinically with children in addition to pharmacological pain interventions (Beyer & Bournaki, 1989).

Central Nervous System Techniques

Relaxation

Pain is often associated with the stress response, which causes anxiety, tension, and muscle contraction. Relaxation is a biobehavioral phenomenon in which the decrease in oxygen consumption, muscle tone, heart rate, respiratory rate, intense slow alpha waves, and occasional theta activity in the brain lead to decreased muscle tension, spasm, fear, and anxiety during painful episodes (Benson, 1975). Most children seem to have learned the ability to relax on their own and can demonstrate relaxation skills from a very young age (e.g., Ross & Ross, 1984). Relaxation reduces pain by regulating pain perception, not pain intensity. The children control the intensity of their reaction to the pain, not the pain itself.

Relaxation is simple, safe, and cost effective. It has consistently been as effective as biofeedback for pain management (Stroebel, 1982) and has been used as a pain management technique with children in a variety of settings (e.g., Larsson & Melin, 1986).

Imagery/Hypnosis

Imagery/hypnosis is a mental representation of reality or fantasy and may use all five senses. It influences the perception of pain through distraction, displacement, distortion, and dissociation, thereby altering the meaning of the pain for the child (Valente, 1991). Guided imagery and hypnosis are generally preceded by some form of relaxation, which is thought to facilitate image development.

Imagery and hypnosis are often used during painful procedures to reduce pain and behaviors indicating distress. Children who use guided imagery regain a sense of personal control, especially when they are encouraged to create their own images. Imagery and hypnosis contribute to reduced muscle tension, anxiety, and pain, thereby reducing the fear and expression associated with pain, as well as the pain itself. Imagery and hypnosis have been used for pain management with children in a number of settings (see Ellis & Spanos, 1994, for a review).

Music

Music is often casually used to lessen the effects of pain among patitents with long-term and life-threatening illnesses (Magill-Levreault, 1993). The therapeutic effect of music may be through a conditioned relaxation response mediated by a change in mood. Music has been used with pediatric oncology patients undergoing lumbar punctures (Rasco, 1992). There are no controlled outcome studies of the effectiveness of music for pain control with a pediatric population.

Distraction

Distraction is the focusing of the child's attention on stimuli other than the pain sensation. Almost any developmentally appropriate activity can qualify as distraction. Pop-up books, storytelling, or puppets provide distraction for younger children. Older children may count objects in the room, say the alphabet, practice breathing exercises, or even watch television. Distraction may increase pain tolerance by placing pain at the periphery of awareness, allowing the child to tune out painful stimuli for a given period of time. There is substantial clinical evidence that distraction is effective in alleviating subjective reports and behavioral evidence of pain (Ross & Ross, 1988).

Biofeedback

Biofeedback is a self-regulation strategy that can be used to control a target physiological parameter such as muscle tension, skin temperature, or electical activity of the brain. A patient can be provided with continuous feedback information about changes in a particular response system. Patients learn to recognize the relevant response system and then learn to produce changes in it by monitoring the signal frequency in a visual display unit. For children, signals are displayed in different ways. For example, a train travels faster as muscle tension increases and slows down when muscle tension decreases. When there is a physiologic change in the monitored parameter, such as decrease in muscle tension, there is also a psychological effect as patients grow in a sense of mastery and control over their pain.

Most research on the effectiveness of biofeedback has been done on adults; however, clinicians report that children are adept at regulating a number of target response systems. In one study, children as young as 3 years old were able to control their pain response (LaBaw & Holton, 1975).

THE FUTURE OF PEDIATRIC PAIN MANAGEMENT

Significant progress has been made in the development of valid, reliable tools for assessing pain in infants and children. Numerous safe and effective options for the treatment of pediatric pain currently exist. Despite these advances, children continue to experience unnecessary pain. An explanation for this inconsistency lies in the inadequate dissemination of knowledge regarding pain management in children (Gonzalez & Gadish, 1990; Schechter & Allen, 1986). It is clear that we are not consistently meeting the needs of children. When asked what was most helpful when undergoing a painful procedure, 99.2% of children reported that having a parent present helped the most (Ross & Ross, 1984). In spite of this information, parents continue to be asked to leave treatment rooms during painful procedures.

Our challenge is to work toward creating interventions to alleviate children's pain. We can reach this goal by continuing to educate those who work with children experiencing pain about the dimensions of pediatric pain, treatment options, the safety and efficacy of pharmacological pain management agents for children, and the availability of effective nonpharmacological techniques for managing pediatric pain. We can also conduct further research on the factors that contribute to the undertreatment of pediatric pain in order to create more effective interventions.

REFERENCES

Acute Pain Management Guideline Panel. (1992). *Acute pain management: Operative or medical procedures and trauma. Clinical practice guideline* (Publication No. 92-0032). Rockville, MD: Agency for Health Care Policy and Research, U.S. Department of Health and Human Services, Public Health Service.

Alex, M. R., & Ritchie, J. B. (1992). Schoolaged children's interpretation of their experience with acute surgical pain. *Journal of Pediatric Nursing, 7,* 171–180.

Anand, K. J. S. (1986). Hormonal and metabolic functions of neonates and infants undergoing surgery. *Current Opinion in Cardiology, 1,* 681.

Anand, K. J. S., Brown, M. J., Bloom, S. R., & Aynsley-Green, A. (1985). Studies on hormonal regulation of fuel metabolism in the human newborn infant undergoing anesthesia and surgery. *Hormonal Research, 22,* 115–128.

Anand, K. J. S., & Hickey, P. R. (1987). Pain and its effects on the human neonate and fetus. *New England Journal of Medicine, 317,* 1321–1329.

Aradine, C., Beyer, J., & Tompkins, J. (1988). Children's perceptions before and after analgesia: A study of instrument construct validity. *Journal of Pediatric Nursing, 3,* 15–23.

Benson, H. (1975). *The relaxation response.* New York: William Morrow.

Beyer, C. R., & Tompkins, J. M. (1988). Children's pain perception before and after analgesia: A study of instruments, construct validity and related issues. *Journal of Pediatric Nursing, 13,* 11–23.

Beyer, J. E., & Aradine, C. R. (1986). Patterns of pediatric intensity: A methodological investigation of a self-report scale. *Clinical Journal of of Pain, 3,* 130–141.

Beyer, J. E., Ashley, L. C., Russell, G. A., & DeGood, D. E. (1983). Patterns of postoperative analgesic use with adults and children following cardiac surgery. *Pain, 17,* 71–81.

Beyer, J. E., & Beyer, M. L. (1985). Knowledge of pediatric pain: The state of the art. *Children's Health Care, 13,* 150–157.

Beyer, J. E., & Bournaki, M. (1989). Assessment and management of postoperative pain in children. *Pediatrician, 16,* 30–38.

Bhatt-Mehta, V., & Rosen, D. A. (1991). Management of acute pain in children. *Clinical Pharmacology, 10,* 667–671.

Brewster, A. B. (1982). Chronically ill hospitalized children's concepts of their illness. *Pediatrics, 69*, 355–362.

Brody, H. (1982). The lie that heals: The ethics of giving placebos. *American Journal of Internal Medicine, 97*, 112–118.

Broome, M. E., Lillis, P. P., McGahee, T. W., & Bates, T. (1992). The use of distraction and imagery with children during painful procedure. *Oncology Nursing Forum, 19*, 499–502.

Broome, M. E., & Slack, J. F. (1990). Influences on nurse's management of pain in children. *Maternal Children Nursing, 1*, 159–162.

Burokas, L. (1985). Factors affecting nurses' decisions to medicate pediatric patients after surgery. *Heart Lung, 14*, 375–379.

Covelman, K. C., Scott, S., Buchanan, B., & Rosman, B. (1990). Pediatric pain control: A family systems model. *Advances in Pain Research Therapy, 16*, 225–236.

Curkovic, B., Vitulic, V., Babic-Naglic, D., & Durrigl, T. (1993). The influence of heat and cold on the pain threshold in rheumatoid arthritis. *Zeitschrift fur Rheumatologie, 52*, 289–291.

Denyes, M. J., Beyer, J. E., Villaruel, A. M., & Neuman, B. M. (1991). Issues in validation of culturally sensitive pain measures for young children (abstract). *Journal of Pain and Symptom Management, 6*, 174.

Dietz, F. R., Mathews, K. D., & Montgomery, W. J. (1990). Reflex sympathetic dystrophy in children. *Clinical Orthopaedics and Related Research, 258*, 225–231.

Dinarello, C. (1984). Interleukia 1. *Reviews of Infections Diseases, 6*(1), 51–95.

Donovan, M. I. (1992). A practical approach to pain assessment. In J. H. Watt-Watson & M. I. Donovan (Eds.), *Pain management: Nursing perspective* (pp. 59–78). St. Louis: Mosby.

Edgar, L., & Smith-Hanrahan, C. M. (1992). Nonpharmacological pain management. In Watt-Watson and M. I. Donovan (Eds.), *Pain management: A nursing perspective* (pp. 162–199). St. Louis: Mosby.

Egdahl, G. (1959). Pitituary-adrenal response following trauma to the isolated leg. *Surgery, 46*, 9–21.

Eland, J., & Anderson, J. (1977). The experience of pain in children. In Jacox, A. (Ed.), *Pain: A sourcebook for nurses and other professionals* (pp. 453–473). Boston: Little, Brown.

Eland, J. M. (1985). The role of the nurse in children's pain. In L. A. Copp (Ed.), *Recent advances in nursing: Vol. 11. Perspectives on pain*. Edinburgh: Churchill Livingstone.

Eland, J. M. (1990b). Pain in children. *Nursing Clinics of North America, 25*, 871–883.

Eland, L. (1991). The use of TENS with children who have cancer pain. *Journal of Pain and Symptom Management, 6*(3), 137–209.

Ellis, J. A., & Spanos, N. P. (1994). Cognitive-behavioral interventions for children's distress during bone marrow aspirations and lumbar punctures: A critical review. *Journal of Pain and Symptom Management, 9*, 96–108.

Fitzgerald, M., & Anand, K. J. S. (1993). Developmental neuroanatomy and neurophysiology of pain. In N. L. Schechter, C. B. Berde, & M. Yaster (Eds.), *Pain in infants and children* (pp. 11–31). Baltimore: Williams & Wilkins.

Fletcher, A. B. (1987). Pain in the neonate. *New England Journal of Medicine, 317*(21), 1347–1348.

Freud, A. (1952). The role of bodily illness in the mental life of children. In R. S. Eissler, H. Hartmann, A. Freud, & E. Kris (Eds.), *The Psychoanalytic study of the child* (Vol. VII, pp. 69–81). New York: International Universities Press.

Gaffney, A., & Duane, E. A. (1987). Children's understanding of the causality of pain. *Pain, 29*(1), 91–104.

Galer, B. S. (1995). Neuropathic pain of peripheral origin: Advances in pharmacologic treatment. *Neurology, 125* (Supp. 9), 517–525.

Gauntlett, I. S. (1987). Analgesic and anesthesia in newborn babies and infants. *Lancet, 1*, 1090.

Goats, G. C. (1994). Massage—the scientific basis of an ancient art: Part 2. Physiological and therapeutic effects. *British Journal of Sports Medicine, 28*, 153–156.

Gonsalves, S., & Mercer, J. (1993). Physiological correlates of painful stimulation in preterm infants. *The Clinical Journal of Pain, 9*, 88–93.

Gonzalez, J., & Gadish, H. (1990). Nurses' decisions in medicating children postoperatively. In D. C. Tyler & E. J. Krane (Eds.), *Advances in pain research therapy* (pp. 37–42). New York: Raven Press.

Goodwin, J., Goodwin, J., & Vogel, A. (1979). Knowledge and use of placebos by house officers and nurses. *Annals of Internal Medicine, 91,* 106–110.

Hester, N. O. (1979). The preoperational child's reaction to immunization. *Nursing Research, 28,* 250–255.

International Association for the Study of Pain. (1979). Pain terms: A list with definitions and notes on usage. *Pain, 6,* 249–252.

Jacox, A., Carr, D. B., Payne, R., et al. (1994). *Management of cancer pain. Clinical practice guideline no. 9 (AHCPR Publication No. 94-0592).* Rockville, MD: Agency for Health Care Policy and Research, U.S. Department of Health and Human Services, Public Health Service.

Johnston, C. C., Stevens, B., Craig, K. D., & Grunau, R. V. E. (1993). Developmental changes in pain expression in premature, full-term, two- and four-month old infants. *Pain, 52,* 201–208.

Jose, P. E. (1990). Just-world reasoning in children's immanent justice judgments. *Child Development, 61,* 1024–1033.

Kaada, B., & Berde, C. (1989). Increase of plasma b-endorphins in connective tissue massage. *General Pharmacology, 20,* 487–489.

Kaplan, M. (1988). Pain, the neonate and the neonatologist. *Journal of Perinatology, 8,* 354–355.

Kehlet, H. (1982). The endocrine-metabolic response to post-operative pain. *Acta Anaesthesiologica Scandinavia, 74,* 173–175.

LaBaw, W. C., & Holton, C. (1975). Use of self-hypnosis in children with cancer. *American Journal of Clinical Hypnosis, 17*(4), 233–238.

Larsson, B., & Melin, L. (1986). Chronic headaches in adolescents: Treatment in a school setting with relaxation training as compared with information-contact and self-registration. *Pain, 25,* 325–336.

Lynn, M. R. (1986). Pain in the pediatric patient: A review of research. *Journal of Pediatric Nursing, 1*(3), 198–201.

Magill-Levreault, L. (1993). Music therapy in pain and symptom managment. *Journal of Palliative Care, 9,* 42–48.

McBride, M. M. (1977). Can you tell me where it hurts? *Pediatric Nursing, 3*(4), 7–8.

McCaffery, M. (1979). *Nursing management of the patient with pain.* Philadelphia: J. B. Lippincott.

McCaffery, M., & Beebe, A. (1989). *Pain clinical manual for nursing practice.* St. Louis: C. V. Mosby.

McGrath, P. A. (1987). An assessment of children's pain: A review of behavioral, physiological and direct scaling techniques. *Pain, 31,* 147–176.

McGrath, P. J., & Craig, D. C. (1989). Developmental and psychological factors in children's pain. *Pediatric Clinics of North America, 36,* 823–836.

Mehta, M. (1986). Current views of noninvasive methods in pain relief. In M. Swerdlow (Ed.), *The therapy of pain* (3rd ed.) (pp. 115–131). Boston: MTP Press.

Mercadante, S., Lodi, F., Sapio, M., Calliagara, M., & Serretta, R. (1995). Long-term ketamine subcutaneous continuous infusion in neuropathic cancer pain. *Journal of Pain and Symptom Management, 10*(7), 564–568.

Messner, J. T., Loux, P. C., & Grossman, L. B. (1979). Intraoperative transcutaneous po2 monitoring in infants (abstract). *Anesthesiology, 51,* S319.

Miller, R. R., & Jick, H. (1970). Clinical effects of meperidine in hospitalized medical patients. *Journal of Clinical Pharmacology, 18,* 180.

Parton, D. A. (1976). Learning to imitate in infancy. *Developmental Psychology, 47,* 14–31.

Perrin, E. C., & Gerrity, P. S. (1981). There's a demon in your belly: Children's understanding of illness. *Pediatrics, 67,* 841–849.

Porter, F. (1989). Pain in the newborn. *Clinical Perinatology, 16,* 549–564.

Pothman, R. (1991). TENS for tension headaches in children. *Pain and Symptom Management*, *6*, 137–209.

Pothman, R., & Goepel, R. (1984). Acupuncture therapy of childhood migraine. In R. Rizzi & M. Visentin (Eds.), *Pain* (pp. 335–339). Padua, Italy: Piccin/Butterworths.

Rasco, C. (1992). Using music therapy as distraction during lumbar punctures. *Journal of Pediatric Oncology Nursing*, *9*, 33–34.

Rogers, A. (1989). Analgesics: The physician's partner in effective pain management. *Virginia Medical*, *116*, 164–170.

Ross, D. M., & Ross, S. A. (1984). Childhood pain: The schoolaged child's viewpoint. *Pain*, *20*, 179–191.

Savedra, M., Gibbons, P., Tesler, M., Ward, J., & Wegner, C. (1982). How do children describe pain? A tentative assessment. *Pain*, *14*, 95–104.

Schechter, N. L., & Allen, D. A. (1986). Physician's attitudes toward pain in children. *Developmental and Behavioral Pediatrics*, *7*, 350–354.

Schechter, N. L., Allen, D. A., & Hansen, M. A. (1986). Status of pediatric pain control: A comparison of hospital analgesic use in children and adults. *Pediatrics*, *77*, 11–15.

Seligman, M. E. P. (1975). *Helplessness: On depression, development, and death.* Freeman: San Francisco, CA.

Stroebel, C. F. (1982). *Qr, the quieting reflex.* New York: G. P. Putnam.

Swaford, L. I., & Allen, D. (1968). Pain relief in the pediatric patient. *Medical Clinics of North America*, *52*, 133.

Tesler, M. D. (1994). Children's pain: Part 1. *Nurseweek*, *7*, 10–11.

Tyler, D. (1992). Post-operative pain management in children. Part 1: History and pain measurement. *Hospital Physician, July*, 38–41.

Valente, A. M. (1991). Using hypnosis with children for pain management. *Oncology Nursing Forum*, *18*, 699–704.

Villaruel, A. M., & Denyes, M. J. (1991). Pain assessment in children: Theoretical and empirical validity. *Advances in Nursing Science*, *14*, 32–41.

Warga, C. (1985). Little swamis. *Psychology Today*, *19*, 16–17.

Watt-Watson, J. H., & Donovan, M. I. (Eds.). (1992). *Pain management: Nursing perspective.* St. Louis: C. V. Mosby.

Webb, C., Stergios, D. A., & Rodgers, B. M. (1989). Patient controlled analgesia as postoperative pain treatment in children. *Journal of Pediatric Nursing*, *4*, 162–171.

Weisenberg, M. (1987). Psychological intervention for the control of pain. *Behavioral Research and Therapeutics*, *25*, 301–312.

Wong, D., & Whaley, L. (1986). *Clinical handbook of pediatric nursing* (2nd ed.). St. Louis: C. V. Mosby.

Yaster, M. (1987). Analgesia and anesthesia in neonates. *British Journal of Pediatrics*, *111*, 394–396.

Yaster, M., & Deshpande, J. K. (1988). Management of pediatric pain with opioid analgesics. *Journal of Pediatrics*, *113*, 421–429.

Zeltzer, L. A., Barr, R. G., McGrath, P. A., & Schechter, N. (1992). Pediatric pain: Interacting behavioral and physical factors. *Pediatrics*, *90*, 816–821.

Zeltzer, L. K., Anderson, C., & Schechter, N. (1990). *Pediatric pain: Current status and new direction.* St. Louis: Mosby-Year Book.

CHAPTER 7

Healthy Adolescent Development
Risks and Opportunities

Nancy Leffert and Anne C. Petersen

INTRODUCTION

Adolescence is a time that is filled with opportunity, challenge, and risk. It is a time of opportunity because the child enters the period generally still possessing the "little girl" or "little boy" body and mind and leaves the second decade of life with a new body, many new skills, and the thinking and reasoning ability to use those new skills in sophisticated ways (Petersen & Leffert, 1995a). Along the way, the adolescent is confronted with many challenges, some of which are risky because they involve making decisions about behaviors that could endanger a healthy lifestyle in the future (Crockett & Petersen, 1993). In this chapter we will examine adolescence as a time of special health risk and opportunity. We will review the concept of adolescence as a developmental transition, critical aspects of development that may contribute to health risks, the domains of adolescent health risk, and opportunities for health promotion during adolescence.

NANCY LEFFERT • Search Institute, 700 South Third Street, Suite 210, Minneapolis, Minnesota 55415.   ANNE C. PETERSEN • Institute of Child Development, University of Minnesota, Minneapolis, Minnesota 55455.

Handbook of Diversity Issues in Health Psychology, edited by Pamela M. Kato and Traci Mann. Plenum Press, New York, 1996.

ADOLESCENCE: A DEVELOPMENTAL TRANSITION

Scholars describe adolescence as the second decade of life and divide it into three subphases: early adolescence (ages 10–14), middle adolescence (15–17), and late adolescence (18–20; e.g., Elliott & Feldman, 1990). Each subphase has its own distinct features. Early adolescence is dominated by puberty, which is also thought to be the time when the actual transition from childhood to adolescence is made. Middle adolescence is what we call to mind when we think of *adolescence* in that it involves an intense preoccupation with peers and the music and attire so often associated with young people. Late adolescence is yet another time of transition when the young person begins to take on the roles and responsibilities of adulthood (Crockett & Petersen, 1993).

The traditional view of adolescence is that it is a time of "storm and stress" (Hall, 1904), a time in which it is considered normative to experience conflicts and stresses in all areas of life (e.g., Blos, 1970; Freud, 1958). Research has clearly demonstrated that a stormy or stressful decade is not the case for *all* adolescents, but instead the experience of a minority of young people (e.g., Douvan & Adelson, 1966; Offer, Ostrov, & Howard, 1981; Rutter, 1980). Adolescence is indeed characterized by change and transition, and it is challenging, but it is not inevitably problematic (Petersen & Leffert, 1995a).

A developmental transition is generally characterized by significant change in biological or social domains of life or both (e.g., Emde & Harmon, 1984). Adolescence is considered a time of transition because of the major changes that take place in all domains of development (e.g., physical, cognitive) and in all social contexts (Petersen, 1988). During this period the young person not only develops physically and sexually to maturity but also continues to develop the skills necessary for adult roles and responsibilities. Adolescents are affected both by the development that has occurred during childhood as well as by the expectations they hold for the future (Lerner, 1987; Petersen, 1987). This is an important concept because it serves to remind us that prior development may affect the resources the young person brings to the period of adolescence. The adolescent is still quite childlike and only gradually develops the physical, cognitive, and social maturity requisite for adult functioning (Crockett & Petersen, 1993). Further, the opportunities and expectations of adulthood, or at least perceptions about these, can motivate or enervate adolescents to prepare for future work roles (Crockett & Petersen, 1993).

The challenge of change in all domains of development can be overwhelmingly stressful to some young people. For example, research has demonstrated that negative outcomes are linked to the experience of simultaneous changes during this period (Petersen, Sarigiani, & Kennedy, 1991; Simmons, Burgeson, Carton-Ford, & Blyth, 1987). This conclusion supports Coleman's (1978) focal theory that developmental tasks can be managed effectively if they occur sequentially, or at least without too many changes occurring at once. The experience of many changes occurring simultaneously is particularly likely to occur during early adolescence, and therefore early adolescence may be a time of particular risk (Petersen & Spiga, 1982).

Biological Development

The physical changes of puberty are dramatic and take place relatively rapidly with a great deal of individual variation in terms of their timing and the tempo (Eichorn, 1975; Petersen & Taylor, 1980; Tanner, 1972). Pubertal change takes place within an already existing endocrine system that was established prenatally but then suppressed until the beginning of puberty (Petersen & Taylor, 1980).

All adolescents experience puberty (except those individual with endocrine disorders that may prevent or interfere with normal puberty) Only the timing and tempo vary (Tanner, 1972). Figure 1 shows gender differences in the timing of pubertal development. Girls may begin puberty as early as 8 years of age and as late as 13½. Boys begin puberty approximately 1½ to 2 years later than girls, beginning as early as 9½ and as late as 13 years of age. The duration of puberty averages 4 years, although it ranges from 1½ to 6 years. During puberty the adolescent experiences genital development, breast development (in girls), pubic and axillary hair development, development of facial hair as well as voice deepening (in boys), changes in the oily secretions of the skin, and rapid gains in both height and weight (Tanner, 1962). Figure 1 shows the sequence of events at puberty, the age ranges of those events, and the gender differences in the timing of their occurrence.

Adolescents today in the United States, Western Europe, and Japan experience puberty earlier than adolescents did 100 years ago (Chumlea, 1982; Frisch, 1990). In addition to earlier puberty, adolescents today are taller, heavier, and appear more mature than their counterparts of previous generations (Chumlea, 1982). The age of menarche was between 15 and 17 years of age 100 years ago; today it averages between 12 and 14 years (Chumlea, 1982; Frisch, 1990; Tanner, 1962). This amounts to a change of approximately 3 to 4 months per decade (Wyshak & Frisch, 1982). Although the age of maturation is more difficult to discern in boys because of the lack of a discrete event that is easily measured, like the onset of menstruation, research indicates that voice deepening has decreased from 18 years of age to 13 or 14 years of age (Chumlea, 1982; Daw, 1970).

Perhaps more compelling than the actual decrease in age of maturation are the hypotheses thought to account for these changes. Researchers posit that this trend is linked with improvements in both prenatal and pediatric health care, nutrition, and living conditions (Chumlea, 1982). It

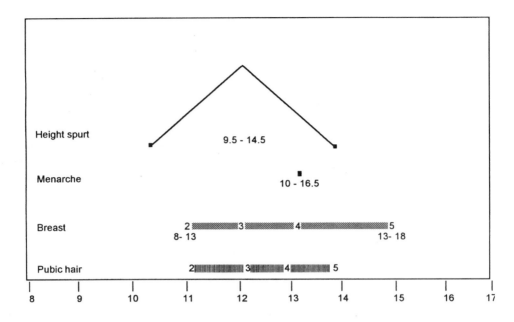

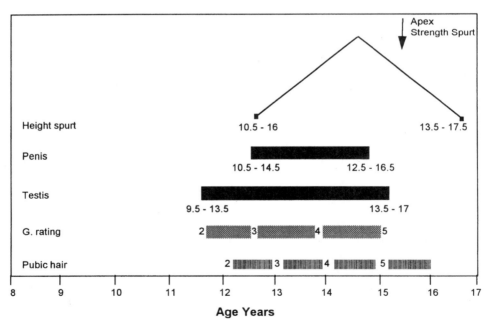

FIGURE 1. Schematic sequence of events at puberty. An average girl (upper) and boy (lower) are represented. The range of ages within which each event charted may begin and end is given by the figures placed directly below its start and finish. (Reproduced with permission by Tanner, 1962.)

has been suggested also, at least in the United States, that this trend has stabilized, as there has been maximum improvement in nutrition.

Cognitive Development

During adolescence the capacity to use formal logic (Inhelder & Piaget, 1958), think hypothetically, and use abstract reasoning all increase (Keating & Clark, 1980). In addition, adolescents become more capable of making decisions (Weithorn & Campbell, 1982), although the ability to make decisions is not always consistent and is affected by novel and stressful contexts. Because adolescents are more likely than older age groups to be in situations that are new to them, they are particularly vulnerable to thinking that is considerably less sophisticated than what they are capable of in situations that are more familiar or comfortable (Crockett & Petersen, 1993; Hamburg, 1986). Like adults, adolescents are susceptible to "hot cognitions" (Hamburg, 1986), thoughts that are emotionally laden and that may interfere with decision-making processes (e.g., Gilligan & Belenky, 1980). These hot cognitions perhaps lead to impulsive behavior that may contribute to the special health risks of adolescence. In these types of situations adolescents may respond impulsively without considering either the consequences of their actions or possible alternative decision options (Furby & Beyth-Marom, 1990). For example, adolescents may have difficulty in negotiating the complexity of social relationships as they pertain to sexuality. They may be overcome by their "feelings." The adult, on the other hand, is better able to make decisions because the novelty of the situation has "worn off" (Petersen & Leffert, 1995b).

Researchers report that by age 14, or by midadolescence, decision-making ability and reasoning is as good as that of adulthood and certainly involves the same flaws (Lewis, 1981; Weithorn & Campbell, 1982). Despite research evidence to the contrary, policies exist that limit adolescents' ability to make decisions and choices that are independent of parental involvement (Adler, 1994; Quadrel, Fischhoff, & Davis, 1993). For example, these policies have affected legislation regarding abortion options or receipt of contraceptive services.

Psychological Development

Self-image and self-esteem are constructs of adolescent psychological development that have been researched a great deal (cf., Harter, 1990). Overall self-esteem increases over the adolescent period (McCarthy & Hoge, 1982; O'Malley & Bachman, 1983), although the increase may follow a decline in self-esteem during early adolescence (Simmons & Rosenberg, 1975). This finding of a dip in self-esteem during early adolescence has not been replicated (Abramowitz, Petersen, & Schulenberg,

1984). Certain aspects of self-image (e.g., physical self-image) evidence different patterns of change (Abramowitz et al., 1984). In addition to the global assessments of self-esteem, researchers have often assessed self-esteem in specific domains, such as physical attractiveness, peer relationships or acceptance, academic competence, athletic competence, and behavior (e.g., Harter, 1990). Although global assessments of self-esteem are typically highly correlated among domains, developmental trends may vary for an individual across domains (e.g., Fend & Schrörer, 1985). This general positive trend contrasts sharply with the popular or media impression that adolescents are falling apart psychologically and with data that show evidence of increased rates of problem behaviors (e.g., Elliott, 1993). The fact that not all adolescents engage or participate in problem behaviors such as delinquency, drug and alcohol use, and precocious sexuality gives at least a partial explanation for the different trends seen in self-esteem (see Petersen & Leffert, 1995a, for more discussion of this issue).

In addition, and consistent with the overall increase in self-esteem, longitudinal studies have shown increasing capacity for autonomy during the course of adolescence (e.g., Steinberg & Silverberg, 1986). Conformity to parental opinion decreases steadily over the course of adolescence. Conformity to peers, however, peaks around age 13 or 14 years of age and then declines during the rest of adolescence (Berndt, 1979).

Psychosocial Development

Important changes occur in adolescence that pertain to psychosocial development. They are influenced by the changes in self-esteem and development of autonomy as well as other aspects of psychological development that affect the adolescent's relationships with both peers and parents.

Parent–Child Relationships

Traditionally, parent–child relationships during adolescence have been characterized as stormy at best. Psychoanalytic models (Blos, 1970; Freud, 1958) have characterized parent–child conflict during adolescence as being a necessary part of autonomy development and the process of individuation. In most cases, research has shown that individuation does not lead to detachment (Crockett & Petersen, 1993). In fact, closeness to parents continues into adulthood (Youniss & Smollar, 1985). However, adolescents report decreased closeness to parents over the adolescent decade (Petersen, Leffert, Miller, & Ding, 1993).

The view that parent-child relationships over the course of adolescence are basically positive does not mean that the relationships are conflict free. In fact, research has shown that conflict increases during early adolescence, an increase that is related to pubertal development

(Hill, Holmbeck, Marlow, Green, & Lynch, 1985; Steinberg, 1981). Conflict reaches a plateau during midadolescence and then declines (Montemayor, 1983). Conflicts that occur between most parents and their adolescent children center on mundane issues (e.g., clothing, clothes, hairstyles; Laursen & Collins, 1994); only approximately 15% of families report severe conflicts that are thought to be related to psychopathology (Montemayor, 1983; Rutter, Graham, Chadwick & Yule, 1976). Generally, these are families in which childhood psychopathology was evident.

Peer Relationships

Peer relationships also change during adolescence. Because adolescents have increased mobility, they move from small neighborhood groups of friends to large school-based groups (cf. Brown, 1990). The peer group not only becomes larger but also changes in complexity compared to the peer relations of children (e.g., Berndt, 1979; Crockett, Losoff, & Petersen, 1984). Adolescents also spend more time engaged in peer relationships.

Although it is popularly thought that peers hold a large degree of influence over adolescent opinions and behaviors, research suggests that peer groups do not dramatically influence values that are considered family based (e.g., religious, educational; Brown, Clasen, & Eicher, 1986). Peers do hold more influence over aspects of adolescent appearance and preferences associated with the teen "culture" (e.g., music). However, peer pressure to participate in problem behaviors often increases over adolescence although not as much as pressure in other areas (Brown, 1982; Brown, Lohr, & McClenahan, 1986). Some young people are more at risk of being influenced by negative peer pressure, particularly early-maturing girls and young people from disrupted families (Magnusson, 1987).

CRITICAL ASPECTS OF ADOLESCENT DEVELOPMENT THAT CONTRIBUTE TO HEALTH RISKS

In addition to the primary changes (e.g., biological, cognitive) that occur during adolescence, a number of other critical aspects of development may influence adolescent health. They generally represent the influence of context on development and provide evidence that simultaneous changes may be excessively challenging for the adolescent and thereby influence health outcomes.

Pubertal Timing

Because young people enter puberty at different times, they may have relatively different experiences when compared to the experiences of their peers. Research has demonstrated that the timing of puberty has impor-

tant influences on other aspects of adolescent development (Ruble &
Brooks-Gunn, 1982). For example, puberty has important effects on self-
esteem and boys tend to generally view puberty more positively than girls
do (e.g., Dorn, Crockett, & Petersen, 1988). Girls often view the changes in
their body shape as increases in fat rather than the development of breast
tissue and hips (Frisch, 1983). This may be related to the cultural ideals of
the slim prepubertal shape (e.g., Faust, 1983; Petersen, Kennedy, & Sullivan, 1991). For example, early maturing girls report more negative body
images (Petersen, Leffert, Graham, Ding, & Overbey, 1994) possibly because they are developing mature body shapes while their peers still have
prepubertal shapes (e.g., Magnusson, 1987; Petersen et al., 1991).

School Transitions

A great deal of evidence has accumulated that suggests that the
transition from elementary school to middle school or junior high can
have negative effects on certain groups of young people (Eccles & Midgley,
1989; Simmons & Blyth, 1987). In the United States this transition generally involves a change to a much larger and more anonymous school that
is farther from home than the neighborhood elementary school. The adolescent must interact with many more peers and teachers, most of whom
do not know the adolescent (Epstein & Karweit, 1983). This transition has
the potential to be challenging or stressful. Research by Eccles and Midgley (1989) has further demonstrated that these teachers are less supportive of autonomy and more demanding of compliant behavior than the
elementary school teachers despite the increased capacities of adolescents relative to children.

Research has demonstrated that academic performance drops with
every school transition (Blyth, Simmons, & Carlton-Ford, 1983) when
compared to the achievement of same-aged peers who are not making a
school transition. The effects are stronger with more transitions or with
other changes occurring at the same time or closely spaced temporally
(Crockett, Petersen, Graber, Schulenberg, & Ebata, 1989). There are also
negative effects on self-esteem, although only for girls (Simmons & Blyth,
1987) and not in all populations (Crockett, 1989; Fenzel & Blyth, 1986).

Parenting Style and Parental Supervision

Parenting style may also affect adolescent health risk. The *authoritative* parenting style as defined by Maccoby and Martin (1983) is one that
combines warmth and control. During adolescence these parents support and encourage the adolescent's bids for increasing autonomy with a
parallel increase in responsibility (Baumrind, 1971). On the other hand,
authoritarian parents are strict disciplinarians, who provide little warmth
or support for autonomy.

Authoritative parenting style is associated with better school performance and psychosocial maturity during adolescence (Steinberg, Elman, & Mounts, 1989) and less substance abuse (Baumrind, 1991). There is some evidence that the effects of authoritative parenting style may be different for African-American families (Steinberg, 1992). Steinberg and colleagues (Steinberg, Dornbusch, & Brown, 1992; Steinberg, Lamborn, Dornbusch, & Darling, 1992) suggest that African-American youth are especially influenced by peers and that this influence may dilute the positive effects of authoritative parenting practices on school work seen in other groups.

One of the hallmarks of adolescent development is the decrease in parental supervision. A shift in responsibility occurs gradually from parents to their sons and daughters, sharing jurisdiction over adolescent activities and responsibilities until entirely borne by the adolescent, usually when the adolescent leaves home (Maccoby, 1984). Adolescents spend progressively more time in the company of their peers with little or no supervision, or a different kind of supervision than typically existed during childhood. This increased autonomy is appropriate, and yet it provides increased exposure to experimentation in health-compromising behaviors (Crockett & Petersen, 1993). For most adolescents, there is probably little risk of involvement in these behaviors as a result of increased autonomy and less supervision. However, certain youth are more likely to socialize with peers who are participating in problem behaviors or deviant peers, all the while increasing their exposure to avenues for misconduct (Crockett & Petersen, 1993; Patterson & Strouthamer-Loeber, 1984).

DOMAINS OF ADOLESCENT HEALTH

Concepts of disease and health have changed over the past decade (Millstein, Petersen, & Nightingale, 1993). Of particular interest here is the notion that adolescents are vulnerable to health-compromising lifestyles (Elliott, 1993). Problem behaviors are the major cause of adolescent illness, accidents, and death (National Center for Health Statistics, 1980). Health trajectories may also be affected by the presence of a chronic illness. The course or complications of an illness may be affected by the normal aspects of adolescent development whether the child developed a chronic illness either before or during adolescence.

Violence and Safety

You cannot pick up a newspaper or news magazine today that does not contain at least one article pertaining to adolescent violence or the safety risks that exist for young people in our schools. Recent evidence suggests a more risky developmental context facing youth today (e.g., Petersen, 1991). Although death as a result of diseases such as cancer or heart disease has declined dramatically over the past 40 years, accidents, homicides, and suicides among adolescents have increased as a cause of mortality during those same 40 years (Petersen, 1991).

As can be seen in Table 1, the United States exceeds the developed countries in deaths among youth between 10 and 14 years of age; only Australia has a slightly higher death rate than the United States for males between 15 and 19 years of age and Canada a slightly higher rate for females between 10 and 14 years of age (Hingson & Howland, 1993). Adolescents in the United States are four to five times more likely to die of a homicide than those young people in other countries. In addition, in recent years these rates have been increasing (Center for the Study of Social Policy, 1991).

This degree of mortality among American youth that is so disparate compared to adolescents in other countries must be examined in relation to increasingly harmful developmental contexts that young people today face. For example, automobile accidents cause approximately three-fourths of the accidental deaths among youth in the United States. Driving at younger ages (usually 15 or 16 years of age) and the availability of firearms accounts, at least in part, for the excessive mortality of youth in the United States (Petersen, 1991). These rates are also higher than those in other countries (Hingson & Howland, 1993; Petersen, 1991). Firearms and drowning result in the rest of accidental death among youths, especially among boys (Gans, Blyth, Elster, & Gaveras, 1990; Hechinger, 1992).

Alcohol in general has a profound effect on adolescent health and specifically accidents and mortality (Tonkin, 1987). The change in the minimum age for purchasing alcohol and the fact that young people are

TABLE 1. Death Rates* for Teenages in Selected Industrialized Nations, 1985

Country	10–14 years		15–19 years	
	Male	Female	Male	Female
United States	18.4	7.8	64.1	23.6
Federal Republic of Germany	9.2	4.5	48.4	15.1
France	13.0	5.9	49.9	18.7
Netherlands	7.2	4.8	27.6	9.0
England and Wales	13.9	5.6	35.6	9.9
Sweden	7.0	4.1	35.0	9.9
Canada	16.6	8.3	55.7	21.1
Japan	6.0	2.1	42.5	7.1
Australia	13.1	5.0	67.1	21.3

*Death rates/100,000.
Source: Reprinted from Hingson & Howland, 1993, by permission.

tempted to drink and drive also accounts for the higher rates of mortality among American young people, compared to youth in other countries with driving being the primary differentiating factor (Petersen, Richmond, and Leffert, 1993).

We do not do a very good job at protecting our youth or keeping them safe (Petersen, Richmond, & Leffert, 1993). Although we sometimes assume, as mentioned above, that adolescents are impulsive and irrational, the strikingly different death rates from one country to another suggest that the variation cannot be primarily attributed to being adolescent.

Sexuality

Rates of adolescent sexual activity rose dramatically during the 1960s and 1970s. Clear links have been demonstrated between the increasing hormonal levels of pubertal development and beginning sexual activity (Katchadourian, 1990; Udry, 1979). Cross-national comparisons suggest that the initiation into sexual activity is quite similar across countries (see Figure 2). There are slight variations in age at initiation and rate of increase from country to country (Department of International Economic and Social Affairs, 1988; Petersen, 1991). Steady increases occur as adolescents get older (Department of International Economic and Social Affairs, 1988), with approximately one-half of all adolescents having had intercourse by the age of 18 (Jones et al., 1986).

Along with these increases have been high rates of nonmarital adolescent childbearing and sexually transmitted diseases (STDs). The United States has the highest teen pregnancy rate of the industrialized nations (Jones et al., 1986). In the 14 years between 1973 and 1987, the pregnancy rate for young adolescents increased 23% (Hechinger, 1992). In 1989 more than two-thirds of all births to teen mothers occurred outside of marriage (compared with 30% in 1970), and 87% of the births to teen mothers from 1985 to 1989 were not planned. Recent research suggests that although rates of sexual activity and childbearing has reached a plateau among older adolescents, rates for younger adolescents have continued to increase. Rates are higher for blacks than whites, although whites have been catching up (Petersen, Richmond, et al., 1993).

Many adolescents in the United States do not use birth control of any kind or delay their use (Zelnik & Kantner, 1980). This is particularly true of early adolescents. For example, Hofferth and Hayes (1987) found that 42% of adolescent girls under the age of 15 delay the use of contraception by more than 12 months after having intercourse for the first time. Only 35% of 15 to 17 year olds and 15% of 18 to 19 year olds delay contraceptive use (Gans et al., 1990).

Cross-national comparisons reveal that young people outside of the United States use contraception more frequently (Jones et al., 1986). This is perhaps a result of the availability of medical/family planning services

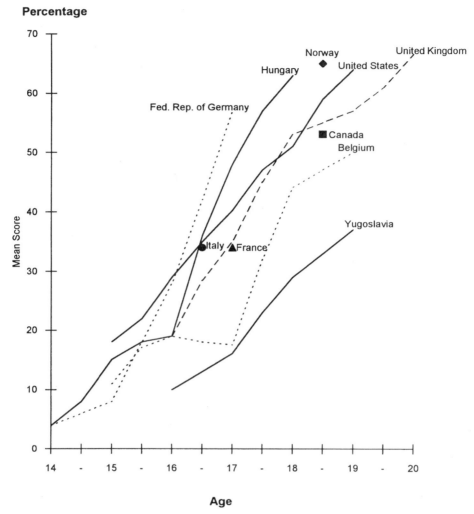

FIGURE 2. Proportion of teenagers who ever had sex, by age, for selected countries. Source: Department of International Economic and Social Affairs, 1988)

to young people in most other countries (Petersen, 1991) either through school-based clinics or because access does not require parental approval. There are other reasons that some adolescents may fail to use contraception. Some adolescents have inaccurate or inadequate information about human sexuality and conception as well as disease processes that can then interfere with their decision making about contraceptive use (e.g., Adler, 1994). Elkind (1984) has suggested that the sense of invulnverability typical of adolescence may also contribute to the lack of contraception as well as adolescent's participation in other problem behaviors. In addition, as mentioned above, emotionally laden situations may compromise decision-making abilities.

The same decision-making and reasoning process affects adolescents' protection against STDs. Gonorrhea is the most common STD among adolescents (Gans et al., 1990). Although easily treated with antibiotics, gonorrhea and the other bacterial STDs can permanently damage the reproductive system if they are left untreated. The most serious STD, acquired immune deficiency (AIDS) is rapidly increasing in the adolescent population (Gans et al., 1990). Although fewer than 1% of people with AIDS are adolescents, members of that age group are at considerable risk in contracting human immunodeficiency virus (HIV) because they tend to have multiple sexual partners and unprotected sex. Between 1987 and 1989, 20% of all AIDS-related deaths were among young people in their 20s, suggesting that they contracted the disease while in adolescence (Gans et al., 1990; Hechinger, 1992; Hein & DiGeronimo, 1989).

Substance Use

Substance use is another domain of adolescent health risk where adolescent decision making plays a role. Forty-five percent of high school seniors in the Untied States have used an illegal substance including marijuana (Johnston, O'Malley, & Bachman, 1993). This rate is the highest among the industrialized nations. Adolescents perhaps use substances, including alcohol, to handle stress. There is also evidence that some youths self-medicate with alcohol or illicit substances in order to stave off a depressive or psychotic episode.

Like sex, drug use has particularly increased among younger adolescents (Johnston et al., 1987; Petersen, Richmond, et al., 1993). For example, in 1990, rates of lifetime use between 12 and 17 year olds were 23% for illicit drugs, 48% for alcohol, and 40% for cigarettes. Heavy drinking in adolescence is especially associated with other problems (Kazdin, 1986).

Chronic Illness and Disability

Cognitive, emotional, and behavioral aspects of individual development during adolescence may affect the course of a chronic illness. For example, in addition to the normative areas of transition during adolescence, the adolescent with Type I or insulin dependent diabetes mellitus (IDDM) must adhere to a treatment regimen. This includes the maintenance of insulin levels, proper diet, regular mealtimes, and adequate exercise (Hanson et al., 1989; White, 1991). However, the adolescent's day-to-day life includes changes in routines established during childhood in both school and home contexts, and the inclusion of longer school days because of involvement in sports or other extracurricular activities. These changes in routine are not necessarily favorable for glycemic control (Leffert, Susman, & Collins, 1993). Perhaps as a way of asserting autonomous decision making relative to parents, adolescents with IDDM are frequently noncompliant with their treatment and dietary regimens (Hamp, 1984). Treatment noncompliance affects the maintenance of diabetic control (White, 1991) and also increases the likelihood of diabetic complications earlier in life because of additional stress put on the circulatory and endocrine systems.

Studies comparing children with diabetes and those without have revealed few psychological differences (Simonds, 1977). However, within group differences have shown more psychological symptoms (e.g., anxiety, depression, behavioral problems) in children with poor metabolic control compared to those children with good metabolic control. One source of these differences may be the compilation or "pile up" of life stresses as the child moves into adolescence. For example, Hanson, Henggeler, Harris, and Moore (1989) report that stress and adherence to the therapeutic regimen are directly associated with metabolic control.

Individual development during the course of adolescence may also be affected by the presence of disability. For example, maturation may be further complicated within the parameters of a chronic illness or disability (Blum, 1988). Pubertal maturation may be delayed or precocious, which may serve to further the isolation of the young person already set apart because of the use of a wheelchair or braces (Blum, 1988).

Psychosocial development may be affected as well. For example, Blum, Resnick, Nelson, and St. Germaine (1991) report that adolescents with spina bifida and cerebral palsy have restricted social lives in terms of best friends or dating. In addition, these young people report close relationships with their parents in which parent–adolescent conflict is absent. Blum et al. (1991) suggest that this perceived harmony in actuality reflects parental overprotectiveness and infantilization, which may serve to ultimately delay normal adolescent development.

Mental Health

Traditional views have portrayed adolescence as a time of storm and stress (Hall, 1904) in which it was considered normal to be moody and preoccupied, and even to be "depressed." Although this may still be the stereotype of adolescence that is reflected by the media, research has not supported this view (Petersen, 1988). The traditional viewpoint is in sharp contrast with research evidence that the majority of adolescents experience no significant psychological difficulties, continue to have close relationships with their families and peers, and develop a healthy sense of themselves by the time they reach adulthood (Petersen, Compas, et al., 1993). These data (e.g., Rutter et al., 1976; Weiner & DelGaudio, 1976) have shown that depression is not a "normal" state of adolescence (Petersen, Compas, et al., 1993) and that adolescents do not "grow out of" psychological disturbances (Petersen, 1993). In fact, studies have shown that the young people that do experience psychological disturbance during adolescence are likely to go on, if left untreated, to have serious psychiatric difficulty in adulthood (e.g., Achenbach, Howell, McConaughy, & Stanger, 1995; Rutter et al., 1976; Weiner & DelGaudio, 1976).

Adolescents may be sufficiently stressed or challenged so that their coping resources are overwhelmed, resulting in various expressions of mental health problems (Klerman, 1993). Although the majority of young people do not experience serious psychological difficulties, there is indeed an increase in the incidence of psychological disorders during adolescence (Rutter et al., 1976). For example, rates of clinical depression or depressive affect increase during adolescence, especially among girls (Achenbach, Howell, Quay, & Conners, 1991; Petersen, Compas, et al., 1993).

THE EFFECTS OF CONTEXT ON PROBLEM BEHAVIORS

Researchers have begun to examine the effects of social contexts on problem behaviors and adolescent development. Social conditions such as poverty may have negative effects on development, behavior (Klerman, 1993), and ultimately health trajectories. For example, Elliott (1993) suggested that lower- and middle-income youth do not differ in the age of initiation of problem behaviors. However, differences emerge in the persistence of these behaviors. Middle-income youth tend to discontinue these behaviors after experimentation with them, and lower-income youth continue them. The continuation of these behaviors may have consequences in terms of the overall health of the adolescent or the trajectory of adult outcomes. Elliott (1993) suggested that lower-income youth lack future life opportunities and consequently engage in high-risk behaviors such as violence, drugs, and precocious or unprotected sex during adolescence.

Research has shown that the problem behaviors that cause health risks during adolescence tend to covary or cluster into a problem behavior lifestyle (Elliott, 1993) or syndrome (Jessor, 1991). Two explanations have been proposed for the covariation of problem behaviors: (1) young people who participate in problem behaviors have a tendency toward deviancy (Donovan & Jessor, 1985; Jessor & Jessor, 1977), and (2) problem behaviors may be causally linked. (For example, an individual may steal in order to support the use of illicit drugs.) Elliott (1993) suggested that both of these factors contribute to the covariation of problem behaviors or the development of problematic lifestyles.

Researchers have suggested that these behaviors are related to the development of problem behavior lifestyles only if they covary during early adolescence. Initiation in late adolescence does not put young people at risk for developing problematic lifestyles (Elliott, 1993). In general, the community or context in which adolescents live provides opportunities to engage in behaviors that may be a risk to health (Crockett & Petersen, 1993). Local peer norms may provide "messages" to young people regarding the realm of appropriate or acceptable behaviors. For example, Brooks-Gunn, Duncan, Klebanov, and Sealand (1993) demonstrated that the prevalence of single-mother households in a neighborhood with few middle-class neighbors affected the rates of school dropout and teenage childbearing. In a community-level analysis, Blyth and Leffert (1995) found that youth with few personal assets benefit (as measured by having fewer risk behaviors) from living in healthy communities. In addition, in accordance with the findings of Elliott (1993), Blyth and Leffert (1995) found that young people living in less healthy communities (as defined by the aggregate number of problem behaviors engaged in by the youth in the community) had more problem behaviors, which began at earlier grade levels and which continued into late adolescence.

PROMOTING ADOLESCENT HEALTH

Adolescence is a transitional time in the life course, one in which there are many opportunities for increased growth. However, the study of early adolescence has demonstrated that negative outcomes are often responses to changes and challenges that accompany the adolescent decade (Petersen, 1993). The many changes that occur during adolescence have important implications for both health risks and health promotion (Crockett & Petersen, 1993). The changes increase the potential exposure to new health risks such as alcohol use and sexual activity.

The occurrence of simultaneous changes in multiple domains may tax the coping capacities of young people and increase the likelihood of participation in health-compromising behaviors (Crockett & Petersen, 1993). For example, Simmons and Blyth (1987) found a linear relationship between added changes (e.g., pubertal change, family changes, school transition) and poorer psychosocial outcomes such as lower self-esteem, more problem behaviors, decrements in achievement or grades. In addition, change during early adolescence has been linked to the emergence of depression in middle adolescence (Petersen, Sarigiani, et al., 1991).

The changes that occur during adolescence may conversely provide opportunities for health promotion. Educators, clinicians, parents, and policy makers may find it useful to capitalize on aspects of development that are ideally suited to either interventions or education. For example, adolescents are interested in all that is happening to them (e.g., Petersen

& Leffert, 1995b) and their new level of cognitive and emotional maturity may be used to facilitate the development of healthy lifestyles (Crockett & Petersen, 1993).

Adolescents' concerns about their physical development and attractiveness may provide the impetus for education regarding a number of health-related topics (Crockett & Petersen, 1993), such as puberty, sexuality, nutrition, exercise, and safe methods of weight control (Carnegie Council on Adolescent Development, 1989). Instructional methods are enhanced because adolescents are better able to comprehend health risks than children are (Crockett & Petersen, 1993). They are also able to think about their behavior and consider its consequences (e.g., Adler, 1994).

Health-promotion efforts need to take into account the developmental differences in reasoning that may be present during the course of adolescence (Crockett & Petersen, 1993). Younger adolescents require more concrete approaches in education whereas older adolescents can take advantage of abstract approaches. Decision-making skills may need to be taught, particularly to younger adolescents (Crockett & Petersen, 1993). Effective decision making and the ability to consider alternative choices (Adler, 1994; Keating, 1990) can be taught to adolescents as young as age 12 (Mann, Harmoni, Power, Beswick, & Ormond, 1988)

Educators interested in health promotion need to take into account the behavior of interest (e.g., substance use, sexuality) and change techniques accordingly. For example, behaviors that are not emotionally laden can be handled on an abstract level. However, "hot" issues may need to include experiential components such as role playing (Crockett & Petersen, 1993). Role playing can help adolescents deal more effectively with novel situations, which are often those situations that involve the greatest risk of participation in problem behaviors. Practice in decision making may also help to improve the adolescent's performance in making alternative choices.

The psychosocial changes that occur during adolescence can also provide avenues for health promotion. For example, providing adolescents with role models in the form of mentorships or apprenticeships will support positive interests and abilities, provide guidance, and challenge young people to seek new options (Crockett & Petersen, 1993; Hamilton & Darling, 1989).

Healthy self-esteem is an important component of positive outcomes in later adolescence and adulthood. Self-esteem is improved when there are opportunities for young people to experience success. It is important to provide areas to perform competently outside of the traditional route of academics, which will serve to engage those young people who are weak in academics but may have other strengths (Crockett & Petersen, 1993; Harter, 1990). Educational opportunities that provide improvement in life skills (Hamburg, 1989) or community service (Scales, 1990) may help to improve adolescent self-esteem. Promoting positive self-esteem and providing role-playing opportunities and practice in decision making may also help young people resist negative peer influence or decrease susceptibility to antisocial influences (Crockett & Petersen, 1993).

The above are but a few examples of how adolescent development may be used to capitalize on both health promotion and interventions targeted to the adolescent decade. Adolescence is a transitional developmental period that is generally positive and full of opportunity. However, adolescence also involves risk. The goal of adolescent health education should be to not only promote positive growth during adolescence but also to help young people avoid problem behaviors or health risks that may compromise their future health and development (Crockett & Petersen, 1993; Perry & Jessor, 1985).

In addition, evidence is accumulating that suggests that interventions should be targeted no later than early adolescence. For example, Elliott (1993) found that rates of alcohol use and sexual involvement become normative by ages 15 and 17, respectively. If the goal of the intervention is to delay onset of problem behaviors, the intervention must take place much earlier. Interventions may require repeated exposure or "boosters" (Petersen, 1993).

This chapter suggests that health-promotion efforts are best served if they consider developmental strengths and competencies. Promotion and interventions should be targeted not only to the cognitive developmental level of adolescents but also should focus on the challenges and concerns that are relevant to this age group. Many promising models of intervention now exist, and researchers are gaining more information on what works (e.g., Bandura, 1988, 1994). Health-promotion efforts that are targeted specifically toward a basic-skills approach to problem solving and managing interpersonal relationships during adolescence are essential (Bandura, 1994; Hamburg, 1989; Petersen, 1993; Price, Cioci, Penner, & Trautlein, 1990) and may ultimately be better suited to generalizing to the adolescent's environment than behavior-specific interventions.

ACKNOWLEDGMENTS

The authors wish to express their thanks to Beverly Nazarian, M.D., for her assistance in the preparation of the chapter.

REFERENCES

Abramowitz, R. H., Petersen, A. C., & Schulenberg, J. E. (1984). Changes in self-image during early adolescence. In D. Offer, E. Ostrov, & K. Howard (Eds.), *Patterns of adolescent self-image* (pp. 19–28). San Francisco: Jossey-Bass.
Achenbach, T. M., Howell C. T., McConaughy, S. H. & Stanger, C. (1995). Six-year predictors

of problems in a national sample of children and youth: I. Cross-informant syndromes. *Journal of the American Academy of Child and Adolescent Psychiatry, 34*(3), 336–347.

Achenbach, T. M., Howell, C. T., Quay, H. C., & Conners, C. K. (1991). National survey of problems and competencies among four-to-sixteen-year-olds. *Monographs of the Society for Research in Child Development, 56.*

Adler, N. (1994). *Adolescent sexual behavior looks irrational—but looks are deceiving.* Washington, DC: Federation of Behavioral, Psychological, and Cognitive Sciences.

Bandura, A. (1988). Self-regulation of motivatin and action through goal ystems. In V. Hamilton, G. H. Bower, & N. H. Frijda (Eds.), *Cognitive perspectives on emotion and motivation* (pp. 37–61). Dordrecht, The Netherlands: Kluwer Academic Publishers.

Bandura, A. (1994). *Self-efficacy: The exercise of control.* New York: Freeman.

Baumrind, D. (1971). Current patterns of parental authority. *Developmental Psychology Monographs, 1,* 1–103.

Baumrind, D. (1991). The influence of parenting style on adolescent competence and substance use. *Journal of Early Adolescence, 11,* 56–95.

Berndt, T. (1979). Developmental changes in conformity to peers and parents. *Developmental Psychology, 15,* 608–616.

Blos, P. (1970). *The adolescent passage.* New York: International Universities Press.

Blum, R. W. (1988). Developing with disabilities: The early adolescent experience. In M. D. Levine & E. R. McAnarney (Eds.), *Early adolescent transitions* (pp. 177–192). Lexington, MA: Lexington Books.

Blum, R. W., Resnick, M. D., Nelson, R., & St. Germaine, A. (1991). Family and peer relationships among adolescents with spina bifida and cerebral palsy. *Pediatrics, 88*(2), 280–285.

Blyth, D. A., & Leffert, N. (1995). Communities as contexts for adolescent development: An empirical analysis. *Journal of Adolescent Research, 100*(1), 64–87.

Blyth, D. A., Simmons, R. G., & Carlton-Ford, S. (1983). The adjustment of early adolescent to school transitions. *Journal of Early Adolescence, 3,* 104–120.

Brooks-Gunn, J., Duncan, G. J., Klebanov, P., & Sealand, N. (1993). Do neighborhoods influence child and adolescent development? *American Journal of Sociology, 99,* 353–395.

Brown, B. B. (1982). The extent and effects of peer pressure among high school students: A retrospective analysis. *Journal of Youth and Adolescence, 11,* 121–133.

Brown, B. B. (1990). Peer groups and peer cultures. In S. S. Feldman & G. R. Elliott (Eds.), *At the threshold: The developing adolescent* (pp. 171–196). Cambridge, MA: Harvard University Press.

Brown, B. B., Clasen, D., & Eicher, S. (1986). Perception of peer pressure, peer conformity, dispositions, and self-reported behavior among adolescents. *Developmental Psychology, 22,* 521–530.

Brown, B. B., Lohr, M. J., & McClenahan, E. L. (1986). Early adolescents perceptions of peer pressure. *Journal of Early Adolescence, 6,* 139–154.

Carnegie Council on Adolescent Development. (1989). *Turning points: Preparing American youth for the 21st century.* Washington, DC: Carnegie Corporation.

Center for the Study of Social Policy. (1991). *Kids count data book: State profiles of child well-being.* Greenwich, CT: Annie E. Casey Foundation.

Chumlea, W. C. (1982). Physical growth in adolescence. In B. B. Wolman, G. Stricker, S. J. Ellman, P. Keith-Spiegel, & D. S. Palermo (Eds.), *Handbooks of developmental psychology* (pp. 471–485). Englewood Cliffs, NJ: Prentice-Hall.

Coleman, J. (1978). Current contradictions in adolescent theory. *Journal of Youth and Adolescence, 7,* 1–11.

Crockett, L. J., Losoff, M., & Petersen, A. C. (1984). Perceptions of the peer group and friendship in early adolescence. *Journal of Early Adolescence, 4,* 155–181.

Crockett, L. J., Petersen, A. C. (1993). Adolescent development: Health risks and opportunities for health promotion. In S. G. Millstein, A. C. Petersen, & E. O. Nightingale

(Eds.), *Promoting the health of adolescents: New directions for the twenty-first century* (pp. 13–37). New York: Oxford University Press.

Crockett, L. J., & Petersen, A. C., Graber, J. A., Schulenberg, J. E., & Ebata, A. (1989). School transitions and adjustment during early adolescence. *Journal of Early Adolescence, 8*, 405–419.

Daw, S. F. (1970). Age of boys' puberty in Leipzig 1727–49 as indicated by voice breaking J.S. Bach's choir members. *Human Biology, 42*, 87–89.

Department of International Economic and Social Affairs (1988). *Adolescent reproductive behavior: Evidence from developed countries* (Population Studies No. 109). New York: United Nations.

Donovan, J., & Jessor, R. (1985). Structure of problem behavior in adolescence and young adulthood. *Journal of Consulting and Clinical Psychology, 53*, 890–904.

Dorn, L. D., Crockett, L. J., & Petersen, A. C. (1988). The relations of pubertal status to intrapersonal changes in young adolescents. *Journal of Early Adolescence, 8*, 405–419.

Douvan E., & Adelson, J. (1966). *The adolescent experience.* New York: Wiley.

Eccles, J. S., & Midgley, C. (1989). Stage/environment fit: Developmentally appropriate classrooms for early adolescents. In R. E. Ames & C. Ames (Eds.), *Research on motivation in education* (Vol. 3). New York: Academic Press.

Eichorn, D. H. (1975). Asynchronization in adolescent development. In S. E. Dragastin & G. H. Elder, Jr. (Eds.), *Adolescence in the life cycle: Psychological change and social context.* (pp. 81–96). Washington, DC: Hemisphere.

Elliott, D. S. (1993). Health enhancing and health compromising lifestyles. In S. G. Millstein, A. C. Petersen, & E. O. Nightingale (Eds.), *Promoting the health of adolescents: New directions for the twenty-first century* (pp. 119–145). New York: Oxford University Press.

Elliott, G. R., & Feldman, S. S. (1990). Capturing the adolescent experience. In S. S. Feldman & G. R. Elliott (Eds.), *At the threshold: The developing adolescent* (pp. 1–14). Cambridge, MA: Harvard University Press.

Elkind, D. (1984). Teenage thinking: Implications for health care. *Pediatric Nursing,* Nov./ Dec., 383–385.

Emde, R. N., & Harmon, R. J. (Eds.). (1984). *Continuities and discontinuities in development.* New York: Plenum Press.

Epstein, J. L., & Karweit, N. L. (Eds.). (1983). *Friends in school.* New York: Academic Press.

Faust, M. S. (1983). Alternative constructions of adolescent growth. In J. Brooks-Gunn & A. C. Petersen (Eds.), Girls at puberty: Biological and psychosocial perspectives (pp. 105 –125). New York: Plenum Press.

Fend, H., & Schrörer, S. (1985). The formation of self-concepts in the context of educational systems. *International Journal of Behavioral Development, 8*, 423–444.

Fenzel, L. M., & Blyth, D. A. (1986). Individual adjustment to school transitions: An exploration of the role of supportive peer relations. *Journal of Early Adolescence, 6*, 315–329.

Freud, A. (1958). Adolescence. *Psychoanalytic study of the child, 13*, 255–278.

Frisch, R. (1983). Fatness, puberty, and fertility: The effect of nutrition and physical training on menarche and ovulation. In Brooks-Gunn & A. C. Petersen (Eds.), *Girls at puberty: Biological and psychosocial perspectives* (pp. 29–49). New York: Plenum Press.

Frisch, R. (1990). The right weight: Body fat, menarche, and ovulation. *Ballière's Clinical Obstetrics and Gynaecology, 4*, 695–701.

Furby, L., & Beyth-Marom, R. (1990). *Risk-taking in adolescence: A decision-making perspective.* Washington, DC: Carnegie Council on Adolescent Development, Carnegie Corporation of New York.

Gans, J. E., Blyth, D. A., Elster, A. B., & Gaveras, L. L. (1990). *America's adolescents: How healthy are they? Vol. 1. Profiles of adolescent health series.* Chicago: American Medical Association.

Gilligan, G., & Belenky, M. F. (1980). A naturalistic study of abortion decisions. In R. Selman & R. Yando (Eds.), *Clinical-developmental psychology* (Vol. 7, pp. 69–90). San Francisco, CA: Jossey Bass.

Hall, G. S. (1904). *Adolescence: Its psychology and its relations to physiology, anthropology, sociology, sex, crime, religion, and education.* New York: Appleton.

Hamburg, B. (1986). Subsets of adolescent mothers: Developmental, biomedical, and psychosocial issues. In B. Lancaster & B. A. Hamburg (Eds.), *School-age pregnancy and parenthood: Biosocial dimensions* (pp. 115–145). New York: Aldine de Gruyter.

Hamburg, B. (1989). *Life skills training: Preventive interventions for early adolescents.* Washington, DC: Carnegie Council on Adolescent Development.

Hamilton, S. F., & Darling, N. (1989). Mentors in adolescents' lives. In K. Hurrelmann & U. Engel (Eds.), *The social world of adolescents: International perspectives* (pp. 121–139). Berlin: Walter de Gruyter.

Hamp, M. (1984). The diabetic teenager. In R. W. Blum (Ed.), *Chronic illness and disabilities in childhood and adolescence* (pp. 217–238). Orlando, FL: Grune & Stratton.

Hanson, C. L., Harris, M. A., Relyla, G., Cigrang, J. A., Carle, D. L., & Burghen, G. A. (1989). Coping styles in youth with insulin dependent diabetes mellitus. *Journal of Consulting and Clinical Psychology, 57,* 644–651.

Hanson, C. L., Henggeler, S. W., Harris, M. A., Burghen, G. A., & Moore, M. (1989). Family system variables and the health status of adolescents with insulin dependent diabetes mellitus. *Health Psychology, 8,* 239–253.

Harter, S. (1990). Self and identity development. In S.S. Feldman & G. R. Elliott (Eds.), *At the threshold: The developing adolescent* (pp. 352–387). Cambridge, MA: Harvard Univerity Press.

Hechinger, F. M. (1992). *Fateful choices: Healthy youth for the 21th century.* New York: Carnegie Corporation of New York.

Hein, K., & DiGeronimo, T. F. (1989). *AIDS: Trading fears for facts. A guide for young people.* Mount Vernon, NY: Consumers Union.

Hill, J., Holmbeck, G., Marlow, L., Green, T., & Lynch, M. (1985). Menarcheal status and parent-child relations in families of seventh-grade girls. *Journal of Youth and Adolescence, 14,* 301–316.

Hingson, R., & Howland, J. (1993). Promoting safety in adolescents. In S. G. Millstein, A. C. Petersen, & E. O. Nightingale (Eds.), *Promoting the health of adolescents: New directions for the twenty-first century* (pp. 305–327). New York: Oxford University Press.

Hofferth, S. L., & Hayes, C. D. (Eds.). (1987). *Risking the future: Adolescent sexuality, pregnancy, and childbearing* (Vol. 2). Washington, DC: National Research Council, National Academy Press.

Inhelder, B., & Piaget, J. (1958). *The growth of logical thinking from childhood to adolescence.* New York: Basic Books.

Jessor, R. (1991). Risk behavior in adolescence: A psychosocial framework for understanding and action. *Journal of Adolescent Health, 12,* 597–605.

Jessor, R., & Jessor, S. (1977). *Problem behavior and psychosocial development: A longitudinal study of youth.* New York: Academic Press.

Johnston, L. D., O'Malley, P. M., & Bachman, J. G. (1987). *National trends in drug use and related factors among American high school students and young adults.* Rockville, MD: National Institute on Drug Abuse.

Johnston, L. D., O'Malley, P. M., & Bachman, J. G. (1993). *Monitoring the future: Questionnaire responses from the nations' high school seniors, 1991.* Ann Arbor, MI: Institute for Social Research, University of Michigan.

Jones, E. F., Forrest, J. D., Goldman, N., Henshaw, S., Lincoln, R., Rosoff, J. I., Westoff, C. F., & Wulf, D. (1986). *Teenage pregnancy in industrialized countries: A study sponsored by the Alan Guttmacher Institute.* New Haven, CT: Yale University Press.

Katchadourian, H. (1990). Sexuality. In S. S. Feldman & G. R. Elliott (Eds.), *At the threshold: The developing adolescent* (pp. 330–351). Cambridge, MA: Harvard University Press.

Kazdin, A. (1986). *Conduct disorders in childhood and adolescence.* Newbury Park, CA: Sage.

Keating, D. P. (1990). Adolescent thinking. In S. S. Feldman & G. R. Elliott (Eds.), *At the threshold: The developing adolescent* (pp. 54–89). Cambridge, MA: Harvard University Press.

Keating, D. P., & Clark, L. V. (1980). Development of physical and social reasoning in adolescence. *Developmental Psychology, 16*, 23–30.

Klerman, L. V. (1993). The influence of economic factors on health-related behaviors in adolescents. In S. G. Millstein, A. C. Petersen, & E. O. Nightingale (Eds.) *Promoting the health of adolescents: New directions for the twenty-first century* (pp. 38–57). New York: Oxford University Press.

Laursen, B., & Collins, W. A. (1994). Interpersonal conflict during adolescence. *Psychological Bulletin, 155*, 197–209.

Leffert, N., Susman, A., & Collins, W. A. (1993). Developmental transitions in parent-adolescent relationships in families with an adolescent with chronic illness. In G. N. Holmbeck (Chair), *Family relationships and psychosocial development in physically impaired and chronically ill children.* Symposium at the biennial meetings of the Society for Research on Child Development, New Orleans, LA.

Lerner, R. M. (1987). A life-span perspective for early adolescence. In R. M. Lerner & T. T. Foch (Eds.), *Biological-psychosocial interactions in early adolescence* (pp. 9–34). Hillsdale, NJ: Erlbaum.

Lewis, C. (1981). How adolescents approach decisions: Changes over grades seven to twelve and policy implications. *Child Development, 52*, 538–544.

Maccoby, E. E. (1984). Middle childhood in the context of the family. In W. A. Collins (Ed.), *Development during middle childhood: The years from six to twelve* (pp. 184–239). Washington, DC: National Academy of Sciences Press.

Maccoby, E. E., & Martin, J. (1983). Socialization in the context of the family: Parent-child interaction. In E. M. Hetherington (Ed.), *Handbook of child psychology: Vol. 4. Socialization, personality, and social development* (pp. 103–196). New York: Wiley.

Magnusson, D. (1987). *Individual development in an interactional perspective: Vol. 1. Paths through life.* Hillsdale, NJ: Erlbaum.

Mann, L., Harmoni, R., Power, C., Beswick, G., & Ormond, C. (1988). Effectiveness of the GOFOR course in decision-making for high school students. *Journal of Behavioral Decision-Making, 1*, 159–168.

McCarthy, J. D., & Hoge, D. R. (1982). Analysis of age effects in longitudinal studies of adolescent self-esteem. *Developmental Psychology, 18*, 372–379.

Millstein, S. G., Petersen, A. C., & Nightingale, E. O. (Eds.). (1993). *Promoting the health of adolescents: New directions for the twenty-first century.* New York: Oxford University Press.

Montemayor, R. (1983). Parents and adolescents in conflict: All families some of the time and some families most of the time. *Journal of Early Adolescence, 3*, 83–103.

National Center for Health Statistics (1980). *Vital Statistics, 86*, 10.

Offer, D., Ostrov, E., & Howard, K. I. (1981). *The adolescent: A psychological self-portrait.* New York: Basic Books.

O'Malley, P. M., & Bachman, J. G. (1983). Self-esteem: Change and stability between ages 13 and 23. *Developmental Psychology, 19*, 257–268.

Patterson, G. R., & Strouthamer-Loeber, M. (1984). The correlation of family management practices and delinquency. *Child Development, 55*, 1299–1307.

Perry, C. L., & Jessor, R. (1985). The concept of health promotion and the prevention of adolescent drug abuse. *Health Education Quarterly, 12*, 169–184.

Petersen, A. C. (1987). The nature of biological-psychosocial interactions. In M. Levine & E. McAnarney (Eds.), *Adolescent transitions* (pp. 123–137). Lexington, MA: Heath.

Petersen, A. C. (1988). Adolescent development. *Annual Review of Psychology, 39*, 583–607.

Petersen, A. C. (1991). *Adolescence in America: Effects on girls.* The 1991 Gisela Konopka Lecture, University of Minnesota, Minneapolis, MN.

Petersen, A. C. (1993). Presidential address: Creating adolescents: The role of context and process in developmental trajectories. *Journal of Adolescent Research, 3*(1), 1–18.

Petersen, A. C., Compas, B., Brooks-Gunn, J., Stemmler, M., Ey, S., & Grant, K. (1993). Depression in adolescence. In R. Takanishi (Ed.), *American Psychologist, 48*(2), 155–168.

Petersen, A. C., Kennedy, R. E., & Sullivan, P. (1991). Coping with adolescence. In M. E. Colten & S. Gore (Eds.), *Adolescent stress: Causes and consequences* (pp. 93–110). Hawthorne, NY: Aldine de Gruyter.

Petersen, A. C., & Leffert, N. (1995a). What is special about adolescence? In M. Rutter (Ed.), *Psychosocial disturbances in young people: Challenges for prevention* (pp. 3–36). London: Cambridge University Press.

Petersen, A. C., & Leffert, N. (1995b). Developmental issues influencing guidelines for adolescent health research. *Journal of Adolescent Health, 17,* 298–305.

Petersen, A. C., Leffert, N., Graham, B., Ding, S., & Overbey, T. (1994). Depression and body image disorders in adolescence. *Women's Health Issues, 4*(2), 98–108.

Petersen, A. C., Leffert, N., Miller, K., & Ding, S. (1993). The role of community and intrapersonal coping resources in the development of depressed affect and depression in adolescence. In *Depression in childhood and adolescence: Developmental issues.* A symposium presentation at the biennial meetings of the Society for Research in Child Development, New Orleans, LA.

Petersen, A. C., & Spiga, R. (1982). Adolescence and stress. In L. Goldberger & S. Breznitz (Eds.), *Handbooks of stress: Theoretical and clinical aspects* (pp. 515–528). New York: Free Press.

Petersen, A. C., & Taylor, B. (1980). The biological approach to adolescence: Biological change and psychosocial adaptation. In J. Adelson (Ed.), *Handbook of adolescent psychology* (pp. 117–155). New York: Wiley.

Petersen, A. C., Sarigiani, P. A., & Kennedy, R. E. (1991). Adolescent depression: Why more girls? *Journal of Youth and Adolescence, 20,* 247–271.

Petersen, A. C., Richmond, J. B., & Leffert, N. (1993). Social changes among youth: The United States experience. *Journal of Adolescent Health, 14,* 632–637.

Price, R. H., Cioci, M., Penner, W., & Trautlein, B. (1990). *School and community support programs that enhance adolescent health and education.* Report prepared for the Carnegie Council on Adolescent Development, Washington, DC.

Quadrel, M. J., Fischhoff, B., & Davis, W. (1993). Adolescent (in)vulnerability. *American Psychologist, 48*(2), 102–116.

Ruble, D. N., & Brooks-Gunn, J. (1982). The experience of menarche. *Child Development, 53,* 1557–1666.

Rutter, M. (1980). *Changing youth in a changing society: Patterns of adolescent development and disorder.* Cambridge, MA: Harvard University Press.

Rutter, M., Graham, P., Chadwick, O., & Yule, W. (1976). Adolescent turmoil: Fact or fiction. *Journal of Child Psychology and Psychiatry, 17,* 35–56.

Scales, P. (1990). Developing capable young people: An alternative strategy for prevention programs. *Journal of Early Adolescence, 10,*420–438.

Simmons, R. G., & Blyth, D. A. (1987). *Moving into adolescence: The impact of pubertal change and school context.* Hawthorne, NY: Aldine.

Simmons, R. G., Burgeson, R., Carlton-Ford, S., & Blyth, D. A. (1987). The impact of cumulative change in earl adolescence. *Child Development, 58,* 1220 –1234.

Simmons, R. G., & Rosenberg, E. (1975). Sex, sex roles, and self-image. *Journal of Youth and Adolescence, 4,* 229–258.

Simonds, J. F. (1977). Psychiatric status of diabetic youth matched with a control group. *Diabetes, 26,* 921–925.

Steinberg, L. (1981). Transformation in family relations at puberty. *Developmental Psychology, 17,* 833–838.

Steinberg, L. (1992). Discussant's comments. In R.K. Silbereisen (Chair), *Psychosocial antecedents of the timing of puberty.* Symposium conducted at the biennial meeting of the Society for Research on Adolescence, Washington, DC.

Steinberg, L., Dornbusch, S., & Brown, B. B. (1992). Ethnic differences in adolescent achievement: An ecological perspective. *American Psychologist, 47,* 723–729.

Steinberg, L., Elman, J. D., & Mounts, N. S. (1989). Authoritative parenting, psychosocial maturity, and academic success among adolescents. *Child Development, 60,* 1424–1436.

Steinberg, L., Lamborn, S. D., Dornbusch, S. M., & Darling, N. (1992). Impact of parenting practices on adolescent achievement: Authoritative parenting, school involvement, and encouragement to succeed. *Child Development, 63,* 1266–1281.

Steinberg, L., & Silverberg, S. (1986). The vicissitudes of autonomy in early adolescence. *Child Development, 57,* 841–851.

Tanner, (1962). *Growth at adolescence.* Springfield, IL: Thomas.

Tanner, J. M. (1972). Sequence, tempo, and individual variation in growth and development of boys and girls aged twelve to sixteen. In J. Kagan & R. Coles (Eds.), *Twelve to sixteen: Early adolescence* (pp. 1–24). New York: Norton.

Tonkin, R. S. (1987). Adolescent risk-taking behavior. *Journal of Adolescent Health Care, 8,* 213–220.

Udry, J. R. (1979). Age at menarche, at first intercourse, and at first pregnancy. *Journal of Biological Science II,* 411–433.

Weiner, I. B., & DelGaudio, A. (1976). Psychopathology in adolescence. *Archives of General Psychiatry, 34,* 98–11.

Weithorn, L. A. & Campbell, S. B. (1982). The competency of children and adolescents to make informed treatment decisions. *Child Development, 53,* 1589–1598.

White, N. R. (1991). Diabetes. In R. M. Lerner, A. C. Petersen, & J. Brooks-Gunn (Ed.), *Encyclopedia of adolescence* (Vol. 1, pp. 232–236). New York: Garland Publishing.

Wyshak, G., & Frisch, R. E. (1982). Evidence for a secular trend in age of menarche. *New England Journal of Medicine, 306,* 1033–1035.

Youniss, J., & Smollar, J. (1985). *Adolescents' relations with mothers, fathers, and friends.* Chicago: University of Chicago Press.

Zelnik, M. & Kantner, J. (1980). Sexual activity, contraceptive use, and pregnancy among metropolitan area teenagers. 1971–1979. *Family Planning Perspectives, 12,* 233–237.

CHAPTER 8

Reversing Disability in Old Age

Becca Levy and Ellen Langer

INTRODUCTION

In his autobiographical novel, *House of God*, medical resident Samuel Shem (1978) described the tendency of physicians in his hospital to call the old patients "gomers." The term *gomer* (or "gome" for short), Shem explains, serves as an acronym for "Get Out of My Emergency Room." The phrase implies than old patients will be annoying and that their health will inevitably decline with a variety of age-related complications. Although Shem wrote his novel in 1978, some hospital house staff still refer to people over the age of 60 as gomes. The doctors who use the term *gome* would defend themselves by pointing out that the term is said tongue in cheek and that they would never use the term in the hearing vicinity of an old patient. We will argue in this paper, however, that the use of the term represents a kind of thinking and behavior that has negative consequences for the health of old people.

Many American health care professionals classify conditions that often have an onset in old age (e.g., osteoporosis) as an inevitable part of the aging process, even though these conditions can be treated or reversed (Manton, 1992; Rowe & Kahn, 1987). Wilkes and Shuchman (1989)

BECCA LEVY • Division on Aging, Harvard Medical School, Boston, Massachusetts 02115.   ELLEN LANGER • Department of Psychology, Harvard University, Cambridge, Massachusetts 02138.

Handbook of Diversity Issues in Health Psychology, edited by Pamela M. Kato and Traci Mann. Plenum Press, New York, 1996.

and Foreman (1994) found that when it comes to old patients many American doctors prefer not to give routine screening tests, such as mammograms, or provide treatments considered standard for younger patients. This form of health rationing does not occur because of the impossibility of treating illnesses in the old. Instead, physicians tend to underestimate the number of years patients are likely to live and assume that if the older patients live much longer, other aspects of their lives, such as cognition, will decline to the point where the illness will not make a difference (Wilkes & Shuchman, 1989). Similarly, mental health professionals tend to feel that the same illnesses they treat in younger clients, such as depression and anxiety, are natural and permanent in their older clients, even though many psychiatric illnesses in old age are treatable (Moses, 1992; Rodeheaver & Datan, 1988).

Where do these assumptions of permanent and inevitable disability in old age come from? It is true that some aspects of some people decline in old age, but people tend to overestimate the correlation between age and disability (Ryan, 1992). The tendency to link old age with physical and mental decline comes in part from the fact that few medical schools and clinical psychology graduate schools require their students to study geriatric medicine or health psychology of old age (Rodeheaver & Data, 1988). But even if health care students read journal articles on aging, they might not become any more enlightened than people who ignore this literature. Many of those who have been writing about gerontology continue to interpret old age as a time of inevitable decline despite the growing number of studies that contradict this long-standing view.

In this chapter we will show that some of the disabilities assumed to occur with natural biological aging never occur among many old people. In the first part, we will explain the disabilities of old age from a social psychological perspective. In the second part, we will examine some of the current research methods that may distort the trends of aging. We will then summarize the research that suggests that many disabilities do not inevitably occur and, when they do occur, frequently can be reversed.

Health psychology of old age has become increasingly important over the last century in large part because of the changes in the major causes of mortality (Taylor, 1986). Before this century, most people died of acute illnesses or diseases with a sudden onset that usually lasted less than 6 months, such as the plague or scarlet fever. Over the last few decades, the advances in health care and medicine have led to preventions and treatments for many of the acute illnesses that ended people's lives in their early adulthood. These advances have led to more elderly living today than ever before. Since the turn of the century, the average life span has almost doubled and the percentage of elders in the population has tripled (United States Bureau of the Census, 1975, 1993). Today most people die of chronic diseases, or illnesses with a slow onset that usually last more than 6 months, such as heart disease and cancer, and often first occur in late adulthood.

Researchers have found an association between some of the chronic illnesses that are particularly prevalent among the aged and social psychological factors. For example, Fawzy (1994) found that he could significantly lower the recurrence and mortality rates of people suffering from skin cancer with a group therapy intervention. In the next section we will explore some of the social psychological mechanisms that contribute to disability in old age. By isolating some of these social psychological factors, researchers and clinicians will be better able to design interventions that prevent or reverse disability by targeting the social psychological dynamics behind disability rather than just the biological symptoms.

DISABILITY MAY NOT BE INEVITABLE: SOCIAL PSYCHOLOGICAL MECHANISMS

Actor–Observer Divergence

Part of the tendency to think of old people as incompetent and disabled comes from the actor–observer divergence. Jones and Nisbett (1971) first coined the term *actor–observer divergence* to refer to the difference in attributional thinking between an actor, who directly experiences an event, and an observer, who watches an event. Actors tend to attribute the causes of events that happen to them to their environments (e.g., I fell because of the large crack in the sidewalk.). Observers, on the other hand, tend to attribute the causes of others' experiences to features internal to the actors (e.g., He fell because he is a clumsy.). Most clinicians and researchers, who frequently are younger than their old patients or subjects, tend to take the observer's perspective and ignore the perspective of the old person (or actor) who may experience events differently. Thus a young psychiatrist may attribute the cause of an old woman's problem, such as depression, to an internal feature, such as a chemical imbalance, rather than an environmental factor, such as her husband just died and she recently broke her hip.

An example of the actor–observer divergence influencing the health of old people is found in the different ways people judge the speeding up of older people's sense of time. Although some elders suffer from insomnia, most elders who complain of sleep disorders experience shifts in circadian rhythms to an earlier cycle. This causes many elders to fall asleep and get up earlier than most young adults (Czeisler et al., 1992). Thus the total number of hours elderly people sleep often does not change, but the particular hours during which they sleep shift. Although it is not yet known why these time changes occur, no harm has been discovered in connection with these changes. Many clinicians and researchers, however, assume that the inevitable decline that accompanies aging causes this developmental change. Some elders also attribute this shift to their progressive deterioration. Other elders take a more adaptive view and blame the environment for their early morning discomfort: if only the rest of the population could get up earlier and open stores, athletic clubs, and libraries earlier, they might feel more in sync with their surroundings.

Rather than letting their old patients know that getting up earlier and feeling time go by faster than when they were young does not necessarily indicate decline, doctors often try to "cure" these changes by prescribing sleeping pills. The elderly are the people to whom sleeping pills are most often prescribed (Foreman, 1993). Although the pills tend to help people sleep later in the short run, they often become harmful in the long run because they can become addictive; in addition, they do not address the change in the internal biological clock. Researchers at Brigham and Women's Hospital in Boston are trying to replace sleeping pills with an alternative treatment of light therapy that should reset the internal biological clock (Czeisler et al., 1986). These researchers and many of the physicians who prescribe sleeping pills have ignored the possibility that early risers can use this extra time in the mornings to their advantage. For example, in China elders frequently meet in parks at 5 a.m. to practice Tai Chi.

Another example of young observers misinterpreting old people's experiences can be seen in the tendency of many young people to attribute old people's inactivity following their retirement to a biological wearing down, rather than a natural response to unchallenging environments and schedules. Problems may arise when people act on the biological interpretation. The young observer who believes that with old age comes a loss of energy and initiative may feel that the older members of society should be placed in routinized environments where they will not become overstimulated or tired out. Several studies suggest that placing elders in environments with little stimulation and not giving them ample control over their daily lives may be harmful (Avorn & Langer, 1982; Langer & Rodin, 1976; Rodin & Langer, 1977).

In their nursing home intervention study, Langer and Rodin (1976) demonstrated that old people may suffer when others make all the decisions for them. The researchers divided the residents of a nursing home into an experimental and a comparison group and encouraged the experimental group members to take more control of their lives by making choices for themselves. For example, the residents decided when and if they wanted to see a movie and where to receive visitors. The experimenters told the comparison group that the staff would take care of everything for them, including the same decisions that their peers in the experimental group made for themselves. Three weeks after the intervention, judges blind to the participants' research groups rated the members of the experimental condition as more active, alert, and happy. Eighteen months later, Rodin and Langer (1977) found that the intervention that required subjects to do more, not less, seemed to increase the length of subjects' lives. Members of the experimental group were half as likely to have died in the intervening months than members of the comparison group.

Despite the dramatic results from the nursing home study, many people still feel it is important to infantalize and minimize stimuli for old adults. For example, a large percentage of Americans think it is important to serve elders bland, easy-to-digest food. Although some elders with specific medical problems need this, most do not. Smell and taste sensitivity tend to decrease in old age (de Graaf, Polet, & Van Staveren, 1994). Thus it would seem more logical to serve elders particularly flavorful meals rather than bland food. Moreover, given that we cannot live forever, perhaps the informed choice of diet should be that of the older patient, regardless of medical condition.

In addition to serving bland foods, the staffs of hospitals and nursing homes often use a condescending tone when communicating with old clients. They frequently avoid sharing personal information, ask them obvious and potentially embarrassing questions, such as, Did you make number one this morning? and adopt a baby talk or "eldertalk" style, which involves simplified speech, a slower rate, and animated tone. Caporael (1981) "content filtered" the tapes of nursing home staff speaking to old residents. When she played the tapes to judges, they assumed that 22% of the taped samples were nursery school workers addressing young children.

The anthropologist Bethel (1992) found the same phenomenon when she studied a Japanese nursing home. Japanese elders probably have a higher status than American elders in relation to younger members of these societies. Politeness theory therefore predicts that Japanese elders should use lower forms of politeness when talking to caregivers, whereas American elders should use higher forms of politeness to address caregivers (Brown & Levinson, 1987). Bethel (1992) noticed that a nursing home staffwoman used the suffix *chan*, normally used for children, when speaking to the old residents. In Japan, however, the old residents returned the use of this suffix when they addressed the staffwoman. We imagine that many institutionalized elders in the United States would not dare to return this condescending tone to their caretakers.

Langer, Rodin, Beck, Wienman, and Spitzer (1979) examined how the lack of self-disclosure of nursing home staff influences elders. In a study of ambulatory nursing home residents, they found that interviewers who used reciprocal self-disclosure were much more effective in cognitively stimulating elders than interviewers who asked questions without offering any personal information. Over the 6-week intervention, residents in the high-reciprocal group showed significantly more improvement on several tests of recall than did the low-self-disclosure group members, who did not differ significantly from a control group that was not visited by the interviewers at all. It would be interesting to see if similar results emerge with an intervention involving varying tone of voice or level of condescension in asking questions. Future research should also address how much eldertalk occurs in noninstitutionalized interactions involving old people (such as in grocery stores, banks, and families) as well as the health implications of this speech style.

Negative Stereotypes of Old Age

Our thoughts and behaviors toward old people are often not willful or conscious, but rather are outcomes of cultural stereotypes about old age. In a meta-analysis of studies about views toward old people, Kite and Johnson (1988) found that even though many ideas about old people exist, most views are negative. Perdue and Gurtman (1990) found that these negative views exist below awareness. They flashed the word *old* or the word *young* on a computer screen at a speed below conscious perception. They found that when they primed their subjects with the word *old*, subjects judged negative words more quickly, and when they primed their subjects with the word *young*, subjects judged positive words more quickly. The authors concluded that the word *old* is more strongly linked to negative beliefs than positive beliefs.

These stereotypes about the inevitable decline of elders probably originate in *premature cognitive commitments*. Chanowitz and Langer (1981) define premature cognitive commitments as rigid beliefs that an individual accepts often after a single exposure. This belief then forms the basis for how subsequent information is assimilated without the individual considering alternative forms the information can take. This unconditional acceptance of information occurs frequently with ideas that initially do not seem relevant to one's life, such as information about aging encountered in childhood. A child may hear about a crippled, senile, old person and allow this image to become the foundation for everything learned about old age (Langer, 1989). Research suggests that childhood exposure to the negative images of old age presented in fairy tales, television, and everyday conversations can influence one's level of activity and alertness in old age (Langer, Perlmuter, Chanowitz, & Rubin, 1988; Rodin & Langer, 1980). Isaacs and Bearison (1986) found that children develop negative stereotypes about old age at around 6 years of age, the same age that they develop negative stereotypes about race and sex.

Langer and Abelson (1974) demonstrated that labels, such as *gome*, can dramatically change how individuals perceive others. They showed the identical video of an interview to two groups of psychotherapists. The researchers told one group that the person interviewed was a job applicant and told the other group that the person interviewed was a patient. These labels changed how subjects perceived the person in the video.

Those in the first group described the interviewee as well-adjusted, whereas those in the second group described the interviewee as maladjusted.

These labels of stereotypes of old age influence how people treat elders and how elders think about themselves. If elders are given the label of helpless, they tend to think of themselves as helpless. This internalized sense of dependency also leads elders to dismiss medical problems as part of the general disabling of aging, even when the problems are environmentally determined, reversible, or both (Ryan, 1992). Avorn and Langer (1982) found that when experimenters encouraged dependency by giving direct assistance, old participants performed worse than when the experimenters verbally encouraged them or left them alone. Showing how stereotypes can be internalized, Langer and Benevento (1978) gave a group of subjects easy arithmetic problems. Then they randomly assigned the subjects to a group of either "assistants" or "bosses" and gave them difficult math problems. Afterwards, when they gave everybody easy problems again, those in the assistant group performed half as well as they had in the first phase of the study.

Unfortunately, nobody has yet discovered how to eliminate or prevent the formation of negative stereotypes of old age. Positive intergenerational contact between old and young individuals, however, seems to reduce the negative stereotypes of the young toward the old (Palmore, 1988). Langer et al. (1988) found that old individuals who grew up with a grandparent function better in old age than a matched set of individuals who did not have the early contact with an elderly person.

The Psychoimmunological Link

An important mediator of the influence of social psychological factors on health appears to be the immune system. Researchers in the growing field of psychoneuroimmunology have documented many important findings related to aging. Adler and Mathews (1994) found that the association between psychological factors and immune competence appears to increase in old age. Rodin (1987) reported that elders may be particularly vulnerable to variables related to control and stress. She gave several reasons for this correlation, including the tendency of the people around elders to assist them with tasks that they formerly performed independently and the loss of friends, family members, and professional relationships that helped make the elders feel competent.

Recent reviews of research in psychoneuroimmunology have found that psychological stress decreases immune competence, whereas feelings of belonging and the presence of support networks increase immune competence (Baron, Cutrona, Hicklin, Russel, & Lubaroff, 1990; Kennedy, Keicolt-Glaser, & Glaser, 1990). Immunologists most often assess immune competency as increased proliferation of lymphocytes (a type of white blood cell) in response to mitogens (foreign matter) or as the ability of natural killer cells to destroy tumors. For example, Bartrop, Luckhurst, Lazarus, Kiloh, and Penny (1977) found that bereaved spouses experienced a lower lymphocyte response to mitogenic stimuli than do control subjects matched by age, sex, and race. In addition, Keicolt-Glaser, Dura, and Speicher (1991) found that Alzheimer's disease caregivers who have good social networks tend to have better immune functioning than those caregivers with poor social networks.

Several studies have found that people who use more negative explanatory styles or who are more likely to consider negative events as internally caused, stable in time, and global in effect (e.g., I lost my keys because I am losing my memory and can't recall anything anymore) tend to report more cases of infectious diseases and experience worse physical health as measured by a physician examination (Peterson & Seligman, 1987; Peterson, Seligman, & Valliant, 1988). Kamen-Siegal, Rodin, Seligman, and Dwyer (1991) studied the relationship between explanatory styles for negative events and immunocompetence in elders. They found that those elders with more pessimistic explanatory styles exhibited lowered immunocompetence. This finding is worrisome because in the United States older people are more likely than younger people to attribute negative events, such as memory failure, to internal and stable causes (Lachman & MacArthur, 1986).

Even though it is possible that lowered immunocompetence causes a pessimistic explanatory style, it seems more likely that sociocultural processes, such as the internalization of negative stereotypes about aging, encourage a pessimistic style among the old that may lead to a lowered immunocompetence. If this reduction in immunocompetence in turn leads to an increase in uncontrollable illnesses among the old, the elevated illness might lead to an even more pessimistic style. Elders need to break out of this cycle by realizing that negative events are not inevitable and not due to the internal, stable, and global nature of the physical and mental decline of old age. They need to realize that most negative events also have a cause that is external, unstable, and specific. For example, when an 85-year-old woman can't find her keys, it could be because her son put a newspaper on top of them rather than because she has started sliding down the slippery slope of memory loss.

RESEARCH METHODS EXAGGERATE DISABILITY

Previous research in health psychology, medicine, and gerontology has supported the tendency to equate becoming old with becoming disabled. Five factors contribute to research results exaggerating, and in some cases creating, the decline. Researchers tend to (1) assume that trends among Americans are universal; (2) assume that all elders are equivalent; (3) rely on cross-sectional rather than longitudinal studies; (4) select research methods that favor younger participants; and (5) avoid studying the most healthy and wealthy old. Scholars of health and aging should keep these tendencies in mind when designing and analyzing studies, and lay people should keep these tendencies in mind when considering the implication of these studies.

Tendency to Assume American Trends Universal

In their review of the literature on the influence of culture on cognition, emotion, and motivation, Markus and Kitayama (1991) point out that many psychological concepts that people assume are universal do not extend beyond the Western subjects studied by Western researchers. Manton (1992) found the same overgeneralizations by Western gerontology researchers about the aging processes of other cultures. He writes that over time many processes and states "associated with human aging and senescence have been redefined, after being better biologically characterized, as 'pathological' because they do not fulfill the critical characteristic of universality" (p. 194). Many changes that have been interpreted as age intrinsic, such as increases in body weight, blood pressure, and serum cholesterol, are now seen as usual in prosperous industrial countries, but not in pastoral and traditional agricultural societies (Rowe & Kahn, 1987). Rossi (1992) found in her cross-cultural research that Western clinicians' assumptions about intense menopausal symptoms may not hold true in other cultures. She found that in societies in which women acquire religious, social, or political power in their postmenopausal years, the women don't dread aging and experience minimal menopausal symptoms.

This tendency to overgeneralize the results of studies of American aged to other cultures applies to cognition as well. For example, we recently found that in cultures that attach more positive labels to the old than in mainstream America, the memory decline, which many Americans take for granted in old age, is lessened (Levy & Langer, 1994). In our cross-cultural study of memory performance and attitudes toward aging we selected two cultures, mainland China and the American deaf community, because research suggests that these cultures hold their old members in high esteem and may be cut off from some of mainstream America's negative stereotypes of old age. We found that the Chinese reported the most positive views toward old age, followed by the American deaf and then the American hearing. As can be seen in Figure 1 and Figure 2, we also found that the pattern of the old participants' memory scores matched the cultural stereotypes. The old Chinese performed the best, followed by the old American deaf, and then the old American hearing. Our results

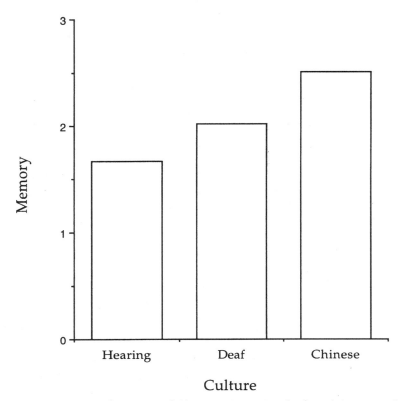

FIGURE 1.   Memory performance of Chinese, American deaf, and American hearing elderly.

suggest that culture may contribute to memory loss (and memory preser-vation) in old age and that American researchers documenting norms of aging should also consider people in other cultures.

Tendency to Assume Elders Homogeneous

With every year, individuals' minds and bodies change in response to numerous combinations of internal and external factors. One might ex-pect that as people age the variation between them should increase, yet many studies rely on designs and statistics that average the scores of elders.

In their 1987 article, "Human Aging: Usual and Successful," Rowe and Kahn began a movement to study successful aging. They advocated conducting research on successful aging by studying the old individuals that perform better than their peers, rather than concentrating on the mean scores of normal adults. As they noted, a certain percentage of the

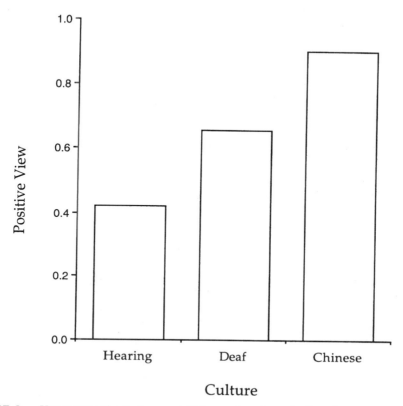

FIGURE 2.   Views toward aging among Chinese, American deaf, and American hearing elderly.

elders in most studies score well above the mean of their same-age peers. The successfully aging elders also often perform at levels equivalent to or better than some of their younger peers and to themselves when they were younger. Most gerontologists still concentrate on studying means and ignore the great heterogeneity of old age when designing and analyzing their research. A study documenting that, on average, forgetfulness increases with age would produce different results from one that considers why some old people maintain photographic memories while others become more forgetful.

Weintraub, Powell, and Whitla (1994) adopted Rowe and Kahn's advice to study successful aging when they conducted their study of more than 1,000 doctors. Weintraub and her colleagues went beyond studying averages. By comparing individuals they found that some doctors over the age of 75 years performed as well as their 35-year-old colleagues on

20 of the 21 subtests of cognitive skills, including memory and visuospatial perception. The only subtest on which the top-scoring old physicians performed uniformly worse than their young peers was analogies. Perhaps the young doctors' more recent exposure to analogies on the S.A.T. accounts for their better scores.

Researchers have also begun to tackle the question of why there is so much variation within old individuals in how they perform. For example, in the area of memory most elders do much better on recognition tasks than on recall tasks and on implicit memory than on explicit memory. Explicit memory, which is measured by most traditional memory tests, requires intentional recall, whereas implicit memory refers to information encoded and retrieved without awareness. By teasing apart this variation within and between elders, researchers should reduce the focus of health professionals on disability in old age.

Tendency to Assume Cross-Sectional Data Reflects Longitudinal Trends

Most researchers of the aged use cross-sectional study designs, in which they simultaneously measure groups of young and old subjects and then compare them. This method allows all participants to be exposed to the same period effects, or particular time in history. Cross-sectional studies, however, risk that one will assume that differences between the groups are due to aging, rather than to cohort differences. For example, one can't attribute the lower scores of older subjects on a math test to cognitive decline when the old cohort received fewer years of math education on average than the younger cohort. One way to avoid cohort effects is to conduct a longitudinal study. In a longitudinal study, researchers follow the same group of people as they age over time. Unfortunately, most researchers cannot afford the money or time required for this type of study.

The results of longitudinal studies often demonstrate the inadequacies of cross-sectional research. For example, Schaie (1993) used both cross-sectional and longitudinal approaches when examining the data from the participants over the age of 60 in the Seattle Longitudinal Study. When considering cross-sectional average differences, he found that all mental abilities studied (e.g., inductive reasoning and spatial orientation) appeared to decline significantly. When he considered individuals longitudinally, however, he found that the majority showed stability or gains. The longitudinal analyses revealed that 15.5% of the old participants showed no decline and more than half showed decline in at most one of the five areas. Some people in the sample even showed improvement. Only 2.3% declined in all five areas. In addition, Schaie found that birth cohort differences accounted for some of the apparent cross-sectional differences.

Manton (1992) also points out that the cohorts that experienced their youth in the beginning of the century may differ dramatically from the cohorts that are young today. For example, most elderly persons alive today reached adulthood before improvements in immunization and the U.S. Surgeon General's reports on the dangers of smoking, cholesterol, and hypertension. Thus, it is possible that the prevalence of chronic diseases among people who are old today is partially due to disease processes initiated before certain immunizations were available and before these people learned about the relationships between certain behaviors and health. Thus, cohorts that have not yet reached adulthood may experience health very differently from those that have already reached old age.

Tendency to Select Research Stimuli That Favor the Young

Several researchers have demonstrated that if stimuli are selected to be relevant to the elderly, or at least not more relevant to the younger subjects, age differences disappear in some memory tasks. Hunley-Dunn and McIntosh (1984) found that in a study of free recall, the young performed better when the stimuli were "young relevant" (i.e., contemporary singers) whereas elders performed better when stimuli were "elder relevant" (i.e., names of big band leaders) or relevant to both (i.e., national politicians). When asked to rate their own performance, however, the old rated their likely performance as worse than the young.

Similarly, Botwinick and Storadt (1980) found that the old performed as well as the young subjects on recall and recognition of sociohistorical events and entertainment when the information dated back to 1910–1919. Perlmutter (1978) also found that even though her older subjects performed worse than the younger subjects on a typical laboratory test involving recall and recognition of word lists, her old subjects performed better than the young with sociohistorical data. This finding held true for all time periods tested, regardless of whether the old were the only ones to have lived through them.

Bias toward old age is not confined to the young. Older adults may also experience a youth-centric view, which can lead to prejudice toward their same-age peers or toward themselves. For example, an old woman who used to enjoy watching television, but who now finds she doesn't have patience for it, might conclude that she can't attend to things anymore. An alternative explanation is that television writers create most shows with young viewers in mind and don't care if it interests an older cohort.

Tendency to Avoid Studying the Most Healthy and Wealthy Old

The healthy and wealthy old do not participate in many studies. The healthy spend little time in nursing homes and hospitals where gerontologists conduct many of their studies. The wealthy do not need the financial rewards offered to research participants and can afford to hire an assistant rather than enter a nursing home if they need help with certain tasks. If elders can afford to stay out of a nursing home, they probably will. If individuals are reasonably disease free until death and do not have an intrinsic interest in volunteering for research studies, they may never become part of our samples. Inadequacies of census data make it hard to know the size of this group. Rowe and Kahn (1987) point out that some studies that take averages not only ignore those in the top ranges but also have means that may be loaded down by old volunteers whose test scores are lowered because they have health complications that are not intrinsic to aging. In our view, including individuals from all socioeconomic classes and health levels in studies should lead to a more accurate and positive image of aging.

REVERSING DISABILITY

Muscle Growth

Although the changes that occur with age are often exaggerated by research methods and are not always negative or in need of reversal (such as the shift in the internal clock), life for older individuals might be easier if some changes could be reversed. For example, people at any age who experience loss in inductive reasoning skills or muscle tone probably would like to reverse these declines. At one time these deficits were assumed to be universal aspects of senescence. Scientists now know that these changes do not always occur and that they can be reversed.

Researchers from the Harvard Medical School and Tufts Center on Aging conducted a dramatic study with residents at the Hebrew Home for the Aged in Boston (Fiatarone et al., 1994). The researchers randomly assigned half of their 100 volunteers, all between the ages of 70 and 98, to 10 weeks of resistance weight training. The control group members participated in other activities, including walking and board games. The weight-training subjects increased their muscle strength by 113%, their ability to climb stairs by 28%, and their walking speed by 11.8%. In an earlier study, the researchers found that some of their older subjects who were formerly wheelchair-bound returned to walking independently after the training (Fiatarone et al., 1990). Physicians and researchers once thought that when muscle mass atrophies after the age of 65, one can never get it back. For example, Schulz, Heckhausen, and Lucher (1991) wrote that "with increasing age, muscle tissue slowly declines in strength, bone, and flexibility" (p. 178). Now doctors and researchers are beginning to realize that muscle tone can be regained.

In another study, Fiatarone et al. (1989) found that healthy elderly subjects who exercise could increase their immune function to the same degree as young subjects. Thus physical ability may make elders less susceptible to the deleterious chain of effects whereby stress lowers immunocompetence, which, in turn, compromises health.

Regular physical activity can also reverse the typical biological markers of aging such as high blood pressure, improper sugar balance, excess body fat, declining bone density, and improper insulin levels. In addition, physical activity has been found to reduce risk of death from most causes (Manton, 1992). Artherosclerosis now appears to be reversible with interventions that draw on good nutrition, exercise, and stress reduction (Ornish et al., 1990). Lindsted, Tonstad, and Kuzma (1991) found in a longitudinal study of 9,800 Seventh Day Adventists that moderate physical activity can reduce the likelihood of mortality in people up to the age of 109.

Brain Plasticity

Another age-related change that can be reversed is the cognitive deterioration thought to be associated with brain shrinkage. In old age the brain loses about 10% of its weight (Terry, Deteresa, & Hansen, 1987). Since the discovery of this shrinkage, most neuroanatomists and psychologists have assumed that it represents the general dying or deterioration of the brain and causes the corresponding loss of cognitive skills in old age. Several discoveries, however, have forced neurologists and psychologists to reconsider this assumption. First, various researchers have demonstrated dramatic neuronal plasticity (or ability of neurons to adapt to environmental changes) in old age, indicating that the brain cells are not just dying (Diamond, 1988).

Cotman and Hoff (1983) demonstrated (by making lesions in the hippocampus of old and young rats) that old rats' brains are as capable as young rats' brains of growing new connections and that no age differences seem to exist in the growth rate of forming new synapses. In humans, researchers have found that during the early stages of Alzheimer's disease, some of the brain regions of old individuals compensate for the loss of neurons by growing new connections (Adams, 1991). Diamond (1988) found that when she put old rats in challenging environments with new toys, their ability to solve mazes increased and their cerebral cortexes grew. When compared to age-matched control rats living in a standard colony, the old rats in the enriched environment exhibited cortexes up to 10% thicker due to the growth of nerve cells and dendrites. Terry, DeTeresa, and Hansen (1987) examined brain slices of people aged 21 to 100 and discovered that although large neurons shrink, the number of small neurons and glia cells actually increase in old age. Thus, although the weight of old people's brains decreases, the number of brain neurons may remain stable and do not lose their ability to grow.

Researchers do not yet understand the meaning of the neuronal changes in old age (Diamond, 1988). Even though these changes could indicate deterioration, they could also indicate increased efficiency. Since these changes occur in all people as they age, even those who improve their physical and cognitive functioning, it is unlikely that these changes result from general deterioration. It is not yet known if slightly different patterns of brain development occur in those who continually challenge themselves into their 80's and 90's. Neurobiologists are studying the brain of Einstein, who died at the age of 76, for clues into how his brain may differ from the brains of others who were less cognitively active during their lifetimes (Diamond, 1988; Greenough, 1994).

Most researchers now agree that these neuronal changes in old age do not lead to inevitable cognitive deterioration. Some medical texts have begun to revise their sections on aging brains, stating that healthy old brains differ little from healthy young brains. This causal link between brain developmental changes and inevitable cognitive decline has been further discredited by the research of Schaie and Willis (1986) and others who have demonstrated that for many people quite a few of their cognitive skills remain stable or improve as they age.

Cognitive Improvement

In a study of elders from the Seattle Longitudinal Study, Willis and Schaie (1986) reversed the decline in two abilities assumed to decline with normal aging: inductive reasoning and spatial orientation. The researchers gave the elders practice and strategy instruction during five 1-hour training sessions. Not only were those who had been stable in these skills over the previous 14 years able to improve, but those who had shown decline improved as well. In fact, 40% of those who previously declined in one or both of these abilities returned to their earlier functioning levels.

Langer et al. (1990) designed an intervention to see if they could reverse some of the markers of aging by putting people into a younger mind-set during a five-day retreat. They told half the participants to imagine that they were living again in 1959 and told the others to reminisce about how things used to be in 1959. The first group spoke in the present tense and used 1959 photographs to identify one another. The control group spoke in the past tense and used recent photographs to identify one another. They found that all improved on a number of measures believed to be markers of aging, such as facial appearance, but the experimental group, encouraged essentially to be younger, improved more on joint flexibility, finger span, sitting height, manual dexterity, vision in the right eye, and the Digit Symbol Substitution subtest from the Wechsler Adult Intelligence Scale.

CONCLUSION

All of these results are encouraging, but considerable research remains to be done to clarify the extent to which all disabilities, even ones still assumed to be permanent, like hearing loss, can be reversed. Intervention studies and research examining old individuals who age successfully in America and other cultures are needed. In fact, we believe that such studies are mandated by the results already obtained. Given the predictions that the life span and percentage of old people will continue to rise over the next couple of decades, it is imperative that researchers of old age change their focus from documenting disability to promoting the abilities of this group, which we all hope to belong to one day.

REFERENCES

Adams, I. (1991). Structural plasticity of synapses in Alzheimer's Disease. *Molecular Neurobiology, 5,* 41–419.

Adler, N., & Mathews, K. (1994). Health psychology: Why do some people get sick and some stay well? *Annual Review of Psychology, 45,* 229–259.

Avorn, J., & Langer, E. (1982). Induced disability in nursing home patients: A controlled trial. *Journal of the American Geriatrics Society, 30,* 397–400.

Baron, R., Cutrona, C., Hicklin, D., Russel, D., & Lubaroff, D. (1990). Social support and immune function among spouses of cancer patients. *Journal of Personality and Social Psychology, 59,* 344–352.

Bartrop, R., Luckhurst, E., Lazarus, L., Kiloh, L., & Penny, R. (1977). Depressed lymphocyte function after bereavement. *Lancet, 1,* 834–836.

Bethel, D. (1992) Life on Obasuteyama, or inside a Japanese institution for the elderly. In T. Lebra (Ed.), *Japanese social organization* (pp. 109–134). Honolulu: University of Hawaii Press.

Botwinick, J., & Storadt, M. (1980). Recall and recognition of old information in relation to age and sex. *Journal of Gerontology, 35,* 70–76.

Brown, P., & Levinson, S. (1987). *Politeness: Some universals in language usage.* New York: Cambridge University Press.

Caporael, L. (1981). The paralanguage of caregiving: Babytalk to the institutionalized aged. *Journal of Personality and Social Psychology, 40,* 876–884.

Chanowitz, B., & Langer, E. (1981). Premature cognitive commitment. *Journal of Personality and Social Psychology, 41,* 1051–1063.

Cotman, C., & Hoff, S. (1983). Synapse repair in the hippocampus: The effects of aging. *Birth Defects, 19,* 119–134.

Czeisler, C., Allan, J., Strogatz, S., Ronda, J., Sanchez, R., Rios, C., Freitag, W., Richardson, G., & Kronauer, R. (1986). Bright light resets the human circadian pacemaker independent of the timing of the sleep–wake cycle. *Science, 233,* 667–671.

Czeisler, C., Dumont, M., Duffy, J., Steinberg, J., Richardson, G., Brown, E., Sanchez, R., Rios, C., & Ronda, J. (1992). Association of sleep–wake habits in older people with changes in output of circadian pacemaker. *Lancet, 340,* 933–936.

de Graaf, C., Polet, P., & Van Staveren, W. (1994). Sensory perception and pleasantness of food flavors in elderly subjects. *Journal of Gerontology: Psychological Sciences, 49,* 93–99.

Diamond, M. (1988). *Enriching heredity: The impact of the environment on the anatomy of the brain.* New York: Free Press.

Fawzy, F. (1994, January). *Psychosocial intervention for individuals with melanoma.* Paper presented at a meeting of the Behavioral Immunology Study Group, Brookline, MA.

Fiatarone, M., Marks, E., Ryan, N., Meredith, C., Lipsitz, L., & Evans, W. (1990). High-intensity strength training in nonogenerians. *Journal of the American Medical Association, 263,* 3029–3034.

Fiatarone, M., Morley, J., Bloom, E., Benton, D., Solomon, G., & Makinodan, T. (1989). The effect of exercise on natural killer cell activity in young and old subjects. *Journal of Gerontology: Medical Sciences, 44*, 37–45.

Fiatarone, M., O'Neill, E., Ryan, N., Clements, K., Solares, G., Nelson, M., Roberts, S., Kehayiuas, J., Lipsitz, L., & Evans, W. (1994). Exercise training and nutritional supplementation for physical frailty in very elderly people. *The New England Journal of Medicine, 330*, 1169–1775.

Foreman, J. (1993, April 26). Trouble sleeping? In later years, our internal clocks change. *The Boston Globe*, p. 39.

Foreman, J. (1994, August 22). Cancer risk rises with age but treatment declines. *The Boston Globe*, pp. 22, 24, 28.

Greenough, W. (1994, May). *Plasticity and environment.* Paper presented at the Harvard Memory distortion conference, Cambridge, MA.

Hunley-Dunn, P., & McIntosh, J. (1984). Meaningfulness and recall of names by young and old adults. *Journal of Gerontology, 39*, 583–585.

Isaacs, L., & Bearison, D. (1986). The development of children's prejudice against the aged. *International Journal of Aging and Human Development, 23*, 175–194.

Jones, E., & Nisbett, R. (1971). The actor and the observer: Divergent perceptions of the causes of behavior. In E. Jones, D. Kanouse, H. Kelley, R. Nisbett, S. Valins, & B. Weiner (Eds.), *Attribution: Perceiving the causes of behavior* (pp. 79–94). Morristown, NJ: General Learning Press.

Kamen-Siegal, L., Rodin, J., Seligman, M., & Dwyer, J. (1991). Explanatory style and cell-mediated immunity in elderly men and women. *Health Psychology, 10*, 229–235.

Keicolt-Glaser, J., Dura, J., & Speicher, C. (1991). Spousal caregivers of dementia victims: Longitudinal changes in immunity and health. *Psychosomatic Medicine, 53*, 345–362.

Kennedy, S., Keicolt-Glaser, J., & Glaser, R. (1990). Social support, stress and the immune system. In B. Sarason, I. Sarason, & G. Pierce (Eds.), *Social support: An interactional view* (pp. 253–266). New York: Wiley.

Kite, M., & Johnson, B. (1988). Attitudes toward older and younger adults: A meta-analysis. *Psychology and Aging, 3*, 233–244.

Lachman, M., & MacArthur, L. (1986). Adulthood and age differences in causal attributions for cognitive, social and physical performance. *Psychology and Aging, 1*, 127–132.

Langer, E. (1989). *Mindfulness.* Reading, MA: Addison-Wesley.

Langer, E., & Abelson, R. (1974). A patient by any other name...: Clinical group differences in labeling bias. *Journal of Consulting and Clinical Psychology, 42*, 4–9.

Langer, E., & Benevento, A. (1978). Self-induced dependence, *Journal of Personality and Social Psychology, 36*, 886–893.

Langer, E., Chanowitz, B., Palmerino, M., Jacobs, S., Rhodes, M., & Thayer, P. (1990). Nonsequential development and aging. In C. Alexander & E. Langer (Eds.), *Higher stages of human development* (pp. 114–136). New York: Oxford University Press.

Langer, E., Perlmuter, L., Chanowitz, B., & Rubin, R. (1988). Two new applications of mindfulness theory: Alcoholism and aging. *Journal of Aging Studies, 2*, 289–299.

Langer, E., & Rodin, J. (1976). The effect of enhanced personal responsibility of the aged: A field experiment in an institutional setting. *Journal of Personality and Social Psychology, 34*, 191–198.

Langer, E., Rodin, J., Beck, P., Weinman, C., & Spitzer, L. (1979). Environmental determinants of memory improvement in late adulthood. *Journal of Personality and Social Psychology, 11*, 2003–2013.

Levy, B., & Langer, E. (1994). Aging free of negative stereotypes: Successful aging in China and among deaf Americans. *Journal of Personality and Social Psychology, 66*, 989–997.

Lindsted, K., Tonstad, S., & Kuzma, J. (1991). Self-report of physical activity and patterns of mortality in Seventh Day Adventists men. *Journal of Clinical Epidemiology, 44*, 355–364.

Manton, K. (1992) The dynamics of aging: Measurement and intervention issues for health and function. *Journal of Cross-Cultural Gerontology, 7*, 185–201.

Markus, H., & Kitayama, S. (1991). Culture and the self: Implications for cognition, emotion and motivation. *Psychological Review, 98*, 224–254.

Moses, S. (1992, August). More clinicians needed to help a graying America. *APA Monitor, 34.*

Ornish, D., Brown, S., Scherwitz, L., Billings, J., Armstrong, W., Ports, T., McLanahan, S., Kirkeeide, R., Brand, R., & Gould, K. (1990) Can lifestyle changes reverse coronary heart disease? *The Lancet, 336*, 129–133.

Palmore, E. (1988). *Facts on aging quiz: A handbook of uses and results.* New York: Springer.

Perdue, C., & Gurtman, M. (1990). Evidence for the automaticity of ageism. *Journal of Experimental Social Psychology, 26*, 199–216.

Perlmutter, M. (1978). What is memory aging the aging of? *Developmental Psychology, 4,* 330–345.

Peterson, C., & Seligman, M. (1987). Explanatory style and illness. *Journal of Personality, 55*, 237–265.

Peterson, C., Seligman, M., & Valliant, G. (1988). Pessimistic explanatory style as a risk factor for physical illness: A 35 year longitudinal study. *Journal of Personality and Social Psychology, 55*, 23–27.

Rodeheaver, D., & Datan, N. (1988). The challenge of double jeopardy: Toward a mental health agenda for aging women. *American Psychologist, 43*, 648–654.

Rodin, J. (1987, October). *The determinants of successful aging.* Paper presented at a meeting of the Federation of the Behavioral, Psychological and Cognitive Sciences, Washington, DC.

Rodin, J., & Langer, E. (1977). Long-term effects of a control relevant intervention with the institutionalized aged. *Journal of Personality and Social Psychology, 35*, 897–902.

Rodin, J., & Langer, E. (1980). Aging labels: The decline of control and the fall of self-esteem. *Journal of Social Issues, 36*, 12–29.

Rossi, A. (1992, August). *Cross-cultural study of menopause.* Paper presented at the meeting of the American Psychological Association, Washington DC.

Rowe, J., & Kahn, R. (1987) Human aging: Usual and successful. *Science, 237*, 143–148.

Ryan, E. (1992). Beliefs about memory across the life span. *Journal of Gerontology: Psychological Sciences, 47*, 41–47.

Schaie, K. W. (1993). The optimization of cognitive functioning in old age: Prediction based on cohort-sequential and longitudinal data. In P. Baltes & M. Baltes (Eds.), *Successful aging: Perspectives from the behavioral sciences* (pp. 94–117). New York: Cambridge University Press.

Schaie, K. W., & Willis, S. (1986). Can intellectual decline in the elderly be reversed? *Developmental Psychology, 22*, 223–232.

Schulz, R., Heckhausen, J., & Locher, J. (1991). Adult development, control and adaptive functioning. *Journal of Social Issues, 47*, 177–196.

Shem, S. (1978). *The house of God: A novel.* New York: R. Marek.

Taylor, S. (1986). *Health psychology.* New York: Random House.

Terry, R., Deteresa, R., & Hansen, L. (1987). Neocortical cell counts in normal human adult aging. *Annals of Neurology, 21*, 530–539.

United States Bureau of the Census. (1975). *Historical statistics of the United States, colonial times to 1970* (p. 10, p. 56). Washington, DC.

United States Bureau of the Census. (1993). *Statistical abstract of the United States: 1993* (113th ed., pp. 15–16). Washington, DC.

Weintraub, S., Powell, D., & Whitla, D. (1994). Successful cognitive aging: Individual differences among physicians on a computerized test of mental state. *Journal of Geriatric Psychiatry, 27*, 15–33.

Wilkes, M., & Shuchman, M. (1989, June 4). What is too old? *New York Times Magazine,* 58–60.

Willis, S., & Schaie, K. (1986). Training the elderly on the ability factors of spatial orientation and inductive reasoning. *Psychology and Aging, 1*, 239–247.

CHAPTER 9

Functional Impairment, Physical Disease, and Depression in Older Adults

ANTONETTE M. ZEISS, PETER M. LEWINSOHN, AND PAUL ROHDE

Elderly adults with physical health problems are frequently reported to be vulnerable to depression. This pattern has been reported for older patients with a wide variety of diseases, including rheumatoid arthritis (Creed & Ash, 1992; Frank et al., 1988), stroke, cancer, Parkinson's disease, Cushing's syndrome, hypothyroidism, vitamin deficiencies (Finch, Ramsay, & Katona, 1992), hypertension, myocardial infarction, and diabetes (Wells, Rogers, Burnam, & Camp, 1993). Other researchers have adopted an epidemiological strategy looking at a variety of physical disease problems in community populations, rather than focusing on single disease categories. Hughes, DeMallie, and Blazer (1993) reported that scores on the Center for Epidemiologic Studies Depression Scale (CES-D; Radloff, 1977) in the elderly are related to both higher mean illness index scores and impaired social support scores. Katona (1992) reported a higher prevalence of depression, compared to that found in other commu-

ANTONETTE M. ZEISS • Geriatric Research Education and Clinical Center, Veterans Affairs Palo Alto Health Care System, Palo Alto, California 94304.   PETER M. LEWINSOHN and PAUL ROHDE • Oregon Research Institute, 1715 Franklin Boulevard, Eugene, Oregon 97403.

Handbook of Diversity Issues in Health Psychology, edited by Pamela M. Kato and Traci Mann. Plenum Press, New York, 1996.

nity studies, in elders attending primary care clinics, acute geriatric admissions, continuing care geriatric patients, and elders with acute hip fractures. One of the most frequently cited references for the idea that physical illness is the strongest correlate of depression in the elderly is a book by Gurland and his colleagues (Gurland et al., 1983). Interestingly, while authors who cite that book almost always emphasize the disease–depression relationship, it is seldom mentioned that the authors (Gurland et al., 1983) included disability and dependence (i.e., indices of functional impairment), along with disease, as determinants of depression in the elderly.

GENERAL ISSUES IN EXAMINING THE RELATIONSHIP OF DEPRESSION TO PHYSICAL DISEASE

Although older adults with disease are more likely to score higher on indices of depression, many questions remain unanswered by the articles cited above. Can depression be reliably diagnosed when there is concurrent disease? What is the direction of the relationship between depression and disease? Do all diseases increase the risk of becoming depressed, or only certain ones? What is it about disease that might increase the risk of becoming depressed? Examining these questions will be the focus of this chapter.

Diagnosing Depression in Patients with Physical Disease

Cohen-Cole and Kaufman (1993) summarized research suggesting an association between disease and depression, but they emphasized the difficulties of diagnosing depression in physically ill patients. For example, some items on self-report scales of depression were answered in a direction suggesting depression simply because of the direct impact of disease. For example, one item on the Beck Depression Inventory (BDI; Beck, Ward, Mendelson, Mock, & Erbaugh, 1961) assesses fatigue (with answers ranging from "I don't get more tired than usual" to "I get too tired to do anything"). Such an item might be answered in the direction of depression by patients with certain debilitating diseases, even if the patient's mood was generally positive. Other potentially confounding items assess impaired sleep, appetite changes, and concern about health.

Cohen-Cole and Kaufman (1993) argued that research examining physical health problems and depression should specify the methodological approach for differentiating illness from depression. They particularly recommended utilizing clinical interviews and research diagnostic criteria for depression, rather than self-report questionnaires or diagnoses based on clinical impressions. Similar conclusions have been drawn by

Schulberg and McClelland (1987). This chapter will emphasize studies utilizing clinical interviews and rigorous diagnostic procedures, although references to studies using self-report measures will be included. When findings conflict, research utilizing careful diagnostic procedures should be weighed more heavily.

Depression Is More Likely in Patients with Disease, but Not Inevitable

Although Cohen-Cole and Kaufman's (1993) review demonstrates a heightened prevalence of depression among patients in many disease categories, they also emphasize that depression is not an inevitable consequence of disease. They argue that, "...the syndrome of major depression is neither statistically nor clinically normal in the medically ill. Many studies applying formal criteria for major depression demonstrate clearly that the majority of patients with physical illness, including terminal cancer, do not meet criteria for major depression" (p. 182). Thus, it is important to consider not only the heightened likelihood of depression in patients with medical disease, but also to consider the factors that might account for variability among patients.

Establishing Causal Relationships

In addition to distinguishing depression from physical disease, it is also important to distinguish functional impairment from physical disease. Functional impairment refers to the loss of ability to take care of one's everyday needs independently in the areas of work, self-care, or important leisure activities. Physical disease increases the likelihood of developing functional impairment, but such loss is not inevitable. In addition, functional impairment can occur in the absence of any specific disease, as with age-related decrements in sensory function. Research seeking to examine the causal relationship between depression and physical disease needs to examine the causal role of functional impairment as well.

Because much of the research has examined physical disease, functional impairment, and depression concurrently (i.e., at the same time), it is impossible to examine the direction of relationships. There are several possible causal patterns. First, depression may predispose one to disease, for example, by impairing adequate health promotion or maintenance behaviors. The second possibility is more frequently, albeit implicitly, considered: that is, the assumption that disease is a precursor to depression. This assumption might occur in three ways: (1) disease might be a direct risk factor for depression through the physiological effect of disease or the physiological impact of medications prescribed for the disease (Gangat, Simpson, & Naidoo, 1986); (2) the effects of disease may be indirect, in that disease might represent a threat to one's mortality or trigger helplessness or hopelessness, leading to depression; (3) disease might increase vulnerability to depression via its impact on functional status, that is, by generating dependence and disrupting valued activities.

These explanations are not mutually incompatible. Depression may predispose individuals to develop chronic disease, and disease may be a risk factor for developing depression. The causal pathways suggested may combine to increase vulnerability to depression. We turn to a theoretical integration that organizes these mutual, bidirectional possibilities into a coherent conceptual framework.

TOWARD A THEORETICAL INTEGRATION

Lewinsohn's Integrative Model of Depression (Lewinsohn, Hoberman, Teri, & Hautzinger, 1985) posits that the chain of events leading to depression is triggered by stressful events (A in Figure 1), which disrupt automatic functioning (B in Figure 1), that is, by events that prevent individuals from using their usual behaviors to carry out routines and accomplish everyday interactions with the environment. This sequence is postulated to be especially disruptive when it results in an increase in negative events and/or a decrease in positive events (see C in Figure 1), resulting in increased vulnerability to depression. This model predicts that disease will lead to depressive onset when it disrupts important functions, such as activities of daily living or engaging in valued activities. Lewinsohn's Integrative Model of Depression also implies that functional declines in the elderly that occur without diagnosable disease (e.g., an age-related decline in hearing or vision) may be risk factors for depression.

The model also provides a framework for understanding how depression increases disease, as the myriad consequences of depression (F in the model) generate a spiral of decreased self-care behaviors. For example, a depressed older adult may not eat adequately, leading to nutritional deficits that precipitate disease. Or a depressed older adult may not take care of personal hygiene, resulting in infections from minor scratches or scrapes. Finally, a depressed older adult who already has some disease may not consistently use health management strategies (e.g., taking medications, exercising, following appropriate diet), leading to significant worsening of disease. Similarly, depression might lead to decreased function in patients beyond the level physically indicated by disease severity. For example, depressed patients may feel hopeless and overwhelmed, and give up dressing or walking, blaming the impairment on the disease when they still have the physical capacity for independent function.

The remainder of this chapter provides an overview of literature on the relationships among disease, functional impairment, and depression

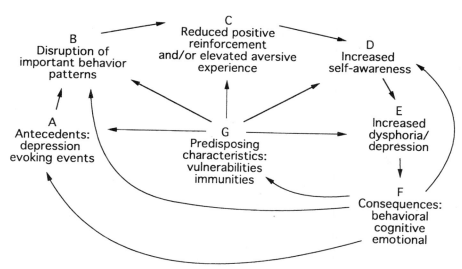

FIGURE 1. Schematic representation of variables involved in the occurrence of unipolar depression.

in the elderly, emphasizing the following hypotheses, each suggested by Lewinsohn's Integrative Model of Depression.

1. Physical disease increases the likelihood of subsequent onset of depression in the elderly only when it is associated with functional impairment.
2. Functional impairment, whether or not it is associated with diagnosable disease, increases the likelihood of subsequent onset of depression.
3. The greater the functional impairment, the greater the risk of onset of depression.
4. Depression can be a risk factor for the development, exacerbation, or both of disease in the elderly.
5. Depression can result in functional impairment at a more extensive level than is physically indicated by disease severity; Roberts (1986) refers to this kind of pattern as "excess disability."

PHYSICAL DISEASE AND DEPRESSION

There are only a few studies addressing the issue of whether disease, independent of functional impairment, increases the risk of depression. Studies that utilized a cross-sectional approach will be discussed first, followed by studies that followed patients longitudinally. The available cross-sectional studies targeted specific disease categories, arthritis and Parkinson's disease. The longitudinal studies, in contrast, combined information across a variety of diseases.

Disease as a Risk Factor for Depression

In a summary of the literature relevant to rheumatoid arthritis, Blalock and DeVellis (1992) conclude that disease severity is not a direct cause of depression: "Studies consistently have found minimal associations between depression and objective measures of disease activity/ severity, including erythrocyte sedimentation rate (ESR) and joint count" (p. 6). Frank and colleagues (1988), in a representative study, also found no relationship between depression, using a diagnosis of dysthymia based on clinical interview criteria, and objective measures of disease activity, including ESR, total joint score, walking time, grip strength, and duration of morning stiffness.

With Parkinson's disease, depression (using a self-report measure only) was reported to occur with elevated prevalence, but to be independent of degree of functional disability (Robins, 1976). Being a neurological disease, Parkinson's may alter brain chemistry in ways that directly affect mood and behavior. Other research suggests that depression in Parkinson's disease patients may be associated with mild intellectual impairment (Mayeux, Stern, Rosen, & Leventhal, 1981). Finally, patients with certain Parkinson's symptoms (bradykinesia, gait disturbance) were more likely to be depressed, whereas patients with tremor as their major symptom were not more likely to be depressed. These results suggest complex relationships between depression and Parkinson's disease, but there is a clear need for studies with clinically based depression criteria, larger samples, and a longitudinal approach to clarify these relationships.

One direct longitudinal look at the relationship of physical disease and depression is available in a report based on the Alameda County Study sample (Seeman, Guralnick, Kaplan, Knudsen, & Cohen, 1989). This sample of over 7,000 community-dwelling adults was followed longitudinally; data were available for 9- and 17-year follow-up periods. These researchers examined a wide spectrum of consequences of physical disease for the 17-year period following the original data collection. Depression was measured using the CES-D. In this study, the number of comorbid medical diseases was not predictive of subsequent depression in the elderly, although it was in younger adults. Although the overall number of diseases did not show a relationship with depression, it is possible that specific diseases might be direct risk factors for depression, for example, Parkinson's disease as discussed above. This issue was not addressed in the Alameda County sample.

Research cited thus far has examined disease in relationship to new episodes of depression; a different approach examined the persistence versus remission of depressive symptoms in elderly community dwelling adults who were depressed at first assessment, using CES-D scores as a criterion (Kennedy, Kelman, & Thomas, 1991). Advanced age and worsening health over a 2-year follow-up period were associated with persistence of depression; improved health was associated with remission. Measures of functional status did not appear to be related to CES-D scores in this study, but little information is presented on the way health and functional impairment measures were obtained.

Depression and Measures Combining Disease and Functional Impairment

Two studies are available that examine the concurrent association of disease presence, functional impairment, and depression. Each study reports significant relationships among these parameters, but both conceptualize disease and functional impairment as a combined variable, so that the unique roles of each cannot be determined.

In the first study, Rapp, Parisi, and Walsh (1988) assessed 150 randomly selected geriatric male medical inpatients, using rigorous criteria to determine depression: Research Diagnostic Criteria (RDC) diagnoses based on Schedule for Affective Disorders and Schizophrenia (SADS) interviews (Spitzer & Endicott, 1977; Spitzer, Endicott, & Robbins, 1978). Rapp et al. showed that depression was associated concurrently with the poorest physical health status. However, the measure of physical health mixed indices of disease presence, disease severity, and functional impairment, so it is impossible to draw conclusions about the extent to which each of these had an independent impact on depression.

In the second study, Smith, Peck, Milano, and Ward (1988) examined the concurrent relationship of depression and disability in 92 rheumatoid arthritis patients. They also examined the role of cognitive distortion as an exacerbating factor, with the expectation that patients who showed cognitive errors, such as catastrophizing (anticipating the outcome of a mildly unpleasant event as catastrophic) or selective attention (noticing only negative events and ignoring positive ones), would respond to stressful disease-related events with more dysphoria. Depression was measured with both the BDI, which (as discussed earlier) includes items that may be endorsed by arthritis patients on the basis of their illness, and the Hamilton Rating Scale for Depression (HRSD; Hamilton, 1960). The HRSD is an interview-based measure that provides a continuous score of depression rather than a diagnosis. In this project, interviewers omitted items on the HRSD when it was clear that subjects were responding on the basis of their arthritis rather than in terms of depression (e.g., not scoring gastric distress if it was clear that this was a side effect of nonsteroidal medication for the arthritis). Subsequent analyses were done separately for the two depression criteria, but results were generally equivalent, so only the overall patterns will be reported here. Cognitive distortion was concurrently associated with elevated depression, even with disease severity controlled. Cognitive distortion was only marginally related to physical disability, as measured by the Health Assessment Questionnaire (HAQ; Fries, Spitz, & Young, 1982), a commonly used measure of functional disability in arthritis patients. In addition, the combination of disease duration, recent disease activity, and disability accounted for 14.5% of the variance in depression; the contributions of the individual components were not reported. Cognitive distortion accounted for another 11% of the variance in depression scores beyond that contributed by disease and disability.

In conclusion, a strong case cannot be made for the hypothesis that having a disease diagnosis per se increases the likelihood of depression in the elderly. Most studies report no such relationship, unless functional impairment is confounded with the disease diagnosis variable. The best available longitudinal study (Seeman et al., 1989) did not find disease presence to predict onset of depression. However, there are no longitudinal studies available that would provide a definitive test of this hypothesis. A definitive test would be to study a sample of aging adults and observe patterns of onset of depression, based on diagnoses derived from clinical interviews, in relation to the diagnosis of new physical diseases. This design would be particularly valuable if the sample contained a sufficiently large number of individuals with specific diseases, such as Parkinson's, which may have direct neurological impact contributing to depression.

This kind of research may be prohibitively expensive to obtain, particularly since the studies looking at concurrent patterns suggest there is no simple, direct relationship between disease and depression. In the absence of such research, it seems wise to examine carefully a rival hypothesis, that is, that functional impairment mediates the relationship between disease and depression.

FUNCTIONAL IMPAIRMENT AND DEPRESSION

There is an extensive body of research that examines the relationship of functional impairment to depression in the elderly. Studies examining the concurrent relationship in samples of patients with a variety of diagnoses will be reported first, followed by longitudinal studies. Our intention is not only to demonstrate a strong, consistent relationship between functional impairment and depression but also to allow conclusions regarding causal relationships.

Concurrent Studies of Mixed Disease Categories

Berkman and colleagues (1986) reported on a sample of 2,806 elderly men and women who were living in the community and who were interviewed as part of the Yale Health and Aging Project. Subjects reported a wide variety of medical diseases, levels of functional disability, and levels of depression, as measured by the CES-D. Berkman et al. found that functional disability was related to every item on the CES-D, not just the somatically oriented items. In addition, the association between age and depressive symptoms was reduced when the researchers included functional disability in a multivariate model to predict depression. Functional disability was far more strongly associated with depressive symptoms than was age. The impact of functional disability was not limited to the somatic items of the scale; functional disability had a pervasive influence across all symptoms of depression.

Mirowsky and Ross (1992) reported on a study of 2,031 adults tested in 1990 and 809 adults tested in 1985. They measured physical dysfunction (e.g., loss of vision, hearing) and malaise (i.e., feeling bad, fatigued), but they did not measure illness directly. They found that loss of function was related to depression and to malaise.

Williamson and Schulz (1992a) examined the relationships among pain, activity restriction, and symptoms of depression in a sample of community-residing elderly adults. Subjects were 228 patients from outpatient geriatric clinics, 55 years of age or older, with a mean age of 72. Only patients with no indication of cognitive impairment (a Folstein Mini-Mental Status Exam score of 25 or more; Folstein, Folstein, & McHugh, 1975) were included, and no patients with a history of psychiatric disorder or alcoholism were included. Data were collected on pain, physical health, depression (using the CES-D), and activity restriction. Functional ability, but not physical illness per se, mediated the relationship between pain and depressed affect and also between physical illness and depressed affect. The authors concluded that both pain and illness are important contributors to functional disability and that disability, in turn, contributes to the development of depression. Restriction of some specific activities (eating behaviors, going shopping, and working on hobbies) was especially strongly related to the relationship between pain and depressed affect.

Lindesay (1991) reported that disease in an elderly community dwelling population was associated with depression. He also examined the relationship of disease to other mental health problems and found associations between disease and cognitive impairment, anxiety, and agoraphobia; simple phobia did not show an increased prevalence in patients with physical disease. Lindesay (1991) examined various hypotheses as explanations of these relationships. The data did not support hypochondriasis or somatization as causal explanations. The possibility that disease may have a direct organic influence on the brain was considered, but could not be tested in this project. The hypothesis that restriction of activity and independence are related to mental health problems received greatest support; strong associations were found between mental health problems and functional impairment.

Only one report considers how functional impairment may differentially affect the psychological well-being of men as compared to women (Penning & Strain, 1994). In a study of 1,406 community-dwelling elders, they examined gender differences in functional disability and reliance on personal assistance and technical aids. They also explored the relationships among the use of personal assistance, functional disability, and subjective well-being. Results included: (1) There was greater disability and somewhat greater use of personal assistance among women and (2) There were differences between men and women in the relationships between both personal and technical resources and subjective well-being, across levels of functional disability. Specifically, for men lower well-being was related to reliance on personal assistance and adaptive devices and to a combination of high levels of disability and receiving personal assistance from others. For women, greater disability was related to lower subjective feelings of well-being, regardless of whether or not they were receiving assistance. According to the authors, "Other things being equal, higher levels of functional disability appear to be somewhat more strongly and negatively related to the subjective well-being of women than of men. However, relying on others and on technical aids when faced with disability is significantly more positively related to subjective well-being among women than men" (p. 207). These results fit the predictions of Lewinsohn's Integrative Model of Depression if women more typically rely on interdependence as a means of coping with life challenges than men, as suggested by the authors (Penning & Strain, 1994). If so, then a need for greater assistance in later life would be less disruptive of patterns of coping for women than for men. Thus Lewinsohn's integrative model predicts that functional impairment to a level requiring use of personal assistance represents the pattern of events leading to depression more for men than for women.

The results reported thus far, based on research combined across various diseases, support the second and third guiding hypotheses of this review: functional impairment increases the likelihood of onset of depression; and the greater the degree of functional impairment, the greater the risk of onset of depression. The next section examines research on these hypotheses done in patients with specific disease diagnoses.

Concurrent Studies of Specific Disease Categories

Diabetes

Littlefield, Rodin, Murray, and Craven (1990) examined the relationships of depression (measured with the BDI), functional impairment measured with the Sickness Impact Profile (SIP; Bergner et al., 1976), and adequacy of social support in 158 adults with diabetes. BDI scores were positively correlated with functional impairment and negatively correlated with adequacy of social support. In addition, social support moderated the impact of impairment on depression: among patients with the most illness-related functional disability, adequate support provided relative protection from depression.

Chronic Obstructive Pulmonary Disease (COPD)

Beck, Scott, Teague, Perez, and Brown (1988) examined patients with COPD and found that, while severity of lung disease was correlated with restriction in tasks of daily living, lung disease was not correlated with emotional factors (e.g., anxiety, depression) on the SCL-90-R. However, restriction in activities was significantly related to reports of higher distress on the SCL-90-R scales of somatization, anxiety, and depression.

Arthritis

In patients with rheumatoid arthritis, self-report depression scores were correlated with pain, duration of morning stiffness, and functional capacity (Chandarana, Eals, Steingart, Bellamy, & Allen, 1987). Murphy, Creed, and Jayson (1988) found that depression was significantly related to weaker grip strength and higher disability according to the HAQ. As in studies reported earlier, they found that depression was not related to severity and activity of rheumatoid arthritis using several indices of disease. Husaini and Moore (1990) studied 600 black community-dwelling elders, some of whom reported osteoarthritis or rheumatoid arthritis. Depression level, measured by the CES-D, and life satisfaction ratings were more negative among those experiencing disability associated with arthritis (days confined to bed or unable to do work or household chores).

Overall, a large amount of the variance in depression among rheumatoid arthritis patients has been shown to be accounted for by measures of functional ability and social stress and isolation, or both. For example, Creed, Murphy, and Jayson (1989) accounted for 74% of the variance in depression scores (using a discriminant function analysis approach) using the combination of grip strength, disability on the HAQ, and social stress. Newman, Fitzpatrick, Lamb, and Shipley (1989) used hierarchical regression to demonstrate very high significant predictability of depression, with most of the predictive power coming from a measure of functional independence and another measure of social contacts. These authors argue that depression in arthritis patients is not a simple function of disease severity; instead, they hypothesize that when disease leads to physical disability and social isolation, patients become depressed.

Parkinson's Disease

In a sample of patients with Parkinson's disease (Gotham, Brown, & Marsden, 1986), depression was significantly associated with both severity of illness and functional disability, although these measures accounted for only a small proportion of the variance in depression. In addition, the depression seen in these patients had some atypical features; depression was characterized by pessimism and hopelessness, decreased motivation and drive, and increased concern with health, whereas guilt, self-blame, and worthlessness were absent. As discussed above, Parkinson's disease may be an exceptional case in which the direct neurological impact of the disease on emotional states needs to be considered.

Longitudinal Studies

One study that provides a detailed longitudinal perspective examined depression among older adults living in long-term care settings, primarily nursing homes (Parmalee, Katz, & Lawton, 1992a). The researchers examined 868 nursing home and congregate apartment residents over a one-year period. At the first assessment (T1), diagnoses of depression were assigned after obtaining scores on the Geriatric Depression Scale (GDS; Yesavage et al., 1983) and conducting a semistructured clinical interview using the SADS - Lifetime version (SADS-L; Endicott & Spitzer, 1978). At T1, depression was related to more impaired cognitive status (measured by the Fuld; Fuld, 1978) and worse physical health (using the Cumulative Illness Rating Scale; Linn, Linn, & Gurel, 1968). By far the strongest relationship at T1 was between depression and functional disability (measured in regard to independence on Activities of Daily Living). To illustrate the magnitude of associations, the F ratios for these measures respectively were 4.40, 5.77, and 45.63. At the second assessment 1 year later (T2), depression was related to cognitive status and strongly related to functional disability, but not related to physical health.

The researchers did not conduct analyses to look at the predictive power of functional disability at T1 in relation to development of depression, but they did examine change in each variable in relation to changes in the other variables. Results indicated that there was a greater increase in disability for the persistently depressed than for the never depressed. The authors concluded that functional disability was the most consistent cross-sectional correlate of depressive state. Because they did not test functional problems at T1 as a predictor of depression at T2, the authors correctly argue that the causal mechanism is unclear, and could be bidirectional.

Another study confirmed one of these findings and extended it by testing a predictive hypothesis (Rapp, Parisi, & Wallace, 1991). Rapp and colleagues reported on 102 geriatric male medical inpatients, followed for one year subsequent to inpatient admission. They found that depression was the most commonly diagnosed psychiatric condition, based on SADS interviews. Most importantly for our purposes, they also found that functional impairment from physical disease was predictive of subsequent psychiatric status, but not the reverse.

A third longitudinal study examined health care utilization. Enrollees in health maintenance organizations (HMOs) were followed over a 1-year period (von Korff, Ormel, Katon, & Lin, 1992). Those selected for this study were 145 patients who were in the top decile of users of ambulatory health care and who exceeded the 70th percentile of HMO norms for depression. Over the 1-year follow-up period, improvement in depression was closely associated with decrease in disability but had only a borderline relationship to disease severity. Unfortunately, predictive relationships were not reported among these variables. Thus the data show that over a prospective period depression and disability covaried, whereas depression and disease severity did not, but the data do not address the causal relationship between depression and disability.

DEPRESSION AS A RISK FACTOR FOR THE DEVELOPMENT OR EXACERBATION OF DISEASE

Can depression be a risk factor for the development or exacerbation of disease in the elderly? Studies examining these questions, which reverses the causal direction usually assumed in studies of disease and depression in the elderly, have reported mixed results.

One longitudinal study (Murphy, Smith, Lindesay, & Slattery, 1988) reported a clear relationship between depression and mortality or disease exacerbation. Depressed and nondepressed elders in the community were followed for 4 years. Consistent with concurrent research findings, those who were initially depressed had more severe health and functional problems. However, over the follow-up period, the depressed group had significantly more deaths, even after controlling for acute and chronic health problems at initial assessment. Koenig, Shelp, Goli, Cohen, and Blazer (1989) also reported that depression resulted in increased mortality, independent of severity of physical illness. In addition, depressed patients consumed more health care resources. Similarly, Saravay, Steinberg, Weinschel, Pollack, and Alovis (1991) found that, even after controlling for physical impairment, depressed patients who were hospitalized for medical conditions stayed longer in the hospital than nondepressed patients.

Roose, Dalack, and Woodring (1991) reviewed literature documenting the association of depression with a greater likelihood of adverse cardiac events, including death due to cardiac problems, in patients with known cardiac disease. Silverstone followed 211 patients with myocardial infarction, subarachnoid hemorrhage, pulmonary embolism, or acute upper gastrointestinal hemorrhage. Following the acute cardiac event, 34% of patients became depressed as measured with the Montgomery-Asberg

Depression Rating Scale (Montgomery & Asberg, 1979). The likelihood of becoming depressed was not related to the initial severity of the illness. However, patients who became depressed had poorer outcomes over a 28-day period following admission: 47% of depressed patients died or had life-threatening complications as opposed to 10% of the nondepressed group.

Other studies do not find that depression predicts worsening health. Colantonio, Kast, and Ostfeld (1992) followed a cohort of 2,812 community dwelling adults over age 65 for a period of 6 years, with the goal of determining whether depression and other psychosocial factors could predict the incidence of new strokes. Depression was assessed with the CES-D; a host of other sociodemographic variables were also collected, including age, sex, medical status, smoking status, and religious attendance. In an initial regression analysis, baseline depression was a significant predictor of stroke, but this effect was not retained once other variables were controlled for (particularly age, sex, hypertension, diabetes, physical function, and smoking).

In a prospective study of nursing home patients that used survival curve analysis procedures (Parmalee, Katz, & Lawton, 1992b), depression, based on SADS diagnosis, was not found to be related to mortality. Initial analyses did show an association with depression, but the effect disappeared when health (measured by the Cumulative Illness Rating Scale) and functional status (Physical Self-Maintenance Scale, Lawton & Brody, 1969) were included.

In summary, the available research suggests that depression may be a precursor to worse health outcomes. This pattern has been shown for cardiac disease, stroke, and in groups of patients with mixed diagnoses. However, studies that have carefully controlled for other variables indicate that the relationship is not robust and may not be a simple causal one. Patients who are depressed also differ in other important ways from patients who are not depressed, and those other variables appear to represent the actual risk factors that predict mortality or other negative health outcomes.

DEPRESSION AS A RISK FACTOR FOR INCREASED FUNCTIONAL DISABILITY

We now turn to our final hypothesis, that is, depression can cause patients to function at a lower level than is physically indicated by the severity of their disease; this increased impairment has been called "excess disability" (Roberts, 1986).

Functional status in rheumatoid arthritis patients was examined in relationship to pain, rheumatologists' ratings of disease, depression (using a self-report measure), and anxiety (Anderson et al., 1988). Depression had a significant relationship with physician ratings of functional status, which the authors interpreted to indicate that depression predicts functional status. Since this study used a concurrent design, the opposite interpretation could be concluded as easily. Dekker, Boot, van der Woude, and Bijlsma (1992) review several similar articles showing that negative affect is associated with higher levels of pain and functional impairment in osteoarthritis patients. Since this relationship has been explained by the impact of functional disability on depression (in longitudinal studies described above), the authors' emphasis on explaining these findings using an excess disability paradigm is not compelling.

Kaplan, Strawbridge, Camacho, and Cohen (1993), utilizing the longitudinal Alameda County Study data previously described in a different study (Seeman et al., 1989), found that depression was a predictor of functional decline over a 6-year follow-up period. Unfortunately, the opposite pattern (that a decline in function predicts depression) was not tested, so the relative strength of the two causal patterns could not be determined. These results do suggest that depression can result in decreased effort and function, a finding congruent with Lewinsohn's Integrative Model of Depression.

In summary, findings are inconclusive. Depression may be a precursor of excess functional disability, but this pattern of results has not been clearly established and replicated.

GENERAL ISSUES REGARDING FUNCTIONAL IMPAIRMENT IN THE ELDERLY

The research reviewed has most consistently supported the conclusion that functional impairment resulting from physical disease is a key mechanism by which disease results in depression. This conclusion suggests three other questions worthy of attention. First, can functional disability be validly measured with the brief self-report questionnaires utilized in most of the studies cited? Second, which diseases are most likely to result in functional decline? Third, does functional impairment in the absence of a specific diagnosable disease (e.g., as a result of age-related sensory decline) also constitute a risk factor for depression? Research relevant to the first two questions will be reviewed and our recent data will be presented to examine the third question.

Assessing Functional Impairment in the Elderly

Two excellent studies examined the quality of self-report measures of functional impairment in older and younger chronically ill patients. Sherbourne and Meredith (1992) examined age differences in the quality of self-report data in 2,304 patients with chronic disease (hypertension, diabetes, heart disease, and depression). The data included indices of reliability, validity, failure to respond to items, and panel retention. Although they noted some problems with both self-report and behavioral measurements, their results showed that self-report data on health and functional impairment could be gathered from older and younger patients without significant loss of information or decrement in data quality.

Myers, Holliday, Harvey, and Hutchinson (1993) also compared self-reports of functional abilities to performance measures. A set of 14 performance tasks, consisting of a range of functional abilities (e.g., simulations of cooking and sweeping) was administered to 99 community-dwelling older adults (aged 60-92) who had previously completed a 50-item instrumental activities of daily living (IADL) questionnaire that had been previously developed and validated (Myers, 1992). A subsample was retested 2 weeks later and reassessed at 1 year; test-retest reliabilities were generally excellent for subjects whose health had not changed significantly over the follow-up period. In addition, both types of measures were related to service needs of the patients, as perceived by care providers. For many measures, the subject's self-report matched the observer's rating, but when discrepancies occurred, they consisted of raters underestimating the difficulty of a task relative to the subject's self-report (the opposite pattern was not found for any activities). Performance measures were not found to be psychometrically superior, more acceptable to respondents, easier to administer, or easier to interpret than questionnaire measures.

Thus research demonstrates that self-report measures of functional status currently in use, although by no means perfect or complete, provide information that is generally equivalent in reliability and validity to more complex and time-consuming behavioral performance measures.

Conditions Leading to Functional Impairment in the Elderly

Spiro and colleagues (1994) examined causes of functional decline in a study of 1,755 men aged 45 to 94. The SF-36, a well-validated measure of health and function (Ware & Sherbourne, 1992), was used to examine functional status; self-reports of the presence of five chronic diseases (hypertension, diabetes, lung disease, arthritis, lower back pain) were also obtained. Age had a negative impact on physical health, but did not have a linear impact on mental health: men in their 60s and 70s had better mental health than did men in their 50s or 80s. Diseases having the most impact on physical functional status were lower back pain, chronic lung disease, and arthritis; these diseases also had the greatest impact on mental health. Diabetes and hypertension had little impact on functional status or on mental health. The total number of chronic diseases was related to all physical function variables and to mental health. The causal relationship between functional decline and mental health could not be tested in this study because a concurrent design was used.

Boult, Kane, Louis, Boult, and McCaffrey (1994) assessed disease and functional status in 6,862 individuals over 70. Diseases most consistently associated with functional impairment were cerebrovascular disease and arthritis; coronary artery disease was close behind. Hypertension, osteoporosis, cancer, obesity, and diabetes were not closely associated with functional status. Kaplan and colleagues (1993) examined factors associated with change in physical functioning in the elderly over a 6-year prospective period, utilizing 356 members of the Alameda County study aged 65 and over. The largest declines in function were associated with hip fracture, stroke, COPD, heart attack, and serious falls. As Boult et al. reported, hypertension, cancer, and diabetes were not closely associated with functional status.

Crimmins and Saito (1993) studied a nationally representative sample of 3,169 community-dwelling people over 70. Subjects were first interviewed in 1984 and again in 1986. Data on disease and functional impairments were obtained both times. Crimmins and Saito concluded that decline in ability to perform specific functions was most likely to occur for those who had a stroke, arthritis, or visual or auditory impairment.

Three out of four of these studies demonstrate that arthritis has a high likelihood of resulting in functional impairment. In addition, in both of the studies that included cerebrovascular disease and stroke, a strong relationship of disease to functional decline was demonstrated. In no case was a problem highly related to functional loss in one study shown to be unimportant in another. Idiosyncratic results, such as the importance of visual and auditory loss for functional impairment in Crimmins and Saito (1993), occurred because a variable was only included in one of the studies.

Crimmins and Saito (1993) did not report which diseases were least associated with functional impairment. Of the three studies reporting such results, all agree that diabetes, cancer, and hypertension were least likely to result in functional decline.

The Impact of Functional Impairment with and without Diagnosable Disease

The hypothesis that functional impairment will be predictive of depression even in the absence of a specific physical disease was examined using a sample of 680 community-dwelling adults over age 50, each measured on at least two occasions, denoted as T1 and T2 (Zeiss, Lewinsohn, Rohde, & Seeley, 1994). This study goes beyond previously reported research in that predictive patterns were tested for a large, representative, community-dwelling population. Health and functional impairment variables were obtained on each occasion, as well as diagnoses of depression based on SADS interviews (Endicott & Spitzer, 1978). All of the subjects included were not depressed at T1.

Physical health for these 680 subjects was determined, using a 30-item checklist on which subjects reported which, if any, medical diseases they were currently experiencing (e.g., arthritis, emphysema, thyroid disease, Parkinson's disease, multiple sclerosis, coronary disease, glaucoma). Of the total sample, 307 subjects (45%) reported no diseases, 231 (34%) reported one disease, and 142 (21%) reported 2 or more diseases. Arthritis was most frequently reported, followed by coronary problems, which were second most frequently reported. Encephalitis, multiple sclerosis, meningitis, and Parkinson's disease were least frequently reported. A composite measure of functional status was developed, using self-report variables of vision, hearing, disabilities, impact of health problems, and ability to walk.

To examine the probability of onset of an episode of depression in subjects not initially depressed at T1, we analyzed the data by the Life Table Method (Anderson et al., 1980; Benedetti, Yuen, & Young, 1985; Kalbfleisch & Prentice, 1980), which generates survival curves showing the pattern of onset of depression over time as well as the overall onset rate. Differences between survival curve patterns for different subsamples were tested by the Mantel-Cox statistic (Mantel, 1966), which tests whether different groups significantly vary in patterns of onset of depression over time.

The primary survival curve analysis was designed to examine the independent and summative effects of disease and functional impairment as risk factors for depression. The survival curve analysis compared four groups: (1) subjects who had no physical disease and reported low functional impairment (referred to as "well, not impaired", N = 230); (2) subjects who had no current physical disease but reported high functional impairment (referred to as "well, impaired", N = 77); (3) subjects who reported disease but low functional impairment (referred to as "ill, not impaired", N = 197); and (4) subjects who reported disease and high functional impairment (referred to as "ill, impaired", N = 176).

The survival curves for the four groups, shown in Figure 2, were significantly different (Mantel-Cox = 18.643, df = 3, p <.0003). As predicted, the two functionally impaired groups had significantly shorter times to onset of depression and higher likelihood of depression compared to the two nonimpaired groups. Survival curves for subjects who had physical disease but were not functionally impaired did not differ from those of subjects who were healthy and not functionally impaired.

Consistent with Cohen-Cole and Kaufman (1993), only a minority of subjects in all conditions became depressed over the time between T1 and T2. Approximately 10% of subjects in the well, not impaired group developed an episode of depression; 11% in the ill, not impaired group; 23% in the ill, impaired group; and 25% in the well, impaired group. Additional analyses confirmed that patients with and without physical disease did not have significantly different survival curves when functional impairment was not considered, nor did having a greater number of medical

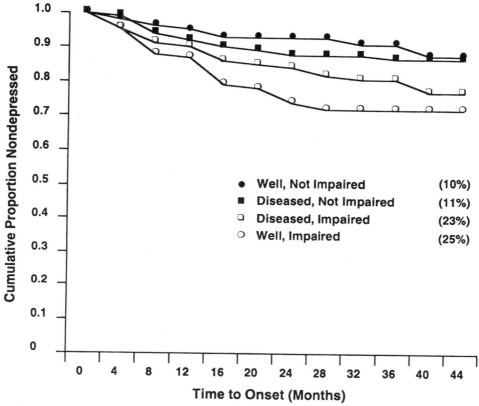

FIGURE 2. Survival curves comparing the four diseased/impaired groups in time to depression onset.

diseases increase the risk of becoming depressed. However, level of functional impairment was a definite risk factor for onset of depression. Over the period in which subjects were followed, about 10% of those with no functional impairment became depressed, about 14% of those in the moderate impairment became depressed, and about 23% of those with high impairment became depressed.

CONCLUSIONS AND CLINICAL IMPLICATIONS

The results of this review and our own research clearly support our first three hypotheses. Loss of ability to engage in usual functional patterns is a significant risk factor for depression (hypothesis 2), and greater impairment increases the risk of future depression (hypothesis 3). The findings reviewed also indicate that disease predicts depression only if it disrupts functional status (hypothesis 1); disease in and of itself is not generally a risk factor for becoming depressed in the elderly. Data are less clear regarding whether depression can exacerbate disease, increase mortality, and lead to excess disability (hypotheses 4 and 5). Some research suggests that each of these patterns may occur, but findings are not definitive.

The results reported provide clear support for Lewinsohn's Integrative Model of Depression. The development of functional impairment, through disease or age-related decline, is exemplary of the antecedent events identified in this model (Figure 1). Functional impairment can be expected to trigger a cascade of events leading to reduced positive reinforcement and increased aversive experience. This pattern may be especially true for men, as the results reported by Penning and Strain (1994) suggest. Once depression has been triggered, it may have additional negative consequences, including further decline in functional ability and self-care behavior. These changes may trigger excess disability, increased disease severity, or mortality, but those relationships have yet to be clearly demonstrated. In evaluating the general utility of Lewinsohn's model, it will be important to test whether these patterns, found in the elderly, are replicated in other age groups.

It is interesting that disease per se is not more clearly a risk factor for depression. There are reasons to expect such a relationship: some diseases may have direct physical effects, and depression has been reported to be a side effect of many medications. There may be certain diseases (e.g., Parkinson's disease) and medications (e.g., propranolol, Gangat et al., 1986) that do directly increase the risk of depression, regardless of degree of functional impairment. Studies seeking to demonstrate such a pattern should identify diseases that seem likely to generate depression based on an understanding of their neurological or physiological impact. Such studies must also utilize a longitudinal methodology to provide conclusive evidence.

While the evidence for the impact of functional impairment on depression in the elderly seems compelling, the critical test of this relationship has not been done. The ideal methodology would follow patients within many disease categories over time, as functional impairment develops, and examine the temporal relationship of illness, impairment, and onset of depression. It may be a long time before funding for such research is available. In the meantime, research should favor longitudinal efforts. It may be especially valuable to emphasize research on patients with arthritis, COPD, stroke, or coronary disease since these conditions often result in significant functional impairment.

The results currently available have important therapeutic implications. Health professionals treating older adults should be sensitive to the fact that those who have functional impairment, with or without a clearly diagnosed disease, are at increased risk for depression. Health professionals should routinely offer patients therapies that reduce functional impairment, such as Occupational Therapy and Physical Therapy modalities. Also, as implied by Lewinsohn's Integrative Model of Depression, health professionals may work with impaired elderly in identifying and implementing new behaviors that are positively reinforcing as an intervention to reduce the risk of depression. While it is admirable that more health professionals are recognizing and treating depression in the elderly, offering antidepressant medications to elders who have medical disease and functional impairment should not be an automatic reaction, although it is one of the most frequent recommendations in the literature cited in this review (e.g., Creed & Ash, 1992; Finch et al., 1992; Parmalee et al., 1992b; von Korff et al., 1992). The potential problems of antidepressant medication in patients with medical disease, particularly tricyclics, have been discussed by Roose, Dalack, and Woodring (1991). Research reviewed here suggests that patients with physical disease need not be depressed if they can maintain or regain physical function and independence in activities of daily living (e.g., Williamson & Schulz, 1992a). Treatment studies examining the efficacy of this approach for treating and preventing depression in older adults with physical disease should be a high research priority.

REFERENCES

Anderson, K. O., Keefe, F. J., Bradley, L. A., McDaniel, L. K., Young, L. D., Turner, R. A., Agudelo, C. A., Semble, E. L., & Pisko, E. J. (1988). Prediction of pain behavior and functional status of rheumatoid arthritis patents using medical status and psychological variables. *Pain, 33*, 25–32.

Anderson, S, Aquier, A., Hauck, W. W., Oakes, D., Vandaele, W., & Weiberg, H. I. (1980). *Statistical methods for comparative studies.* New York: Wiley.

Beck, A. T., Ward, C. H., Mendelson, M., Mock, J., & Erbaugh, J. (1961). An inventory for measuring depression. *Archives of General Psychiatry, 4*, 561–571.

Beck, J. G., Scott, S. K., Teague, R. B., Perez, F. I., & Brown, G. A. (1988). Correlates of daily impairment in COPD. *Rehabilitation Psychology, 33*, 77–84.

Benedetti, J., Yuen, K., & Young, L. (1985). Life tables and survival functions. In W. J. Dixon (Ed.), *BMDP statistical software* (pp. 557–594). Berkeley: University of California Press.

Bergner, M., Bobbitt, R. A., Kressel, S., Pollard, W. E., Gilson, B. S., & Morris, J. R. (1976). The sickness impact profile: Conceptual formulation and methodology for the development of a health status measure. *International Journal of Health Services, 6*, 393–415.

Berkman, L. F., Berkman, C. S., Kasl, S., Freeman, D. H., Leo, L., Ostfeld, A. M., Cornoni-Huntley, J., & Brody, J. A. (1986). Depressive symptoms in relation to physical health and functioning in the elderly. *American Journal of Epidemiology, 124*, 372–388.

Blalock, S. J., & DeVellis, R. F. (1992). Rheumatoid arthritis and depression: An overview. *Bulletin on the Rheumatic Diseases, 41*, 6–8.

Boult, C., Kane, R. L., Louis, T. A., Boult, L. & McCaffrey, D. (1994). Chronic conditions that lead to functional limitation in the elderly. *Journal of Gerontology: Medical Sciences, 49*, M28–M36.

Chandarana, P. C., Eals, M., Steingart, A. B., Bellamy, N., & Allen, S. (1987). The detection of psychiatric morbidity and associated factors in patients with rheumatoid arthritis. *Canadian Journal of Psychology, 32,* 356–361.

Cohen-Cole, S. A., & Kaufman, K. G. (1993). Major depression in physical illness: Diagnosis, prevalence, and antidepressant treatment (A ten-year review: 1982–1992). *Depression, 1,* 181–204.

Colantonio, A., Kast, S. V., & Ostfeld, A. M. (1992). Depressive symptoms and other psychosocial factors as predictors of stroke in the elderly. *American Journal of Epidemiology, 136,* 884–894.

Creed, F., & Ash, G. (1992). Depression in rheumatoid arthritis: aetiology and treatment. *International Review of Psychiatry, 4,* 23–34.

Creed, F., Murphy, S., & Jayson, M. V. (1989). Measurement of psychological disorders in RA. *Journal of Psychosomatic Research, 34,* 79–87.

Crimmins, E. M., & Saito, Y. (1993). Getting better and getting worse: Transitions in functional status among older Americans. *Journal of Aging and Health, 3,* 3–36.

Dekker, J., Boot, B., van der Woude, L. H. V., & Bijlsma, J. W. J. (1992). Pain and disability in osteoarthritis patients: A review of biobehavioral mechanism. *Journal of Behavioural Medicine, 15,* 189–214.

Endicott, J., & Spitzer, R. L. (1978). A diagnostic interview for affective disorders and schizophrenia. *Archives of General Psychiatry, 35,* 837–844.

Finch, E. J. L., Ramsay, R., & Katona, C. L. E. (1992). Depression and physical illness in the elderly. *Clinics in Geriatric Medicine, 8,* 275–287.

Folstein, M. F., Folstein, S., & McHugh, P. R. (1975). "Mini-mental state": A practical method for grading the cognitive state of patients for the clinician. *Journal of Psychiatric Research, 12,* 189–198.

Frank, R. G., Beck, N. C., Parker, J. C., Kashani, J. H., Elliot, T. R., Haut, A. E., Smith, E., Atwood, C., Brownlee-Duffeck, M., & Kay, D. R. (1988). Depression in rheumatoid arthritis. *Journal of Rheumatology, 15,* 920–925.

Fries, J. F., Spitz, P. W., & Young, D. Y. (1982). The dimensions of health outcomes: The health assessment questionnaire disability and pain scales. *Journal of Rheumatology, 9,* 789–793.

Fuld, P. A. (1978). Psychological testing in the differential diagnosis of the dementias. In R. Katzman, R. Terry, & K. L. Bick (Eds.), *Alzheimer's diseases: Senile dementias and related disorders* (pp. 185–193). New York: Raven Press.

Gangat, A. E., Simpson, M. A., & Naidoo, L. R. (1986). Medication as a potential cause of depression. *South African Medical Journal, 70,* 224–226.

Gotham, A. M., Brown, R. G., & Marsden, C. D. (1986). Depression in Parkinson's disease: A quantitative and qualitative analysis. *Journal of Neurology, Neurosurgery, and Psychiatry, 49,* 381–389.

Gurland, B., Copeland, J., Kuriansky, J., Kelleher, M., Sharpe, L., & Dean, L. (1983). *The mind and mood of aging.* New York: Haworth Press.

Hamilton, M. (1960). A rating scale for depression. *Journal of Neurology, Neurosurgery, and Psychiatry, 23,* 36–62.

Hughes, D. C., DeMallie, M. D., & Blazer, D. G. (1993). Does age make a difference in the effects of physical health and social support on the outcome of a major depressive episode? *American Journal of Psychiatry, 150,* 728–733.

Husaini, B. A. & Moore, S. T. (1990). Arthritis disability, depression, and life satisfaction among black elderly people. *Health and Social Work, 15,* 253–260.

Kalbfleisch, J. D., & Prentice, R. L., (1980). *The statistical analysis of failure time data.* New York: Wiley.

Kaplan, G. A., Strawbridge, W. J., Camacho, T., & Cohen, R. D. (1993). Factors associated with change in physical functioning in the elderly: A six-year prospective study. *Journal of Aging and Health, 5,* 140–153.

Katona, C. L. E. (1992). The epidemiology of depression in old age: The importance of physical illness. *Clinical neuropharmacology, 1* (Suppl. 1), 281A–282A.

Kennedy, G. J., Kelman, H. R., & Thomas, C. (1991). Persistence and remission of depressive symptoms in late life. *American Journal of Psychiatry, 148,* 174–178.

Koenig, H. G., Shelp, F., Goli, V., Cohen, J., & Blazer, D. G. (1989). Survival and health care utilization in elderly medical inpatients with major depression. *Journal of the American Geriatrics Society, 37,* 599–606.

Lawton, M. P. & Brody, E. M. (1969). Assessment of older people: Self-maintaining and instrumental activities of daily living. *The Gerontologist, 9,* 179–188.

Lewinsohn, P. M., Hoberman, H., Teri, L., & Hautzinger, M. (1985). An integrative theory of depression. In S. Reiss & R. R. Bootzin (Eds.), *Theoretical issues in behavior therapy* (pp. 331–359). New York: Academic Press.

Lindesay, J. (1991). The guy's/age concern survey: Physical health and psychiatric disorder in an urban elderly community. *International Journal of Geriatric Psychiatry, 5,* 171–178.

Linn, B. S., Linn, M. W., & Gurel, L. (1968). Cumulative illness rating scale. *Journal of the American Geriatrics Society, 16,* 622–626.

Littlefield, C. H., Rodin, G. M., Murray, M. A., & Craven, J. L. (1990). Influence of functional impairment and social support on depressive symptoms in persons with diabetes. *Health Psychology, 9,* 737–749.

Mantel, N. (1966). Evaluation of survival data and two new rank order statistics arising in its consideration. *Cancer Chemotherapy Reports, 50,* 163–170.

Mayeux, R., Stern, Y., Rosen, J., & Leventhal, J. (1981). Depression, intellectual impairment and Parkinson disease. *Neurology, 31,* 645–650.

Mirowsky, J., & Ross, C. E. (1992). Age and depression. *Journal of Health and Social Behavior, 33,* 187–205.

Montgomery, S. A., & Asberg, M. (1979). A new depression scale designed to be sensitive to change. *British Journal of Psychiatry, 134,* 282–289.

Murphy, E., Smith, R., Lindesay, J., & Slattery, J. (1988). Increased mortality rates in late life depression. *British Journal of Psychiatry, 152,* 347–353.

Murphy, S., Creed, F., & Jayson, M. I. V. (1988). Psychiatric disorder and illness behaviour in rheumatoid arthritis. *British Journal of Rheumatology, 27,* 357–363.

Myers, A. M. (1992). The clinical Swiss Army knife: Empirical evidence on the validity of IADL functional status measures. *Medical Care, 30* (Suppl.), MS96–111.

Myers, A. M., Holliday, P. J., Harvey, K. A., & Hutchinson, K. S. (1993). Functional performance measures: Are they superior to self-assessments? *Journal of Gerontology: Medical Sciences, 48,* M196–M206.

Newman, S. P., Fitzpatrick, R., Lamb., R., & Shipley, M. (1989). The origins of depressed mood in rheumatoid arthritis. *Journal of Rheumatology, 16,* 740–744.

Parmalee, P. A., Katz, I. R., & Lawton, M. P. (1992a). Depression and mortality among institutionalized aged. *Journal of Gerontology: Psychological Sciences, 47,* P3–P10.

Parmalee, P. A., Katz, I. R., & Lawton, M. P. (1992b). Incidence of depression in long-term care settings. *Journal of Gerontology: Medical Sciences, 47,* M189–M196.

Penning, M. J., & Strain, L. A. (1994). Gender differences in disability, assistance, and subjective well-being in later life. *Journal of Gerontology: Social Sciences, 49,* S202–208.

Radloff, L. (1977). The CES-D Scale: A self-report depression scale for research in the general population. *Applied Psychological Measurement, 1,* 385–401.

Rapp, S. R., Parisi, S. A., & Wallace, C. E. (1991). Comorbid psychiatric disorders in elderly medical patients: A 1-year prospective study. *Journal of the American Geriatrics Society, 39,* 124–131.

Rapp, S. R., Parisi, S. A., & Walsh, D. A. (1988). Psychological dysfunction and physical health among elderly medical inpatients. *Journal of Consulting and Clinical Psychology, 56,* 851–855.

Roberts, A. H. (1986). Excess disability in the elderly: Exercise management. In L. Teri & P. M. Lewinsohn (Eds.), *Geropsychological assessment and treatment: Selected topics* (pp. 87–119). New York: Springer.

Robins, A. H. (1976). Depression in patients with parkinsonism. *British Journal of Psychiatry, 128,* 141–145.

Roose, S. P., Dalack, G. W., & Woodring, S. (1991). Death, depression, and heart disease. *Journal of Clinical Psychiatry, 52,* 34–39.

Saravay, S. M., Steinberg, M. D., Weinschel, B., Pollack, S., & Alovis, N. (1991). Psychological comorbidity and length of stay in the general hospital. *American Journal of Psychiatry, 148,* 324–329.

Schulberg, H. C., & McClelland, M. (1987). Depression and physical illness: The prevalence, causation, and diagnosis of comorbidity. *Clinical Psychology Review, 7,* 145–167.

Seeman, T. E., Guralnick, J. M., Kaplan, G. A., Knudsen, L., & Cohen, R. (1989). The health consequences of multiple morbidity in the elderly. *Journal of Aging and Health, 1,* 50–66.

Sherbourne, C. D., & Meredith, L. S. (1992). Quality of self-report data: A comparison of older and younger chronically ill patients. *Journal of Gerontology: Social Sciences, 47,* S204–S211.

Silverstone, P. H. (1990). Depression increases mortality and morbidity in acute life-threatening medical illness. *Journal of Psychosomatic Research, 34,* 651–657.

Smith, T. W., Peck, J. R., Milano, R. A., & Ward, J. R. (1988). Cognitive distortion in rheumatoid arthritis: Relation to depression and disability. *Journal of Consulting and Clinical Psychology, 56,* 412–416.

Spiro, A., Miller, D., Clark, J., Kressin, N., Bosse, R., & Kazis, L. (1994). Quality of life in adulthood: Effects of age and illness. Poster presented at American Psychological Association, Los Angeles.

Spitzer, R. S., & Endicott, J. (1977). *The schedule for affective disorders and schizophrenia—change (SADS-C) interview.* New York: New York Psychiatric Institute.

Spitzer, R. S., Endicott, J., & Robbins, E. (1978). Research diagnostic criteria: Rationale and reliability. *Archives of General Psychiatry, 35,* 773–782.

von Korff, M., Ormel, J., Katon, W., & Lin, E. H. B. (1992). Disability and depression among high utilizers of health care: A longitudinal analysis. *Archives of General Psychiatry, 49,* 91–100.

Ware, J. E., & Sherbourne, C. D. (1992). The MOS 36-Item short-form health survey (SF-36): I. Conceptual framework and item selection. *Medical Care, 30,* 473–483.

Wells, K. B., Rogers, W., Burnam, M. A., & Camp, P. (1993). Course of depression in patients with hypertension, myocardial infarction, or insulin-dependent diabetes. *American Journal of Psychiatry, 150,* 632–638.

Williamson, G. M., & Schulz, R. (1992a). Pain, activity restriction, and symptoms of depression among community-residing elderly adults. *Journal of Gerontology: Psychological Sciences, 47,* P367–P372.

Williamson, G. M., & Schulz, R. (1992b). Physical illness and symptoms of depression among elderly outpatients. *Psychology and Aging, 7,* 343–351.

Yesavage, J. A., Brink, T. L., Rose, T. L., Lum, O., Huang, V., Adey, M. B., & Leirer, V. O. (1983). Development and validation of a geriatric depression rating scale. *Journal of Psychiatric Research, 17,* 31–49.

Zeiss, A. M., Lewinsohn, P. M., Rohde, P., & Seeley, J. R. (1994). The relationship of physical illness and functional impairment to depression in the elderly. Paper presented at Association for Advancement of Behavior Therapy, San Diego, CA.

PART III

GENDER AND SEXUAL ORIENTATION ISSUES IN HEALTH PSYCHOLOGY

CHAPTER 10

Why Do We Need a Health Psychology of Gender or Sexual Orientation?

TRACI MANN

Why study the health psychology of females separately from males, and homosexuals separately from heterosexuals? In this chapter I argue that a careful study of the health psychology of gender and sexual orientation can have several benefits. Research on specific populations can lead to interventions that are tailored to particular groups, and these targeted interventions tend to be more effective than interventions created for a wider audience (Price, Cowen, Lorion, & Ramos-McKay, 1989). For instance, when quitting smoking, different problems arise for men than for women. Interventions to help people quit smoking will therefore be most effective if they are tailored specifically to either men or women (Chesney & Nealy, this volume).

Research on specific populations can also shed light on the health and wellness of these different groups, leading to an increased knowledge of the particular health issues that people of each group face. This is particularly important for groups that have been understudied, such as women and homosexuals.

There are, however, several risks to studying specific populations, and these risks require that researchers approach this work carefully.

TRACI MANN • Health Risk Reduction Projects, UCLA Neuropsychiatric Institute, 10920 Wilshire Boulevard, Suite 1103, Los Angeles, CA 90024.

Handbook of Diversity Issues in Health Psychology, edited by Pamela M. Kato and Traci Mann. Plenum Press, New York, 1996.

Researchers must keep in mind that the goal is not to study difference for difference's sake, but to study differences so that effective interventions can be designed for all people. Studying the differences between groups, however, may mask the differences that exist within groups, potentially leading to stereotypes and stigma. Researchers must remember that even within groups there is heterogeneity and that specific groups are being studied because they are easy to target for interventions. Another risk to studying specific populations is that one might collect data that may shed a negative light on a particular group. Although this is a legitimate worry, the real danger would be to let this fear prevent researchers from studying ways to promote the health of people of different groups.

In the hands of sensitive researchers, a health psychology of gender and sexual orientation can lead to enormous rewards. Studying these populations separately is the best way to create effective interventions that are uniquely suited to each group's specific health needs. And in a time of limited resources, targeting specific groups is one way to reduce the costs of health promotion interventions. In the upcoming pages, I will (1) define relevant terms, (2) discuss some differences in the health of heterosexual men and women and homosexual men and women, and (3) describe several types of explanations for the health differences between people of the different groups.

DEFINITIONS

Gender

Different researchers use the words *sex* and *gender* in different ways. In general, the term *sex differences* refers to reliable biological distinctions between males and females. Anatomical differences, hormonal differences, and brain differences are examples of sex differences. The term *gender differences,* on the other hand, refers to differential behaviors that are learned as appropriate for either males or females in a particular society (Lott, 1994). These behaviors are assumed to be socialized throughout life and are not necessarily related to, or even based upon, sex differences. Of course, it is not always clear whether to attribute a particular distinction to sex or to gender, and in those cases, by convention, differences will be attributed to gender.

When looking at health differences between men and women, it is often difficult to tell whether the differences are based on biology (sex differences) or culture (gender differences). For example, at every age, boys and men have higher mortality rates than girls and women (Strickland, 1988). Is this a biological difference or a social difference? Clearly, prebirth mortality differences must be biological. The causes of mortality differences throughout the rest of the life span, however, are harder to pinpoint. Some researchers argue that biological differences caused by genes (Ramey, 1982), hormones (Hamilton, Parry, & Blumenthal, 1988), or the absorption of toxins (Calabrese, 1985) lead to the differential mortality for men and women. Others argue that the mortality difference is based on lifestyle (Hamburg, Elliot, & Parron, 1982). Finally, some researchers argue that an interaction of biological and lifestyle factors accounts primarily for the differential mortality of men and women (e.g., Matthews, 1989).

Sexual Orientation

Sexual orientation has been defined by researchers according to three different criteria: same-gender sexual behavior, self-identification as lesbian or gay, and membership in the lesbian or gay communities. These categories may overlap, but it is also possible for people to be categorized differently based on the differing dimensions. Rothblum (1994) argues that the nature of the research question should determine which dimension to emphasize.

Sexual Behavior

Rothblum (1994) claims that much of the heterosexual public has defined sexual orientation by a person's sexual behavior. That is, they define a person as a homosexual if that person engages in same-gender sexual behavior. Defining homosexuality this way may lead to the inclusion or exclusion of people from the homosexual category for seemingly inappropriate reasons. For instance, many people engage in same-gender sexual behavior but do not consider themselves to be homosexuals. In addition, many people consider themselves to be homosexuals but for various reasons do not engage in same-gender sexual behavior. Lesbian couples, in particular, are less likely to engage in sexual behavior than gay male couples, married heterosexual couples, or cohabiting heterosexual couples (Blumstein & Schwartz, 1983). If researchers, however, are studying the health consequences of various forms of sexual behavior, then the behavioral criterion is the appropriate choice of classification.

Self-Identity

The American Psychological Association Committee on Lesbian and Gay Concerns (CLGC) distinguishes between self-identity and sexual behavior (CLGC, 1991). According to the dimension of self-identity, people are considered to be homosexuals if they identify themselves as gays or lesbians. As mentioned above, this group will not completely overlap with the group of people who engage in same-gender sexual behaviors. Self-identified gays and lesbians are considered especially desirable to include in research samples, particularly in epidemiologic research, since they are considered to be the most representative of the homosexual population (Rothblum, 1994). Self-identified gays and lesbians, however, are harder to locate than are homosexuals who participate in the lesbian or gay communities.

Participation in Community

A third dimension of homosexuality is participation in lesbian and gay community groups. Most existing research on homosexuals has used this dimension of homosexuality in recruiting subjects (Albro & Tully, 1979), probably because it is the easiest group to locate. Researchers simply recruit subjects from various community groups. Recruiting from community groups, however, yields a nonrepresentative sample of the homosexual population, since it only includes the lesbians and gay men who are most open about their sexual orientation. In addition, samples collected this way tend to be biased toward young, white, college-educated subjects (Albro & Tully, 1979). Research about societal acceptance of homosexuals or about being a homosexual who is "out," however, should focus on people from this sample of visible homosexuals.

DIFFERENCES IN HEALTH OUTCOMES

There are many differences in health outcomes between men and women, and between heterosexuals and homosexuals. All these differences require that the health of each group be studied individually. In general, health differences between these groups fall into three main categories: differences in *which* illnesses occur, differences in *how often* illnesses occur, and differences in the relationships among risk factors and illnesses. These categories of differences will be reviewed in turn.

Differences in the Occurrence of Illnesses

Some illnesses are specific to people of one sex. Obviously, particular illnesses of the reproductive system only occur in people of one sex. If only men are studied, no information will be learned about women's reproductive systems. This seems obvious, and yet, up until recently, women were excluded from many research samples. Even when women are included in samples, health outcomes specific to women are not necessarily studied. For example, when women were first enrolled in clinical studies of AIDS, researchers did not look at the effect of AIDS on women's gynecological health. Women were being studied, but health outcomes that only occur in women were not (Faden, 1994).

Differences in the Frequency of Illnesses

Many health problems occur with different frequency among men and women, homosexuals, and heterosexuals. Women are more likely than men to have most self-reported chronic conditions and all acute illnesses (except injuries) (Wingard, Cohn, Kaplan, Cirillo, & Cohen 1989). Higher proportions of women than men have diabetes, rheumatoid arthritis, lupus, anemia, osteoporosis, and respiratory and gastrointestinal problems (Strickland, 1988). Males, on the other hand, have higher proportions of congenital conditions, such as hemophilia and muscular dystrophy (Travis, 1988).

Although most measures of morbidity show that women are sick more than men, more men than women die of each of the twelve leading causes of death (Wingard, 1984). And as mentioned earlier, in almost all societies women have higher life expectancies than men (World Bank, 1991). One researcher explained this paradox by positing that men are sick less often, but when they are sick they have more severe illnesses. Women, on the other hand, are more frequently ill, but not with life-threatening illnesses (Verbrugge, 1989). Consider the following examples of differential frequencies of illness between various groups of people.

A review of existing research on lesbian health suggests that breast, ovarian, and endometrial cancers are more frequent among lesbians than among heterosexual women (O'Hanlan, 1995). Why are lesbians at higher risk for these cancers than heterosexual women? Without a health psychology of gender and sexual orientation—without studying lifestyle factors of heterosexual women and homosexual women separately—this question cannot be answered.

The incidence of lung cancer is higher in males than in females, but the rate among females is rising rapidly (Waldron, 1988). Researchers attribute the rise in lung cancer in females to their increased smoking in recent years, whereas men's smoking is decreasing (Waldron, 1988).

The incidence of HIV infection is much higher in homosexual males than in heterosexual males and is on the rise in heterosexual females. Interventions to prevent the spread of HIV will most likely be more effective if they are tailored to the differing needs, interests, and circumstances of people in these different groups. For example, it is often difficult for women to convince their sexual partners to use condoms, so women need to be taught techniques to accomplish this. Heterosexual men, on the other hand, do not have to convince a partner to use a condom, so interventions for them need not primarily focus on persuading a partner. Interventions for homosexual men will be different from interventions for women as well as those for heterosexual men.

Finally, heterosexual women are more likely to have eating disorders than heterosexual men, whereas the situation reverses for homosexuals:

Gay men are more likely to have eating disorders than lesbians (Herzog, Norman, Gordon, & Pepose, 1984). What accounts for these differences?

Differences in the Relationships among Risk Factors and Illnesses

Several risk factors for illness differ in their impact on the health of males and females. Women appear to be less affected by high blood cholesterol than men, possibly because estrogen may to some extent protect women from cardiovascular disease (Bush et al., 1987). Diabetes, however, is a stronger risk factor for heart disease in women than it is in men (Barrett-Connor, Cohn, Wingard, & Edelstein, 1991). There is also some evidence that there is a stronger association between cigarette smoking and lung cancer for women than for men, indicating a higher susceptibility to lung cancer among female smokers than male smokers (Risch et al., 1993).

POSSIBLE EXPLANATIONS FOR HEALTH DIFFERENCES

There are many possible explanations for the health differences between males and females, and between heterosexuals and homosexuals. These explanations range from strictly biological ones to behavioral ones to interactions between the two. In this section, various categories of explanations for health differences are discussed.

Biological Differences

Several health differences between males and females can be linked to biology. Any differences in health that are based on differential amounts or types of hormones in the system can be attributed to biology. For example, differences due to the protective effects of estrogen are biological. Similarly, researchers have speculated that testosterone can elevate the body's response to many stressors (Travis, 1988).

Differences based on genetics are also possible because females have an XX chromosome pairing while males have an XY pairing. The X chromosome carries much more information than the Y chromosome, and since information that could lead to abnormal development tends to be carried on a recessive X chromosome, differential health effects can occur in males and females (Travis, 1988). In females, the information is typically suppressed by information on the other X chromosome (the dominant one), so the female most likely becomes nothing more than a carrier. In males, however, information on the Y chromosome cannot overrule information on the X chromosome, so the abnormal information is more likely to be expressed. This leads to a male predominance of such congenital conditions as hemophilia, meningitis, muscular dystrophy, and mental retardation (Travis, 1988).

Males and females also differ in how drugs and toxins affect them. They differ in gastrointestinal absorption, enzymatic activation, and tissue distribution of ingested chemicals (Calabrese, 1985). Because of these differences, females contract lead poisoning more readily than males (Roels, Balis-Jacques, Buchet, & Lauwerys, 1979), have a fivefold greater risk of developing hypothyroid conditions from lithium medication than males (Lloyd, Rosser, & Crowe, 1973), and are at higher risk of benzene intoxication than males (Sato, Nakajima, Fujiwara, & Murayama, 1975).

Some researchers have speculated that there may be biological differences between heterosexuals and homosexuals (Levay, 1993). It is not clear whether these differences are a cause or a consequence of homosexuality, or if they have any impact on the health outcomes discussed here.

Interaction with the Medical System

Men tend to use the medical system less often than women. Across most age categories, men have a lower frequency of physician office visits than women (U.S. Bureau of the Census, 1990). Men are also less likely than women to notice symptoms or to report symptoms to their doctors (Pennebaker, 1982). Men may underuse the medical system because they do not tend to notice symptoms. In addition, men may not want to take off from work or may not be able to take off from work to see a physician. They may not be as likely as women to have yearly checkups, whereas women tend to see gynecologists regularly. Unlike women, men may not be forced into contact with physicians while taking care of children. In any case, this underuse of the medical system could lead to later detection of illnesses or to minor illnesses being untreated.

Not only do men and women respond differently to the medical system, but the medical system responds differently to men and women. For certain identical groups of symptoms, women are more likely than men to be diagnosed with mental or nervous disorders. Doctors are more likely to attribute women's symptoms to a psychological disorder (Travis, 1988). In addition, physicians may be less likely to diagnose women with conditions that they consider to be "men's diseases." In one study, women with the same symptoms of heart disease as men were only one-tenth as likely as men to be referred for tests to see if bypass surgery was necessary (Tobin et al., 1987).

Lesbians and gay males underuse the medical system, but they have entirely different reasons for doing so than do heterosexual males. Lesbians have less access to the medical system than most women because they are less likely to have insurance from a spouse's employment. Gay men, particularly because of the AIDS epidemic, feel stigmatized by the medical community and discriminated against by insurance companies and subsequently are not eager to see physicians (Kass, Faden, Fox, & Dudley, 1992). Lesbians report that they are afraid to tell physicians their sexual orientation for fear of how the physician will react. In addition, many lesbians report that they experienced hostility when they revealed their sexual orientation to their physician (Smith, Johnson, & Guenther, 1985). Clearly, interventions designed to get people to make greater use of the medical system must be different for homosexuals than for heterosexuals.

Social Roles, Stress, and Coping

Women and men differ in the amount of stress they feel, the way they cope with stress, and their satisfaction with their social roles. Women are less likely than men to be employed, more likely to be unhappy, and report a higher level of stress (Verbrugge, 1989). In addition, there is substantial evidence that marriage disproportionately benefits men (Levenson, Carstensen, & Gottman, 1993). Not only do husbands report higher levels of marital satisfaction than do wives (Skolnick, 1986), but married men report higher satisfaction (Steil, 1984), lower rates of mental health problems (Russo, 1985), and lower rates of physical health problems than single men (Helsing, 1981). Married women, on the other hand, report the opposite: lower satisfaction (Steil, 1984) and higher rates of mental health problems (Russo, 1985) than single women. Finally, unhappily married women report more physical symptoms than both men (regardless of marital status) and happily married women (Levenson, Carstensen, & Gottman, 1994).

Looking at homosexual couples may help to clarify the gender differences in the effects of marriage on health and satisfaction (Rothblum, 1994). The factors that are assumed to put married women at risk for mental health problems may not do so for lesbian or gay couples. Lesbians in committed relationships do not usually take on the role of homemaker or mother (though more and more lesbian couples are having children either through adoption or through artificial insemination). If, for example, lesbians reported higher satisfaction with their relationships than do heterosexual women, it could mean that the roles of homemaker and mother provide stress and reduce satisfaction for heterosexual women. Another possibility is that the effects of relationships on mental health may be based not on the individual's gender, but on the individual's partner's gender: Perhaps good mental health is promoted if one is in a relationship with a woman but compromised if one is in a relationship with a man. Looking at the satisfaction of gay male couples would shed further light on this issue. Studying both heterosexual and homosexual couples is essential for understanding what underlies the effects of relationships on health.

Finally, lesbians and gay males have to cope with many stressors that are unique to homosexuals. They have to cope with being a member of a stigmatized group and with revealing their sexual orientation to others ("coming out"). Once a homosexual has come out, several stressors emerge, including the discrimination that continues to exist against homosexuals. And unlike people of ethnic minorities, who typically come from homes in which their parents are of the same ethnic minority, most homosexuals do not come from homes in which their parents are members of the same minority group (homosexuals) as them. Therefore, most homosexuals are not able to learn to cope with being gay by watching their parents and relatives. In addition, many lesbians and gay men are misunderstood or disparaged by members of their own families.

In terms of stressors, gay males who are members of the gay community have to cope with both the emotional and physical stress of the HIV epidemic. Members of the gay community, whether or not they have HIV themselves, frequently have to cope with multiple bereavement, as well as caretaking for sick friends, including friends who have been abandoned by their families. Having HIV on top of these other stressors significantly increases the psychological burden.

High-Risk Behavior

It has been argued that "as much as 50% of mortality from the ten leading causes of death in the United States today can be traced to aspects of lifestyle" (Hamburg, Elliot, & Parron, 1982). For example, cigarette smoking increases risk for cancer, heart disease, and stroke, which are the top three causes of death in the United States. Males consistently have higher risk scores than females associated with lifestyle factors, which include smoking, alcohol use, harmful dietary habits, use of illicit drugs, and physical daring (Waldron, 1988). Men are hospitalized more than women for injuries (Travis, 1988), although they are hospitalized less than women for virtually every other condition.

A higher percentage of lesbians and gay men use alcohol, marijuana, and cocaine than the general population (McKirnan & Peterson, 1989). Reasons for this may include that homosexuals are under increased stress because they are members of a marginalized group, or that gay bars and clubs remain the primary social outlet for homosexuals. In addition, a national survey of 1,925 lesbians found that almost one third of the sample used tobacco on a daily basis (Bradford, Ryan, & Rothblum, 1994). Because people in these different groups engage in high-risk behaviors for different reasons, interventions to prevent high-risk behaviors will be more effective if they take these differences into account.

CONCLUSION

In this chapter, I have described general differences in health between males and females, and between heterosexuals and homosexuals. I have also described possible reasons for these differences, ranging from purely biological explanations to purely psychological ones. From the information in this chapter, it is clear that a health psychology of gender and sexual orientation is necessary if researchers are to provide effective health care interventions for heterosexual males and females as well as for homosexual males and females.

The chapters in this section each describes a problem or situation that is unique to one of these populations, either heterosexual women or men, gay men, or lesbians. Each author makes it clear why it is important to consider these groups separately, describes important health outcomes relevant to the group, and proposes solutions that are tailored directly to members of each group.

In Chapter 11, Margaret Chesney and Jill Nealy discuss the rising problem of smoking among heterosexual women. They argue that because women and men smoke for different reasons and quit for different reasons, interventions to help people stop smoking need to be tailored specifically to either men or women. They describe strategies for interventions to prevent smoking initiation and foster smoking cessation among women.

In Chapter 12, Michael Copenhaver and Richard Eisler discuss one factor that may explain differential health problems in men: masculine gender role stress. They propose that social requirements for men to be masculine prevent them from taking care of themselves, from getting emotinal support, and from seeking medical care. They also argue that the masculine gender role leads to stress, anger, and cardiovascular reactivity, all of which compromise men's health. They describe three intervention strategies to help men prevent these problems.

In Chapter 13, Gary Grossman talks about different ways to help gay men cope with being HIV positive. Grossman focuses on gay men in the gay community because they have a different coping task than do people who are not in contact with other people with HIV. In addition, gay men in the gay community are likely to have to cope with bereavement as well as their own health problems.

In Chapter 14, Katherine O'Hanlan, a gynecologic oncologist, discusses the particular health issues of the lesbian population. She focuses on the effects of cultural homophobia as an obstruction to adequate recognition and provision of the psychological and medical health needs of lesbians, and she describes the unique health demography of lesbians. She describes several changes that need to be made by society in general, and by physicians in particular, in dealing with lesbian patients.

REFERENCES

Albro, J., & Tully, C. (1979). A study of lesbian lifestyles in the homosexual micro-culture and the heterosexual macro-culture. *Journal of Homosexuality, 4,* 331–344.

Barrett-Connor, E., Cohn, B., Wingard, D., & Edelstein, S. (1991). Why is diabetes mellitus a stronger risk factor for fatal ischemic heart disease in women than in men? *Journal of the American Medical Association, 265,* 627–631.

Blumstein, P., & Schwartz, P. (1983). *American couples.* New York: William Morrow.

Bradford, J., Ryan, C., & Rothblum, E. (1994). National lesbian health care survey: Implications for mental health care. *Journal of Consulting and Clinical Psychology, 62,* 228–242.

Bush, L., Connor, B., Cowen, D., Criqui, H., Wallace, D., Suchindran, M., Tyroler, A., & Rifkind, M. (1987). Cardiovascular mortality and noncontraceptive use of estrogen in women: Results from the lipid research clinics program follow-up study. *Circulation, 6,* 1102–1109.

Calabrese, E. (1985). *Toxic susceptibility: Male/female differences.* New York: Wiley Interscience.

Committee on Lesbian and Gay Concerns. (1991). Avoiding heterosexual bias in language. *American Psychologist, 46,* 973–974.

Faden, R. (1994). *Perspectives on research issues for women.* Paper presented at the American Psychological Association Conference on Psychosocial and Behavioral Factors in Women's Health: Washington, DC.

Hamburg, D., Elliot, G., & Parron, D. (1982). *Health and behavior: Frontiers of research in the biobehavioral sciences.* Washington, DC: National Academy Press.

Hamilton, J., Parry, B., & Blumenthal, S. (1988). The menstrual cycle in context: II. Human gonadal steroid hormone variability. *Journal of Clinical Psychology, 49,* 480–484.

Helsing, K. (1981). Factors associated with mortality after widowhood. *American Journal of Public Health, 71,* 802–809.

Herzog, D., Norman, D., Gordon, C., & Pepose, M. (1984). Sexual conflict and eating disorders in 27 males. *American Journal of Psychiatry, 141,* 989–990.

Kass, N., Faden, R., Fox, R., & Dudley, J. (1992). Homosexual and bisexual men's perceptions of discrimination in health services. *American Journal of Public Health, 82,* 1277–1279.

LeVay, S. (1993). *The sexual brain.* Cambridge, MA: The MIT Press.

Levenson, R., Carstensen, L., & Gottman, J. (1993). Long-term marriage: Age, gender, and satisfaction. *Psychology and Aging, 8,* 301–313.

Levenson, R., Carstensen, L., & Gottman, J. (1994). Influence of age and gender on affect, physiology, and their interrelations: A study of long-term marriages. *Journal of Personality and Social Psychology, 67,* 56–68.

Lloyd, G. G., Rosser, R. M., & Crowe, M. J. (1973). Effect of lithium on thyroid in man. *Lancet, 2,* 619.

Lott, B. (1994). *Women's lives: Themes and variations in gender learning.* Pacific Grove, CA: Brooks/Cole Publishing Company.

Matthews, K. (1989). Interactive effects of behavior and reproductive hormones on sex differences in risk for coronary heart disease. *Health Psychology, 8,* 373–387.

McKirnan, D., & Peterson, P. (1989). Alcohol and drug use among homosexual men and women: Epidemiology and population characteristics. *Addictive Behaviors, 14,* 545–553.

O'Hanlan, I. (1995). Lesbian health and homophobia: Perspectives for the treating obstetrician/gynecologist. *Current Problems in Obstetrics, Gynecology, and Fertility, 18,* 97–133.

Pennebaker, J. (1982). *The psychology of physical symptoms.* New York: Springer-Verlag.

Price, R., Cowen, E., Lorion, R., & Ramos-McKay, J. (1989). The search for effective prevention programs: What we learned along the way. *American Journal of Orthopsychiatry, 59*, 49–58.

Ramey, E. (1982). The natural capacity for health in women. In P. Berman & E. Ramey (Eds.), *Women: A developmental perspective* (pp. 3–12). (NIH Publication No. 82-2298). Washington, DC: U.S. Department of Health and Human Services.

Risch, H., Howe, G., Jain, M., Burch, J., Holowaty, E., & Miller, A. (1993). Are female smokers at higher risk for lung cancer than male smokers? *American Journal of Epidemiology, 5*, 281–293.

Roels, H. A., Balis-Jacques, M. N., Buchet, J. P., & Lauwerys, R. R. (1979). The influence of sex and of chelation therapy on erythrocyte protoporphyrin and U-ALA in lead exposed workers. *Journal of Occupational Medicine, 21*, 527–539.

Rothblum, E. (1994). "I only read about myself on bathroom walls": The need for research on the mental health of lesbians and gay men. *Journal of Consulting and Clinical Psychology, 62*, 213–220.

Russo, N. (1985). *A national agenda to address women's mental health needs.* Washington, DC: American Psychological Association.

Sato, A., Nakajima, T., Fujiwara, Y., & Murayama, N. (1975). Kinetic studies on sex difference in susceptibility to chronic benzene intoxication with special reference to body fat content. *British Journal of Industrial Medicine, 32*, 321–328.

Skolnick, A. (1986). *The psychology of human development.* San Diego: Harcourt Brace Jovanovich.

Smith, E., Johnson, S., & Guenther, S. (1985). Health care attitudes and experiences during gynecologic care among lesbians and bisexuals. *American Journal of Public Health, 75*, 1085.

Steil, J. (1984). Marital relationships and mental health: The psychic costs of inequality. In J. Freeman (Ed.), *Women: A feminist perspective* (pp. 113–123). Palo Alto, CA: Mayfield Press.

Strickland, B. (1988). Sex-related differences in health and illness. *Psychology of Women Quarterly, 12*, 381–399.

Tobin, J., Wassertheil-Smoller, S., Wexler, J., Steingart, R., Budner, N., Lense, L., & Wachspress, J. (1987). Sex bias in considering coronary bypass surgery. *Annals of Internal Medicine, 107*, 19–25.

Travis, C. (1988). *Women and health psychology.* Hillsdale, NJ: Lawrence Erlbaum Associates.

U.S. Bureau of the Census. (1990). *Statistical abstracts of the United States: 1990* (110th ed.). Washington, DC: Author.

Verbrugge, L. (1989). The twain meet: Empirical explanations of sex differences in health and mortality. *Journal of Health and Social Behavior, 30*, 282–304.

Waldron, I. (1988). Gender and health related behavior. In D. Gochman (Ed.), *Health behavior: Emerging research perspectives* (pp. 193–208). New York: Plenum Press.

Wingard, D. (1984). The sex differential in morbidity, mortality, and lifestyle. *Annual Review of Public Health, 5*, 433–458.

Wingard, D., Cohn, B., Kaplan, G., Cirillo, P., & Cohen, R. (1989). Sex differentials in morbidity and mortality risks examined by age and cause in the same cohort. *American Journal of Epidemiology, 130*, 601–610.

World Bank. (1991). *World development report, 1991.* Washington, DC: Author.

CHAPTER 11

Smoking and Cardiovascular Disease Risk in Women
Issues for Prevention and Women's Health

MARGARET A. CHESNEY AND JILL B. NEALEY

Recent years have seen increased attention to women's health. Within this relatively new field, topics range from conditions that are unique to women such as menopause to coronary heart disease, which is the leading cause of death among women. The role of gender in the etiology, diagnosis, treatment, and prevention of disease is far more than that of a sociodemographic variable that simply mediates the effects of other factors on outcome. Gender is a dynamic construct that interacts with psychological, social, physical, and behavioral factors in influencing disease risk, expression, course, and prognosis. Health-related behaviors, such as smoking, are embedded in the complex network of psychological, social, physical, and behavioral factors that differ for men and women. Understanding risks to women's health and the behaviors that contribute to this risk is like studying a mosaic. It is necessary to step back and view the behavior in context; only then can we see the full picture and effectively intervene to prevent disease.

In this chapter on women's health, we will focus on smoking, the single most preventable cause of morbidity and mortality in women today.

MARGARET A. CHESNEY • School of Medicine, University of California, San Francisco, San Francisco, California 94061.   JILL B. NEALEY • Department of Psychology, University of Utah, Salt Lake City, Utah 84112.

Handbook of Diversity Issues in Health Psychology, edited by Pamela M. Kato and Traci Mann. Plenum Press, New York, 1996.

Not only is smoking a significant risk factor, but it provides an excellent illustration of the importance of studying health-related behaviors in context. In the first section, we discuss prevalence rates for smoking among adult and adolescent women, drawing contrasts with men. In the second section, we describe the health consequences of smoking for women, focusing on cardiovascular disease. In the third section, we review the complex dynamic influences of psychological, social, physiological, and behavioral factors on smoking among women. In the final section, we offer suggestions for interventions and discuss the implications for health policy.

SMOKING PREVALENCE AMONG ADOLESCENT AND ADULT WOMEN

Smoking prevalence was first recorded by the National Cancer Institute in 1955, when it was determined that 24.5% of American women and 52% of American men smoked (United States Department of Health and Human Services [USDHHS], 1988). While the prevalence of smoking among males has steadily decreased from that first estimate, the rate of smoking among women rose to a high of 40% in 1977, before beginning its decline (USDHHS, 1989). Alarmingly, the most recent estimates available for smoking prevalence have shown that smoking among women may once again be on the rise, having increased from 22.8% (21.6 million) in 1990 to 23.5% (22.2 million) in 1991 (Centers for Disease Control and Prevention [CDC], 1993). This estimate represents an increase of 600,000 of American women who smoke cigarettes. Approximately one-third of these women can be expected to die prematurely from tobacco-related causes.

After decades of men having a higher prevalence of smoking than women, there is a convergence in the rates of smoking between the sexes (Biener, 1988). This shift in trends is due to both a lower rate of smoking cessation and a higher rate of smoking initiation among women compared to men (Chesney, 1991). The next section will review these differential rates of cessation and initiation.

Smoking Cessation Rates Lower among Women Than among Men

Most evidence indicates that the rate at which women stop smoking is lower than that for men (Harris, 1983; Remington et al., 1985). The percentage of male former smokers compared to female former smokers is higher for every age group between 25 and 65, but lower for people between 20 and 24 (USDHHS, 1989). For example, in a study of 50- and 60-year-old men and women who were identified as heavy smokers at adolescence, 63% of the men had quit smoking versus only 27% of the women (Clausen, 1982). In addition, of those people who had not quit, 25% of the women never attempted quitting compared with just 6% of the men.

While the majority of studies point to higher cessation rates among men, not all studies have observed this differential (Waldron, in press). Jarvis (1984) has also pointed out that higher cessation rates among men do not take into account the numbers of men who have switched to other forms of tobacco use (i.e., smokeless tobacco, cigars, pipes, snuff). When former smokers who had switched to other forms of nicotine were reclassified as smokers, the discrepancy in the quit ratio between males and females was diminished from 8.6 to 2.2 percentage points. Even with this reappraisal, the rate of smoking cessation is still increasing at a faster rate in men than it is in women. Reasons underlying these different rates will be discussed later in this chapter.

Smoking Initiation Rates Higher among Women Than among Men

The rates at which adolescent and young adult women and men initiate smoking is alarming. It is estimated that 3,000 new smokers are recruited in the United States each day (Pierce, Fiore, Novotny, Hatziandreu, & Davis, 1989). The majority of these new smokers are young, as indicated by the fact that 87% of smokers started smoking before the age of 18 (CDC, 1993). Smoking prevention programs to combat these striking rates of smoking initiation are conducted in high schools, targeting juniors and seniors. Between 1976 and 1981, the percentage of high school seniors who smoked declined from 29% to 20%, but little decline has occurred since that time (USDHHS, 1989). According to a 1993 report on approximately 50,000 high school students from across the United States (USDHHS, 1993), 29.9% of high school seniors had smoked within the last 30 days, and 19.0% smoked daily. Contrary to rates for adults, the prevalence of smoking among adolescent girls is greater than or equal to that among boys. Higher rates among girls were first observed in 1976 (Gilchrist, Schinke, & Nurius, 1989). These differences between girls and boys continued until 1988 when the gender differences in prevalence rates seemed to level off (USDHHS, 1993).

Women have started smoking at progressively younger rates. For women smokers born between the years of 1935 and 1939, 76% started smoking before reaching the age of 20. For women born between 1960 and 1964, this number rises to 84% (USDHHS, 1989). Not only is the age of initiation decreasing, but the number of female smokers classified as heavy smokers is increasing. From 1965 to 1985 the percentage of women smokers who smoke more than 25 cigarettes a day rose from 13% to 23% (Stoto, 1986).

THE CONSEQUENCES OF SMOKING

Cigarette smoking is a major cause of morbidity and mortality among women. It is associated with increased risk for cardiovascular disease, cancer, and chronic obstructive pulmonary disease. Smoking exacts a further toll in its adverse impact on reproductive health. These adverse consequences of smoking will be reviewed in this section. It is important to note that cigarette smoking is a core behavior that correlates with other risk behaviors (Castro, Newcomb, McCreary, & Baezconde-Garbanati, 1989). Compared to nonsmokers, smokers often show patterns of unhealthy behaviors including excessive alcohol and coffee consumption, nonuse of seat belts, and more frequent drunk driving episodes (Carmody, Brischetto, Matarazzo, O'Donnell, & Connor, 1985). There are established social traditions that support these patterns of risk behavior, as demonstrated by the fact that bars and taverns are among the few public places in communities to permit smoking, reinforcing the association between smoking and alcohol consumption.

The burden of smoking on health is assessed in terms of increased rates of diseases and reduced quality of life. The burden of smoking is also felt indirectly. It is estimated that across their lifespan, smokers use the health care system 50% more than nonsmokers (Chesney, 1991). Cigarette smoking is also associated with reduced productivity. Compared to nonsmokers, smokers have higher rates of absenteeism and shorter work days. That is, smokers work an average of 30 minutes less per day, devoting this lost time to smoking breaks and integrating smoking with work tasks (Luce & Schweitzer, 1978; Shimp, 1986). Thus the total costs and consequences of smoking among women as well as men extend from individual health to the welfare of social groups.

Smoking and Cardiovascular Disease

Smoking is one of the most significant risk factors for cardiovascular disease, the leading cause of death for women and the condition responsible for approximately one-half of all deaths in the United States. Smoking one pack of cigarettes a day is estimated to increase one's risk of coronary heart disease by two and one-half times the rate for nonsmokers (USDHHS, 1983). For example, in a study of female nurses between 30 and 55 years of age by Willett and colleagues (Willett, Hennekens, Bain, Rosner, & Speizer, 1981), the rate of myocardial infarction for smokers was found to be three times greater than that experienced by women who had never smoked. In another study, the association between smoking and myocardial infarction in 4,397 women under age 50 were evaluated. The risk of myocardial infarction for smokers was found to be 5.5 times that experienced by nonsmokers (Rosenberg et al., 1983). It is estimated that in the absence of other risk factors, 70% of myocardial infarction among women under 50 are attributable to smoking (Slone et al., 1981).

Cigarette smoking was found to be associated with the extent of coronary occlusion in female heart disease patients (Barboriak, Anderson, & Hoffmann, 1984). The mean occlusion score for women who smoked one or more packs a day for 20 years was almost twice that found for nonsmoking women. Again, this difference was more pronounced in women under the age of 50. In addition, smoking poses a greater risk for coronary occlusion in women than it does in men (Chesney, 1991). Smoking among women is also associated with adverse events following coronary artery bypass surgery, including early mortality (i.e., death less than 30 days postsurgery). The relative risk for early mortality was 5.6% in women, and 2.4% in men (Ramstrom et al., 1993).

There is growing evidence of a synergistic effect of concurrent smoking and oral contraceptive (OC) use on development of cardiovascular disease (Salonen, 1982; Stadel, 1981). Use of OC among nonsmoking premenopausal women increases the risk of fatal coronary heart disease two-fold, whereas among women who smoke, OC use raises the risk 13-fold (Jonas, Oates, Ockene, & Hennekens, 1992). The potentially beneficial use of hormone replacement therapy (HRT) in postmenopausal women may also be negated by smoking. The protective effect of HRT for prevention of first-time occurrence of myocardial infarction (MI) has been reported to extend only to nonsmokers (Mann, Lis, Chukwujindu, & Chanter, 1994). The odds ratio for first MI for nonsmokers was 0.70 and 1.05 for smokers.

Smoking also increases cardiovascular disease risk by lowering the age of onset of menopause. Epidemiological data suggest that the naturally occurring estrogen levels found in premenopausal women reduce risk for cardiovascular disease. It is estimated that smoking causes women to reach spontaneous menopause 1 to 2 years earlier than normal. This increase in onset of menopause has been shown to be dose-dependent, with heavy smokers having the earliest onset at 48, moderate smokers at 49, and nonsmokers at the average age of 50 years (Jick, Porter, & Morrison, 1977). Thus cigarette smoking indirectly increases risk for cardiovascular disease by lowering the age of menopause and removing the presence of these protective hormones (Hartz et al., 1987; Kannel & Thomas, 1982).

Smoking and Lung Disease

The risk associated with coping for morbidity and mortality extends far beyond its effects on cardiovascular disease. Of particular public health significance, smoking is a major cause of lung cancer, the leading cause of cancer deaths among women in the United States. It is estimated that well over 150,000 people died of lung cancer in 1994. Among these, approximately one third were women. The rate of lung cancer deaths in both men and women has risen steadily since it was first recorded in 1950, and while the death rate due to lung cancer is still higher in men, a convergence in the rates for men and women are predicted to mirror that which is occurring in rates of smoking (Russell & Epstein, 1988). Similar patterns exist for laryngeal cancer, which has also been linked to cigarette smoking. Chronic obstructive pulmonary disease (COPD), a condition resulting from chronic damage to the lungs (Harris, 1983), is significantly associated with smoking. Like the death rate due to lung cancer, the number of deaths attributable to COPD is on the rise. Also, as with lung cancer, the decreasing death rate for COPD among men compared with the increasing rate in women provides dramatic evidence of the adverse consequences of smoking on women's health.

Smoking and Reproductive Health

Smoking is associated with increased rates of spontaneous abortion, reduced fertility, increased rates of fetal and neonatal deaths, and a greater incidence of premature birth (Feng, 1993; Russell & Epstein, 1988). Perhaps the most documented consequence of smoking during pregnancy is on fetal birth weight, with children born to smoking mothers weighing an average 200 grams less than those born to nonsmoking mothers (USDHHS, 1980). Recent research also documents adverse effects on newborn children from nonsmoking mothers who are exposed to "secondhand" or "passive" smoke (i.e., ambient cigarette smoke exhaled by a smoker living in their environment; Eliopoulos et al., 1994).

MOTIVATIONS FOR SMOKING INITIATION AND MAINTENANCE: BARRIERS TO CESSATION

As evidence of the dangers of smoking increases and social pressure against smoking mounts, why does smoking among women continue? The answer to this question is complex and multidimensional. In this section, we will address the motivations underlying smoking from four perspectives: psychological, social, behavioral, and physiological. It is important to note that these four perspectives are not mutually exclusive but rather create a dynamic context surrounding the initiation of smoking, attempts to quit, and the struggle to maintain smoking cessation.

Psychological Motivations: The Effect of Negative Affect

It has been proposed that some women continue to smoke in an effort to control emotional discomfort, tension, and stress (Ockene, 1993). The link between these indexes of negative affect and smoking is not new.

Both laboratory and self-report studies have consistently shown that smokers smoke more when under stress. These findings have led to the belief that smoking is a coping mechanism for managing stress. Investigators have found that women, more than men, report smoking in response to negative affect (Livson & Leino, 1988; USDHHS, 1980; USDHHS, 1989). The specific reasons for the negative affect and smoking among women are not clear. Compounding this association, women report more problems coping with stress than men (Grunberg, Winders, & Wewers, 1991) and have been observed to have fewer alternatives for coping with negative affect than men (Brandon, Tiffany, Obremski, & Baker, 1990). If smoking is a coping mechanism for managing stress, the combination of women reporting smoking in response to negative affect more often than men, and women having fewer alternatives for coping may contribute to women's lower cessation rates.

Negative affect is also a precursor to smoking relapse (Marlatt & Gordon, 1980; Shiffman, 1982). A survey of smokers who had relapsed or felt "at risk" for relapse revealed that 71% of all smoking crises were brought about by negative affect (Shiffman, 1982). Similarly, Brandon et al. (1990) reported that 66% of cessation lapses occurred during negative affect states. Specific mood states reported by participants included anxiety, anger, and depression (Shiffman, 1982).

Associations between negative mood and relapse led to the assumption that stressful events lead to negative moods, which in turn trigger relapse. In a study investigating this relationship, stressful events were not found to lead to relapse (Hall, Havassy, & Wasserman, 1990). Rather, this study confirmed that higher levels of negative moods (independent of stress) and more physical symptoms predict relapse. Smokers' expectations regarding their ability to deal with stress in the absence of nicotine and their beliefs about the stress-reducing capabilities of smoking predict relapse (Shadel & Mermelstein, 1993). Those with high expectations about their ability to handle stress without the use of nicotine have a lower chance of relapse, whereas those with strong beliefs about the coping benefits of smoking are more likely to relapse. This finding is supported by evidence that former smokers who did not relapse had higher coping resources than those who did relapse (Bliss, Garvey, Heinhold, & Hitchcock, 1989). Unfortunately, these studies did not examine differential effects of gender.

Depression, as an important component of negative affect, is associated with smoking and failure at smoking cessation (Hall, Munoz, Reus, & Sees, 1993). Studies using the Center for Epidemiologic Studies Depression (CES-D) scale to measure depression find significant associations between the level of depression and prevalence of smoking (Anda et al., 1990; Perez-Stable, Marin, Marin, & Katz, 1990). Consistent with this finding, individuals with a history of major depressive disorder are over-represented in smoking cessation trials (Glassman et al., 1988; Hall et al.,

1993). For instance, studies evaluating depression among clients entering a smoking treatment clinic found lifetime prevalence rates for major depressive disorder ranging from approximately 30% to 45% (Hall, Munoz, & Reus, 1990; Hall, Munoz, & Reus, 1991), while lifetime expectancy of major depressive disorder is approximately 20% in women and 10% in men (Kaplan & Saddock, 1988).

Studies of adolescents suggest that depressed mood is both a current correlate and a precursor to smoking. Specifically, the association between depression and smoking is observed among adolescents who are smokers (Covey & Tam, 1990), and depressed mood assessed during adolescence also predicts smoking 9 years later (Kandel & Davies, 1986). Research is needed to examine the extent to which these associations are influenced by gender, particularly given the evidence of the link between negative affect and smoking among women.

For some time, the research literature on smoking has emphasized the importance of psychological characteristics, other than depression, in the initiation, persistence, and cessation of smoking. Low self-esteem, anxiety, and anger have been shown to predict failure in cessation and a tendency among former smokers toward relapse (Hall et al., 1993). Early investigations focused on neurotic behavior as a hallmark of smokers (Eysenck, 1973; Guilford, 1966). Those who typically begin and maintain smoking were reported to be extroverted, anticonformist, and rebellious (e.g., Barefoot, Dodge, Peterson, Dahlstrom, & Williams, 1989; Spielberger, 1986). In a recent study, data collected on a sample of college men revealed that higher levels of impulsiveness, sensation seeking, and hostility predicted smoking more than 2 decades later. Conversely, low hostility scores during college were associated with success in smoking cessation (Lipkus, Barefoot, Williams, & Siegler, 1994). Unfortunately, similar longitudinal studies have yet to be undertaken with women.

Smoking and Social Norms for Thinness

Social norms have a significant impact on smoking by women. The influence of the women's movement (USDHHS, 1989) and changes in the acceptability of women as smokers are cited as key factors in the sustained prevalence of smoking among women. Advertising has played on the associations of smoking to lower weight and independence in an effort to maintain and build a market for cigarette use among women.

Recent research has revealed that the fear of weight gain is an important barrier to smoking cessation in both men and women (Grunberg, 1986). Given our culture's preoccupation with thinness in women (Ogden, 1992) it is not surprising that women use smoking as a strategy to control weight (Klesges & Klesges, 1988). This is particularly true of adolescent girls and young adult women. Approximately one-fourth of the smokers in a high school sample (Camp, Klesges, & Relyea, 1993) and one-third of those in a college sample (Klesges & Klesges, 1988) specifically stated that they use smoking to control weight. Women made up the majority in both of these weight-concerned groups.

Concerns about weight gain create a barrier to smoking cessation. Among former smokers, weight gain and increased appetite are often cited as causes of relapse (Klesges & Klesges, 1988; Pirie, Murray, & Luepker, 1991). Indeed, these concerns are reinforced as women gain an average of 6 pounds upon cessation of smoking (USDHHS, 1990). Women who did not return to smoking after intervention gained significantly more weight, but were less concerned about weight gain and were more physically active than women who relapsed (Streater, Sargent, & Ward, 1989). Similarly, Hall and colleagues found that women who had not relapsed 1 year after a smoking cessation program had gained significantly more weight than those who relapsed (Hall, Ginsberg, & Jones, 1986). Taken together, these findings suggest that women who successfully quit smoking gain weight but are less concerned about that gain than their unsuccessful counterparts.

While many recent interventions attempt to inhibit weight gain from smoking cessation, in a recent analysis of the published studies, Perkins challenges current thinking that preventing weight gain due to smoking cessation thwarts relapse (Perkins, 1994). Perkins calls attention to the fact that the addition of weight control components to cessation interventions rarely succeeds in either maintaining lower levels of weight or in increasing rates of maintained cessation. In some instances, the additional attention to weight control increases smoking relapse (Hall, Tunstall, Vila, & Duffy, 1992; Pirie et al., 1992).

Postcessation weight gain may be unavoidable given that cessation removes the physiologic effect of nicotine on body weight (Perkins, 1994). Nicotine lowers body weight to an amount below normal by affecting metabolic rate or energy expenditure. Upon cessation, the suppression of weight by nicotine is removed and body weight returns to the presuppression, normal level. This "set point theory" is supported by evidence that smoking onset lowers weight to an amount equivalent to the gain seen by former smoker's postcessation (Noppa & Bengtsson, 1980). These findings suggest that rather than design interventions that have concurrent weight control components, it would be beneficial to help smokers understand the weight suppression effects of nicotine and to jointly establish a plan for addressing any weight gain following smoking cessation.

Smoking and Independence

The portrayal of smokers as independent, glamorous people has encouraged smoking among young women. Advertisements depict female smokers as attractive, slender, sophisticated, and emancipated. The profile of young adult and adolescent female smokers is different from that of young male smokers, and thus one would assume that females' motivations to initiate smoking would be different (Gilchrist et al., 1989; USDHHS, 1980). In recent years, surveys of young female smokers indicate that they are self-confident, social, sophisticated and extroverted, whereas young male smokers tend to be socially insecure and report using cigarettes as a display of masculinity (USDHHS, 1989).

It is evident that the tobacco industry takes these differing characteristics into account as they create motivation for smoking. Advertisements in magazines are tailored to present male smokers as masculine and female smokers as feminine, attractive, and self-confident. The success of these advertisements can be gauged by examining the impressions young people have of smokers. In a study of sixth graders, women who smoked were rated as more attractive and more desirable as friends than nonsmoking women, but men who smoked were rated as less attractive or desirable as friends (Barton, Chassin, Clark, & Sherman, 1982).

While the tobacco industry continually denies they have targeted their advertising to appeal to adolescent girls and young women, evidence of the correlation in the rise of smoking prevalence and advertisement campaigns is unmistakable. Cigarette advertising in women's magazines increased rapidly in 1967 (Warner & Goldenhar, 1992), and this increase corresponded with an immediate rise in smoking prevalence rates for women of all ages (Pierce, Lee, & Gilpin, 1994). A recent analysis of the correlation between smoking initiation by adolescent girls and advertising targeted to women showed that prevalence rates increased markedly starting in the late 1960s with the introduction of two brands of cigarettes for women (Pierce et al., 1994). Prevalence rates peaked around 1973 and finally dropped slightly in 1974, two years after the ban on cigarette advertising in the electronic media took effect. Borrowing a slogan used by one of the tobacco companies, advertising has indeed helped women "come a long way" toward equality in morbidity and mortality due to cigarettes.

Physiological Motivation: Addiction and Withdrawal

Nicotine meets the criteria for an addictive drug and as such exerts a significant role in the maintenance of smoking behavior and issues of relapse (Henningfield & Nemeth-Coslett, 1988). Nicotine positively reinforces smoking behavior through stimulation of nicotine receptors in the brain, providing immediate, rewarding consequences that elicit cravings to smoke (Hughes et al., 1984). Unfortunately, these effects go beyond the elicitation of simple cravings by forming tolerance and addiction, although some individuals are more susceptible to nicotine addiction than others. The specific mechanisms to explain these differences in susceptibility are not well understood (Pomerleau, Collins, Shiffman, & Pomerleau, 1993). Physiological differences in susceptibility to nicotine addiction may explain why one-third to one-half of the people who try cigarettes go on to become regular smokers, while the others either stop smoking or smoke intermittently (McNeil, 1991).

Two important factors seem to mediate addiction to nicotine: initial sensitivity to the drug and the development of acute pharmacodynamic tolerance. Vulnerability to nicotine dependence may be contingent upon constitutional differences in nicotine sensitivity (Pomerleau et al., 1993). According to the sensitivity model, individuals who have high innate sensitivity are thought to be more susceptible to tolerance and addiction. High sensitivity to nicotine, coupled with other factors that foster continuation of smoking behaviors (e.g., advertising campaigns, or individuals in the social environment who encourage smoking), facilitates addiction. This model, which posits an innate sensitivity to nicotine as a factor in the development of addiction, may shed light on studies showing a genetic component for smoking behavior. Hughes (1986) reviewed 18 twin studies, finding heritability rates for tobacco use ranging from 28% to 84% (with a mean of 53%).

In addition to the positively rewarding features of the physiological responses to nicotine and the impact these responses have on maintaining smoking, the physiological responses to withdrawal from smoking serves as a barrier to smoking cessation (Henningfield & Keenan, 1993). The presence of withdrawal symptoms is a well known cause of relapse following smoking cessation. While some studies show that withdrawal symptoms are more pronounced in women than men (Gritz & Jarvik, 1978; Shiffman, 1979; USDHHS, 1989), others have failed to validate such findings, by either reporting no difference between men or women (Gunn, 1986; Svikis, Hatsukami, Hughes, Carroll, & Pickens, 1986) or by indicating that withdrawal symptoms are greater in men (Pirie et al., 1991). Taken together, there is not yet a sound basis to indicate that physiological withdrawal symptoms are more severe in women than men.

Regardless of gender differences, the influential role of physiological factors in maintaining smoking behavior and creating a barrier to cessation cannot be overlooked in planning smoking cessation programs. These physiological factors are responsible for the development of various nicotine replacement strategies to aid in smoking cessation, such as the nicotine patch or chewing gum. These alternative strategies vary in the dose of nicotine they deliver. Likelihood of success using these systems may be diminished if the systems fail to deliver enough nicotine to prevent severe symptoms of nicotine withdrawal in addicted individuals.

Behavioral Motivations

By the time young people reach the seventh grade, the majority believe that smoking is dangerous to one's health (Evans, 1976). However, many adolescents between 12 and 14 years of age experiment with smoking and roughly 4% to 5% smoke regularly. Clearly, there are behavioral or social factors or both, that take precedence over adolescents' knowledge about the dangers of smoking. There are a myriad of behavioral models that can be used to explain motivations for a young person to experiment with cigarette smoking. For the sake of brevity we will discuss only two: Bandura's (1977) social learning theory and Erickson's (1963) theories of psychosocial development.

Of the behavioral models, Bandura's (1977) social learning theory is perhaps the most applicable to the processes of initiation and maintenance of smoking behavior. The processes of conditioning and imitation, which are central to this theory, are directly relevant to both the initiation of smoking behaviors and its maintenance in the face of adverse consequences. The positive and negative consequences of smoking can be conveyed through vicarious learning and used as a model for future behavior and expectation. Social reinforcement, normally in the form of peer pressure, is assumed significant for maintenance of early smoking behavior (Presti, Ary, & Lichtenstein, 1992), especially as some form of reinforcement is needed to overcome the usually negative first experience with cigarettes (Bewley, Bland, & Harris, 1974). Social cues often provide the appropriate stimulus conditions to facilitate smoking maintenance after an individual's smoking patterns have been established. Events such as coffee breaks or gatherings in social settings elicit and reinforce continued smoking behavior (Castro et al., 1989). These behavioral inducers are significant barriers to cessation efforts.

Theories about stages of psychosocial development may also be important in smoking initiation. Adolescence is a time characterized by conflicts and identity formation. These conflicts may explain why role models shift from parents and teachers (who are exhorting the dangers of smoking) to peers (who are seen to reject parental norms). The advertising agencies have emphasized this theme by creating coupons that can be redeemed for items that reinforce a peer uniform, such as leather jackets and hats, all carrying a cigarette logo.

Also relevant to the discussion of theories of behavioral motivation is the awareness that people's perceptions regarding their vulnerability to disease affects their health behavior (Chesney, 1993). Evidence indicates that women today are primarily concerned about breast cancer and do not know that heart disease is their leading cause of death (Gallup Organization, 1994). If women underestimate their risk for lung and heart diseases, it is unlikely that they will pay attention to prevention messages or alter behaviors that, while putting them at risk, also have reinforcing value in terms of weight, stress, and image.

IMPLICATIONS FOR INTERVENTION

Interventions to prevent initiation of smoking and foster smoking cessation among women are clearly a top priority in health psychology and medicine. That behavioral and biomedical scientists have focused considerable research and intervention efforts on smoking for decades with little headway suggests that we need to change our approach (Leventhal & Cleary, 1980). Most interventions have only a 10% to 25% success rate, measured at 6 months to a year after the intervention (Lando & McGovern, 1985; Ockene, Hymowitz, Sexton, & Broste, 1982). The data presented in this chapter indicate that we might improve these rates by addressing smoking from a multidimensional, contextual perspective, rather than seeking a single mechanism or key to change. Moreover, the gender differences in initiation and cessation rates, social influences, and motivational factors indicate that this new contextual perspective must take gender into account.

Prevention of Smoking Initiation among Women

Efforts to prevent initiation of smoking should address the psychological motivations, social influences, physiological effects, and behavioral consequences of smoking. These factors encourage young people to first experiment with and later to maintain smoking. Thus behavioral interventions to prevent smoking must strive to identify strategies that neutralize these forces. One innovative program (Altman, in press) encouraged students to increase their awareness of the influences of advertising on their smoking behavior and the power of their social environments to create barriers to successful smoking cessation. In addition to enlightening the young people about these influences and barriers, the program created experiences for participants to gain confidence in their ability to shape the environment or render themselves less vulnerable to its influence. These experiences included the development of antismoking billboards to counter the advertising promoting cigarettes to young women and men, and creation of antismoking "rap" videos highlighting adverse factors about smoking that the young people identified. Given what we know about the differential factors leading to smoking among young women and men, innovative programs could be designed to specifically target issues for young women, including concerns about weight and image.

Smoking Cessation

The studies of gender differences in smoking cessation rates, reasons for relapse, and motivations to smoke suggest that smoking cessation programs should be developed specifically for women. In particular, these programs will need to grapple with barriers facing women, including weight gain and coping with negative affect. Early efforts to address these barriers by adding dimensions to interventions, including weight control programs, actually appear to have led to diminished effects (Perkins,

1994). Other strategies need to be developed and evaluated in clinical trials. Possibilities include staging of interventions. For example, a program that begins with training in alternative strategies for coping with negative affect. After the coping training is complete, the smoking cessation aspect of the program is then implemented. With alternative skills for coping, women smokers may overcome the barrier to smoking cessation created by negative affect.

Cessation Program Delivery

The majority of people who have successfully quit smoking have done so on their own (Fiore et al., 1990). Women, more than men, endorse a belief that smokers should stop smoking without the assistance of a formal program (Cappotelli & Orleans, 1985). These gender differences suggest that new venues of program delivery be explored, including the use of television or other forms of telecommunications for in-home behavior change. Such interventions could be tailored to individual reasons for reliance on cigarettes, personal motivations for change, and personalized strategies for progressing to cessation. Research on gender differences in smoking cessation strategies suggests that stepped approaches, beginning with decreased smoking, may be more effective in women, while sudden cessation may be more effective in men (Blake et al., 1989).

One of the most important targets for intervention is pregnant women. While it is estimated that 40% of smoking women stop smoking during pregnancy, postpartum relapse is high, with more than 50% of women relapsing within 3 months postdelivery and 70% by 1 year (Fingerhut, Kleinman, & Kendrick, 1990; Williamson, Serdula, Kendrick, & Binkin, 1989). These rates of relapse remain high even when special interventions for pregnant smokers have been offered (Ershoff, Mullen, & Quinn, 1989; Sexton & Hebel, 1984). The practice of returning to smoking following pregnancy illustrates the importance of understanding motivations for smoking. If a pregnant woman's primary reason for cessation is protecting her child during her pregnancy, rather than general health, she will likely return to smoking following delivery or breast feeding, particularly if she is concerned with losing weight. An opportunity for maintaining pregnancy-induced cessation may exist by emphasizing the ongoing risk to infants exposed to second-hand smoke. In addition, the higher frequency with which pregnant women and women with young children must be seen by the health care system as providing more opportunities for intervention and follow-up support.

Interventions in Primary Care

It is estimated that physicians and health care workers have contact with 70% of all smokers and 78% of all women each year (Ockene, 1993).

This means that 18 million of the 22 million annual female smokers could be reached through physician contact. Considerable research evidence has shown that physician intervention can have a significant impact on the smoking behavior of their patients (i.e., Kottke et al., 1988; Lindsay et al., 1994; Wilson et al., 1988), with the effect related to the thoroughness of the intervention (Kottke, Battista, DeFriece, & Brekke, 1988). As with other intervention strategies, the message delivered to patients is important. Cessation rates have been enhanced through a patient-centered approach tailored to personalizing risk perception and to helping women understand and disarm their own reasons for smoking (Ockene, 1993). Coordinated referrals between physicians and other medical care settings to provide assistance and reinforcement may also increase the effectiveness of physician interventions. While some physicians already discuss smoking behavior with patients, special training of physicians to present brief interventions could increase the likelihood of success (Kottke et al., 1988; Wilson et al., 1988).

POLICY AND SMOKING PREVENTION

In a society as easily lead by popular images and personalities as ours, it is important to consider the possibilities of changing some of the larger, underlying causes for smoking motivation. Society's unhealthy regard for thinness is an obvious target for such change. These values could be publicly examined and the advertising media could be encouraged to move away from promoting thinness as an ideal, in general, and the link between smoking and weight control, in particular.

As our understanding of the complexity of the issues grows, so does the need for a thoughtful, multidimensional approach. Models of the past have proven that striving to identify single mechanisms that explain smoking in all men and women will achieve only limited success. Interventions based on these models have only achieved limited success.

Successful smoking cessation for women necessitates an approach that tailors the complexities that exist among women as well as men. As we formulate interventions for women as a group, we must not allow ourselves to look at gender unidimensionally. As Russo (1987) urges, understanding the role of gender in the etiology, diagnosis, treatment, and prevention of disease requires viewing gender not just as a predictor variable, but also as a dynamic construct that varies across social class and ethnic group, and works in a complex interaction with psychological, social, physical, and behavioral factors. Smoking, other cardiovascular risk factors, and other adverse health behaviors exist in a complex network that is, as noted earlier in this chapter, like a mosaic. To understand the mosaic, we must begin by standing back to get the full picture. To change the mosaic, we must recognize the forces that maintain smoking for women and design programs that redirect these forces to support smoking cessation, improved health, and higher quality of life.

ACKNOWLEDGMENTS

The authors wish to express their appreciation to Ashley Wilder Smith for her assistance and insightful suggestions on this chapter.

REFERENCES

Altman, D. B. (in press). Strategies for community health intervention: Promises, paradoxes, pitfalls. *Psychosomatic Medicine.*

Anda, R., Williamson, D., Escobedo, L., Mast, E., Giovino, G., & Remington, P. (1990). Depression and the dynamics of smoking: A national perspective. *Journal of the American Medical Association, 264,* 1541–1545.

Bandura, A. (1977). *Social learning theory.* Englewood Cliffs, NJ: Prentice-Hall.

Barboriak, J., Anderson, A., & Hoffmann, R. (1984, March). Smoking and coronary artery occlusion in female heart patients. Presented at the American Heart Association Conference on Cardiovascular Disease Epidemiology, Tampa, FL.

Barefoot, J., Dodge, K., Peterson, B., Dahlstrom, W., & Williams, R. (1989). The Cook–Medley hostility scale: Item content and ability to predict survival. *Psychosomatic Medicine, 51,* 46–57.

Barton, J., Chassin, L., Clark, C., & Sherman, S. (1982). Social image factors as motivators of smoking initiation in early and middle adolescence. *Child Development, 53,* 1499–1511.

Bewley, B., Bland, J., & Harris, R. (1974). Factors associated with the starting of cigarette smoking by primary school children. *British Journal of Preventive and Social Medicine, 28,* 37–44.

Biener, L. (1988). Coping and adaptation. In R. Barnett, L. Biener, & G. Baruch (Eds.), *Gender and stress* (pp. 332–349). New York: Free Press.

Blake, S., Knut-Inge, K., Pechacek, T., Folsom, A., Leupker, R., Jacobs, D. R., & Mittlemark, M. (1989). Differences in smoking cessation strategies between men and women. *Addictive Behaviors, 14,* 409–418.

Bliss, R., Garvey, A., Heinhold, J., & Hitchcock, J. (1989). The influence of situation and coping on relapse crisis: Outcomes after smoking cessation. *Journal of Consulting and Clinical Psychology, 57,* 443–449.

Brandon, T., Tiffany, S., Obremski, K., & Baker, T. (1990). Postcessation cigarette use: The process of relapse. *Addictive Behavior, 15,* 105–114.

Camp, D., Klesges, R., & Relyea, G. (1993). The relationship between bodyweight concerns and adolescent smoking. *Health Psychology, 12,* 24–32.

Cappotelli, H., & Orleans, C. (1985). Partner support and other determinants of smoking cessation maintenance among women. *Journal of Consulting and Clinical Psychology, 53,* 455–460.

Carmody, T., Brischetto, C., Matarazzo, J., O'Donnell, R., & Connor, W. (1985). Co-occurrent use of cigarettes, alcohol, and coffee in healthy, community-living men and women. *Health Psychology, 4,* 323–335.

Castro, F., Newcomb, M., McCreary, C., & Baezconde-Garbanati, L. (1989). Cigarette smokers do more than just smoke cigarettes. *Health Psychology, 8,* 107–129.

Centers for Disease Control and Prevention (1993). Cigarette smoking among adult—United States, 1991. *Morbidity and Mortality Weekly Report, 42,* 230–233.

Chesney, M. A. (1991). Women, work-related stress, and smoking. In M. Frankenhaeuser, U.

Lundberg, & M. Chesney (Eds.), *Women, work, and health* (pp. 139–155). New York: Plenum Press.

Chesney, M. A. (1993). Behavioral barriers to cardiovascular health in women. In Wenger, N. (Ed.), *Women and cardiovascular disease* (pp. 55–60). New York: LaJacque Publishing.

Clausen, J. (1982). Teenage personality and smoking: Longitudinal studies. In *1982 directory: On-going research in smoking and health* (pp. 164–165). Washington, DC: U.S. Department of Health and Human Services, Public Health Service.

Covey, L., & Tam, D. (1990). Depressive mood, the single-parent home, and adolescent cigarette smoking. *American Journal of Public Health, 80,* 1330–1333.

Eliopoulos, C., Klein, J., Phan, M., Knie, B., Greenwald, M., Chitayat, D., & Koren, G. (1994). Hair concentrations of nicotine and cotinine in women and their newborn infants. *Journal of the American Medical Association, 271,* 621–623.

Erickson, E. H. (1963). *Childhood and society* (2nd ed.). New York: W. W. Norton.

Ershoff, D., Mullen, P., & Quinn, V. (1989). A randomized trial of a serialized self-help smoking cessation program for pregnant women. *American Journal of Public Health, 79,* 182–187.

Evans, R. (1976). Smoking in children: Developing a social psychological strategy of deterrence. *Journal of Preventative Medicine, 5,* 122–127.

Eysenck, H. (1973). Personality and the maintenance of the smoking habit. In W Dunn (Eds.), *Smoking behavior: Motives and incentives.* Washington, DC: Winston.

Feng, T. (1993). Substance abuse in pregnancy. *Current Opinion in Obstetrics and Gynecology, 5,* 16–23.

Fingerhut, L., Kleinman, J., & Kendrick, J. (1990). Smoking before, during, and after pregnancy. *American Journal of Public Health, 80,* 541–544.

Fiore, M., Novotny, T., Pierce, J., Giovino, G., Hatziandreu, E., & Newcomb, P. (1990). Methods used to quit smoking in the United States: Do cessation programs help? *Journal of the American Medical Association, 263,* 2760–2764.

Gallup Organization (1994). *1993 Ortho women's health research poll: A national survey.* Raritan, NJ: Ortho.

Gilchrist, L., Schinke, S., & Nurius, P. (1989). Reducing onset of habitual smoking among women. *Preventative Medicine, 18,* 235–248.

Glassman, A., Stetner, F., Walsh, B., Raizman, P., Fleiss, J., & Cooper, T. (1988). Heavy smokers, smoking cessation, and clonidine: Results of a double-blind, randomized trial. *Journal of the American Medical Association, 259,* 2863–2866.

Gritz, E., & Jarvik, M. (1978). Nicotine and smoking. In L. Iverson, S. Iverson, & S. Snyder (Eds.), *Handbook of psychopharmacology* (pp. 426–464). New York: Plenum Press.

Grunberg, N. (1986). Behavioral and biological factors in the relationship between tobacco use and body weight. In E. Katkin & S. Manuck (Eds.), *Advances in behavioral medicine* (pp. 97–129). Greenwich, CT: JAI Press.

Grunberg, N., Winders, S., & Wewers, M. (1991). Gender differences in tobacco use. *Health Psychology, 10,* 143–153.

Guilford, J. (1966). *Factors related to a successful abstinence from smoking: Final report.* Washington, DC: U.S. Public Health Service, Division of Chronic Diseases, Bureau of State Services.

Gunby, P. (1994). Legal challenge to medically correct smoking bans. *Journal of the American Medical Association, 271,* 577.

Gunn, R. (1986). Reactions to withdrawal symptoms and success in smoking cessation clinics. *Addictive Behaviors, 11,* 49–53.

Hall, S., Ginsberg, D., & Jones, R. (1986). Smoking cessation and weight gain. *Journal of Consulting and Clinical Psychology, 54,* 342–346.

Hall, S., Havassy, B., & Wasserman, D. (1990). Commitment to abstinence and acute stress in relapse to alcohol, opiates, and nicotine. *Journal of Consulting and Clinical Psychology, 58,* 175–181.

Hall, S., Munoz, R., & Reus, V. (1990). Smoking cessation, depression and dysphoria. In L. Harris (Ed.), *Problems of drug dependence 1990: Proceedings of the 52nd Annual Scientific Meeting: The Committee on Problems of Drug Dependence, Inc* (pp. 502–504). Rockville, MD: National Institute on Drug Abuse.

Hall, S. M., Muñoz, R. F., & Reus, V. I. (1994). Cognitive behavioral intervention increases abstinence rates for depressive history smokers. *Journal of Counseling and Clinical Psychology, 62,* 141–146.

Hall, S., Muñoz, R., Reus, V., & Sees, K. (1993). Nicotine, negative affect, and depression. *Journal of Consulting and Clinical Psychology, 61,* 761–767.

Hall, S., Tunstall, C., Vila, K., & Duffy, J. (1992). Weight gain prevention and smoking cessation: Cautionary findings. *American Journal of Public Health, 82,* 799–803.

Harris, J. (1983). Cigarette smoking among successive birth cohorts of men and women in the United States during 1900–80. *Journal of the National Cancer Institute, 71,* 473–479.

Hartz, A., Kelber, S., Borkowf, H., Wild, R., Gillis, B., & Rimm, A. (1987). The association of smoking with clinical indicators of altered sex steroids: A study of 50,145 women. *Public Health Reports, 102,* 254–259.

Henningfield, J., & Keenan, R. (1993). Nicotine delivery kinetics and abuse liability. *Journal of Consulting and Clinical Psychology, 5,* 743–750.

Henningfield, J., & Nemeth-Coslett, R. (1988). Nicotine dependence: Interface between tobacco and tobacco-related disease. *Chest, 93,* 37S–55S.

Hughes, J. (1986). Genetics of smoking: A brief review. *Behavior Therapy, 17,* 335–345.

Hughes, J., Hatsukami, D., Pickens, R., Krahn, D., Malin, S., & Luknic, A. (1984). Effect of nicotine on the tobacco withdrawal syndrome. *Psychopharmacology, 83,* 82–87.

Jarvis, M. (1984). Gender and smoking: Do women really find it harder to give it up? *British Journal of Addiction, 79,* 383–387.

Jick, H., Porter, J., & Morrison, A. (1977). Relation between smoking and age of natural menopause. *Lancet, i,* 1354.

Jonas, M., Oates, J., Ockene, J., & Hennekens, C. (1992). Position statement: Statement on smoking and cardiovascular disease for health care professionals. *Circulation, 86,* 1664–1669.

Kandel, D., & Davies, M. (1986). Adult sequelae of adolescent depressive symptoms. *Archives of General Psychiatry, 43,* 255–262.

Kannel, W., & Thomas, H. (1982). Sudden coronary death: The Framingham study. *Annals of the New York Academy of Sciences, 383,* 3–21.

Kaplan, H., & Saddock, B. (1988). *Synopsis of psychiatry: Behavioral sciences, clinical psychiatry.* Baltimore: Williams and Wilkins.

Klesges, R., & Klesges, L. (1988). Cigarette smoking as a dieting strategy in a university population. *International Journal of Eating Disorders, 7,* 413–419.

Kottke, T. E., Battista, R. N., DeFriese, G. H., & Brekke, M. L. (1988). Attributes of successful smoking cessation interventions in medical practice: A meta-analysis of 39 controlled trials. *Journal of the American Medical Association, 259,* 2882–2889.

Lando, H., & McGovern, P. (1985). Nicotine fading as a nonaversive alternative to broad spectrum tests. *Addictive Behaviors, 10,* 153–161.

Leventhal, H., & Cleary, P. D. (1980). The smoking problem: A review of the research and theory in behavioral risk modification. *Psychological Bulletin, 88,* 370–405.

Lindsay, E. A., Ockene, J. K., Hymowitz, N., Giffen, C., Berger, L., & Pomrehn, P. (1994). Physicians and smoking cessation. *Archives of Family Medicine, 3,* 341–348.

Lipkus, I., Barefoot, J., Williams, R., & Siegler, I. (1994). Personality measures as predictors of smoking initiation and cessation in the UNC alumni heart study. *Health Psychology, 13,* 149–155.

Livson, N., & Leino, E. (1988). Cigarette smoking motives: Factorial structure and gender differences in a longitudinal study. *International of Addictions, 23,* 535–544.

Luce, B., & Schweitzer, S. (1978). Smoking and alcohol abuse: A comparison of their economic consequences. *New England Journal of Medicine, 298,* 569–571.

Mann, R., Lis, Y., Chukwujindu, J., & Chanter, D. (1994). A study of the association between hormone replacement therapy, smoking and the occurrence of myocardial infarction in women. *Journal of Clinical Epidemiology, 47,* 307–312.

Marlatt, G., & Gordon, J. (1980). Determinants of relapse: Implications for the maintenance of behavior change. In P. Davidsen & S. Davidsen (Eds.), *Behavioral medicine: Changing health lifestyles* (pp. 474–482). New York: Brunner/Mazel.

McNeil, A. (1991). The development of dependence on smoking in children. *British Journal of Addiction, 86,* 589–592.

Noppa, H., & Bengtsson, C. (1980). Obesity in relation to smoking: A population study of women in Goteborg, Sweden. *Preventive Medicine, 9,* 534–543.

Ockene, J. (1993). Smoking among women across the life span: Prevalence, interventions, and implications for cessation research. *Annals of Behavioral Medicine, 15,* 135–148.

Ockene, J., Hymowitz, N., Sexton, M., & Broste, S. (1982). Comparison of patterns of smoking behavior change among smokers in the multiple risk factor intervention trial (MRFIT). *Preventive Medicine, 11,* 621–638.

Ogden, J. (1992). *Fat chance! The myth of dieting explained.* New York: Routledge, Chapman & Hall.

Perez-Stable, E., Marin, G., Marin, B., & Katz, M. (1990). Depressive symptoms and cigarette smoking among Latinos in San Francisco. *American Journal of Public Health, 80,* 1500–1502.

Perkins, K. (1994). Issues in the prevention of weight gain after smoking cessation. *Annals of Behavioral Medicine, 16,* 46–52.

Pierce, J., Fiore, M., Novotny, T., Hatziandreu, E., & Davis, R. (1989). Trends in cigarette smoking in the United States: Projections to the year 2000. *Journal of the American Medical Association, 261,* 61–65.

Pierce, J., Lee, L., & Gilpin, E. (1994). Smoking initiation by adolescent girls, 1944 through 1988. *Journal of the American Medical Association, 271,* 608–611.

Pirie, P., McBride, C., Hellerstedt, W., Jeffrey, R. Hatsukami, D., Allen, S., & Lando, H. (1992). Smoking cessation in women concerned about weight. *American Journal of Public Health, 82,* 1238–1243.

Pirie, P., Murray, D., & Luepker, R. (1991). Gender differences in cigarette smoking and quitting in a cohort of young adults. *American Journal of Public Health, 81,* 324–327.

Pomerleau, O., Collins, A., Shiffman, S., & Pomerleau, C. (1993). Why some people smoke and others do not: New perspectives. *Journal of Consulting and Clinical Psychology, 61,* 723–731.

Presti, D., Ary, D., & Lichtenstein, E. (1992). The context of smoking initiation and maintenance: Findings from interviews with youths. *Journal of Substance Abuse, 4,* 35–45.

Ramstrom, J., Lund, O., Cadavid, E., Thuren, J., Oxelbark, S., & Henze, A. (1993). Multiarterial coronary artery bypass grafting with special reference to small vessel disease and results in women. *European Heart Journal, 14,* 634–639.

Remington, P., Forman, M., Gentry, E., Marks, J., Hogelin, G., & Trowbridge, F. (1985). Current smoking trends in the United States: The 1981–1983 behavioral risk factor surveys. *Journal of the American Medical Association, 253,* 2975–2978.

Rosenberg, L., Miller, D., Kaufman, D., Helmrich, S., Vad de Carr, S., Stoley, P., & Shapiro, S. (1983). Myocardial infarction in women under 50 years of age. *Journal of the American Medical Association, 250,* 2801–2806.

Russell, P., & Epstein, L. (1988). Smoking. In E. Blechman & K. Brownell (Eds.), *Handbook of behavioral medicine for women* (pp. 369–383). Elmsford, NY: Pergamon.

Russo, N. (1987). Position paper. In A. Eichler & D. Parron (Eds.), *Women's mental health: Agenda for research.* Rockville, MD: National Institute of Mental Health.

Salonen, J. (1982). Oral contraceptives, smoking and risk of myocardial infarction in young women: A longitudinal population study in Eastern Finland. *Acta Medica Scandinavica, 212,* 141–144.

Sexton, M., & Hebel, J. (1984). A clinical trial of change in maternal smoking and its effect on birth weight. *Journal of the American Medical Association, 251*, 911–915.

Shadel, W., & Mermelstein, R. (1993). Cigarette smoking under stress: The role of coping expectancies among smokers in a clinic-based smoking cessation program. *Health Psychology, 12*, 443–450.

Shiffman, S. (1979). The tobacco withdrawal syndrome. *NIDA Research Monograph, 23*, 158–184.

Shiffman, S. (1982). Relapse following smoking cessation: A situational analysis. *Journal of Consulting and Clinical Psychology, 50*, 71–86.

Shimp, D. (1986). Nonsmokers' rights in the workplace: A new look. *American Lung Association Bulletin, 3*, 3–6.

Slone, D., Shapiro, S., Kaufman, D., Rosenberg, L., Miettinen, O., & Stolley, P. (1981). Risk of myocardial infarction in relation to current and discontinued oral contraceptive use. *New England Journal of Medicine, 305*, 420–424.

Spielberger, C. (1986). Psychological determinants of smoking behavior. In R. Tollison (Ed.), *Smoking and society: Toward a more balanced assessment* (pp. 89–134). Lexington, MA: Health & Co.

Stadel, B. (1981). Oral contraceptives and cardiovascular disease. *New England Journal of Medicine, 305*, 672–677.

Stoto, M. (1986). *Changes in adult smoking behavior in the United States: 1955 to 1983.* Cambridge, MA: Harvard University, Institute for the Study on Smoking Behavior and Policy, John F. Kennedy School of Government.

Streater, J., Sargent, R., & Ward, D. (1989). A study of factors associated with weight change in women who attempt smoking cessation. *Addictive Behaviors, 14*, 523–530.

Svikis, D., Hatsukami, D., Hughes, J., Carroll, K., & Pickens, R. (1986). Brief report: Sex differences in tobacco withdrawal syndrome. *Addictive Behaviors, 11*, 459–462.

United States Department of Health and Human Services (1980). *The health consequences of smoking for women: A report of the surgeon general.* Washington, DC: Public Health Service, Office of the Assistant Secretary of Health, Office on Smoking and Health.

United States Department of Health and Human Services (1983). *The health consequences of smoking—cardiovascular disease: A report of the surgeon general* (DHHS Publication No. PHS 84-50204). Washington, DC: U.S. Government Printing Office.

United States Department of Health and Human Services (1988). *The health consequences of smoking—nicotine addiction: A report of the surgeon general.* Washington, DC: U. S. Government Printing Office.

United States Department of Health and Human Services (1989). *Reducing the health consequences of smoking, 25 years of progress.* Washington, DC: Author.

United States Department of Health and Human Services (1990). *The health benefits of smoking cessation: A report of the surgeon general.* Rockville, MD: Author.

United States Department of Health and Human Services (1993). *National survey results on drug use from the monitoring the future study, 1975–1992.* Washington, DC: U.S. Government Printing Office.

Waldron, I. (in press). Patterns and causes of gender differences in smoking. *Social Science and Medicine.*

Warner, K., & Goldenhar, L. (1992). Targeting of cigarette advertising in US magazines, 1959–1986. *Tobacco Control, 1*, 25–30.

Willett, W., Hennekens, C., Bain, C., Rosner, B., & Speizer, F. (1981). Cigarette smoking and non-fatal myocardial infarction in women. *American Journal of Epidemiology, 113*, 575–582.

Williamson, D., Serdula, M., Kendrick, J., & Binkin, N. (1989). Comparing the prevalence of smoking in pregnant and non-pregnant women, 1985–1986. *Journal of the American Medical Association, 261*, 70–74.

Wilson, D., Taylor, D., Gilbert, J., Best, J., Lindsay, E., Willms, D., Singer, J. (1988). A randomized trial of a family physician intervention for smoking cessation. *Journal of the American Medical Association, 260*, 1570–1574.

CHAPTER 12

Masculine Gender Role Stress
A Perspective on Men's Health

MICHAEL M. COPENHAVER AND RICHARD M. EISLER

INTRODUCTION

Over the past decade there has been unprecedented interest in fostering improved health practices through lifestyle change and stress reduction. This interest is reflected in the popular literature as well as in health-related research. Whereas the burden of health-related problems was once imposed by infectious diseases, today many serious health problems result from unhealthy life styles (Baffi, Redican, Sefchick, & Impara, 1991). As interest in health research has grown, so has attention to identifying factors that make distinctive populations of individuals uniquely vulnerable to various forms of stress and illness.

One relatively recent area of intrigue is research on gender differences in prevention of illness and maintenance of well-being. While lifestyles and health behaviors affect the vitality of all individuals to some extent, it is important to understand how men's and women's health is

MICHAEL M. COPENHAVER and RICHARD M. EISLER • Department of Psychology, Virginia Polytechnic Institute and State University, Blacksburg, Virginia 24060.

Handbook of Diversity Issues in Health Psychology, edited by Pamela M. Kato and Traci Mann. Plenum Press, New York, 1996.

affected by the distinctive ways in which each sex experiences, reacts to, and copes with life's stressors. Increasingly, work in the fields of psychology, medicine, public health, and education has begun to identify andexamine factors that may underlie differential vulnerabilities of men and women to various health problems.

There is growing empirical evidence of the deleterious effects of masculine gender role scripts on men's health. In reviewing the mortality rates of both sexes throughout the life span, Harrison, Chin, and Ficarrotto (1989) concluded that biological factors alone could not explain the shorter life expectancy of men relative to women subsequent to childhood. Interestingly, Waldron and Johnson (1976) had previously estimated that 75% of the sex difference in life expectancy could be accounted for by high-risk behaviors including smoking, alcohol abuse, and propensity toward violent or dangerous activities. These high-risk behaviors are consistent with men's gender roles.

As an indication of the enormity of sex differences in stress-related physical health, one need only examine large-scale measures including premature mortality, lethal illness, and hazardous life-styles (Cleary, 1987; Harrison et al., 1989; Levant, 1990). In the United States, men live approximately 7 fewer years, on average, than do women. The rate of death is higher for men than women at all ages and in all leading causes of death (Verbrugge, 1985). Some of these data suggest that gender-related lifestyles may underlie the differential death rates. For example, between the ages of 15 and 24, men die at three times the rate of women, largely because of the higher rates of violent deaths (e.g., accidents, homicide, suicide) among males during this time of life (Cleary, 1987). Further, Waldron and Johnson (1976) presented statistics showing that men die of lung cancer nearly six times as often as women, and die of cirrhosis of the liver twice as often as women, suggesting that relatively greater smoking and drinking among men accounts for the increased male death rates. Men also have approximately double the rate of death due to heart disease than women.

Thus of the seven leading causes of premature death among men, it could be argued that all appear directly or indirectly related to acquired psychosocial characteristics associated with the masculine gender role. For instance, men's higher rates of coronary artery disease have been attributed to greater numbers of male smokers and the lethal aspects of the Type A coronary-prone behavior pattern associated with masculinity (e.g., anger and competitiveness). In addition, men show significantly greater incidence of cirrhosis of the liver due to alcohol abuse. More men drink alcohol than women, and more importantly, more men than women drink to excess by a ratio of 4:1 (Cahalan, 1970). It seems likely that heavy alcohol consumption serves as a manifestation of the masculine toughness and as a coping strategy that does not violate male norms. Thus the relative excess of male deaths due to cirrhosis of the liver from alcohol abuse is not surprising given this context.

With respect to general lifestyle issues, men are socialized to engage in more high-risk employment (e.g., fire fighting) and high-risk leisure activities (e.g., bungee cord jumping) to validate their masculinity. High-risk activities may contribute significantly to the higher male death rates in accidents of all kinds (Harrison et al., 1989; Waldron & Johnson, 1976). Finally, the greater vulnerability of males to death by suicide or homicide may be interpreted, in part, as a result of the male predisposition to masculine action-oriented coping strategies such as physical aggression and violence.

A number of epidemiologists and mental health researchers have examined the relationship between gender and the vulnerability to various mental health problems (Cleary, 1987; Franks & Rothblum, 1983; Widom, 1984). Robins et al. (1984) conducted a large-scale epidemiological study to examine the lifetime prevalence rates of DSM–III psychiatric disorders. The results indicate that men, in contrast to women, were far more prone to antisocial personality disorder and drug and alcohol abuse.

Other researchers (e.g., Widom, 1984) have cited evidence that men are much more involved than women in violent crime including armed robbery, spouse and child abuse, and rape. Based on these findings, it appears that men possess a lower threshold for aggressive coping responses than do women. Interestingly, although aggression and coercive use of force are regarded as repugnant in the commission of criminal acts, violence and aggressive behavior are applauded in other contexts including sports contests, military operations, and business competitions. Thus much of the social program of masculine behavior for men requires the use of culturally sanctioned male coping styles of competitiveness, aggressiveness, and an offensive rather than a cooperative approach to solving problems.

By virtue of their gender role socialization, men have learned to rely on coping behaviors that may increase their risk of injury, ill health, and early mortality. It is therefore necessary to examine how specific "masculine" gender role attitudes and behaviors may contribute to men's health problems. Advances in this area of health psychology will allow researchers and practitioners to better educate the public and to develop prevention and intervention strategies specifically tailored to the health needs of men.

The present chapter provides a discussion of how the construct of masculinity relates to men's health issues and describes recent efforts to examine the factors thought to underlie the distinctive vulnerabilities of men. In addition, suggestions are made as to how health-oriented interventions might be modified to better address men's awareness and comprehension of their health requirements.

MASCULINITY AND THE STUDY OF MEN'S HEALTH

The idea that masculine gender role socialization might predispose men to different kinds of health problems than women may be seen as an application of sociocultural and psychosocial models to the etiology of men's health disorders. Central to this notion is the individual's acquisition of either a masculine or feminine gender identity, which is enacted primarily through a masculine or feminine gender role (Franklin, 1988). For instance, many people in our culture believe that it is not masculine for men to display emotions such as fear or sadness, except on rare occasions; however, most people have little difficulty accepting as masculine a man's expression of anger.

Masculinity then, like femininity, is acquired and regulated by the individual through his or her learned beliefs and expectations. Thus becoming masculine with respect to one's thoughts, expression of one's feelings, and behavioral repertoires requires extensive sociocultural education. The development of masculinity is promoted by the developing male's interactions with adult role models, his peers, and major societal institutions. Because masculine beliefs and behaviors are so pervasive among men both within and across cultures, people are often surprised to learn that many of these beliefs and behaviors have cultural roots.

Foundation of the Masculine Gender Role Stress Paradigm

The notion that masculine traits such as dominance and competitiveness are imposed on men by the culture rather than through innate biological forces or through developmental needs was advanced by Pleck (1981) in his book *The Myth of Masculinity*. In this provocative work, Pleck asserted that there is no innate need for humans who are biologically male to develop masculine attributes. However, because men wish to obtain valued social approval and to avoid social condemnation, most men maintain displays of masculine behavior and masculine ways of coping.

Previous paradigms of sex role development held that development of masculine attributes in males was essential for their mental health and psychological adjustment. To counter the "masculinity is healthy for men" argument, Pleck (1981; 1995) asserted and refined what he termed the gender role strain paradigm (GRS). In this model, Pleck outlined some of the dangers of believing that masculinity is inherently desirable and healthy for men. For example, the masculine ideas that men should not give in to pain or should be able to consume large quantities of alcohol have provided obvious health risks for large numbers of young men eager to prove their masculinity.

The implications of Pleck's (1981; 1995) work for our gender role stress theory can be summarized as follows: (a) men have been externally

directed by societal expectations to live up to culturally imposed definitions of masculinity, (b) the struggle to attain these masculine characteristics may frequently have undesirable health consequences for many,
if not most, men and (c) the routine deployment of masculine strategies
for managing life's problems may produce dysfunctional solutions and
emotional distress for many men.

In an attempt to explain how some men within a given culture become
strongly "sex-types," Bem (1981) introduced the notion of gender schema
to describe a way of processing information according to gender dichot-
omies defined by one's culture. She proposed that sex-typed masculinity
originates from a man's tendency to encode and organize information
about the world and himself in terms of his culture's definitions of male-
ness and femaleness. Thus a person's self-concept becomes interwoven
with culturally approved, sex-typed distinctions.

Bem's (1981) gender schema theory implies that sex-typed (masculine or feminine) attitudes and behaviors are learned as one processes
information primarily according to society's mandates of what is appropriate for one's own sex. For example, the adults in a child's world may
seldom note how *nurturantly* a little boy behaves or how *stoically* a little
girl behaves. As a result of such influences, the male child quickly learns
to behave in ways that are largely consistent with his male gender schema
(stoically rather than nurturantly). Although it may seem natural for men
to develop masculine attributes, recent research (e.g., Eisler & Skidmore,
1987; Eisler, Skidmore, & Ward, 1988; Lash, Eisler, & Schulman, 1990)
suggests that for many men, adherence to the traditional masculine
schema may lead to increased feelings of anger and stress, and in turn, to
poor health outcomes.

Masculine Gender Role and Men's Stress

Appraisal theories of stress help to clarify the ways in which men and
women differ in their evaluation of events as stressful. These theories are
based on the notion that a person's cognitive appraisal of threat (Lazarus,
1991) is the pivotal mechanism that links environmental events to emotional arousal, and, if prolonged, to stress. Lazarus and colleagues (Lazarus & Folkman, 1984; Lazarus, 1991) developed a model of stress appraisal, emotional arousal, and coping that is particularly relevant to
gender and stress. According to these investigators, the interaction between one's cognitive appraisal of the situation combined with the evaluation of one's ability to cope with the situation defines the stress process.

Gender ideology may influence one's appraisal of a situation as being
either challenging or threatening. The belief that one has the ability or
skill to deal with a threat will result in less perceived stress than the belief
that one is not up to the task. Thus if a man, in accord with his masculine
gender ideology, believes that he is not equipped to deal with a crying

infant, he will experience greater stress than a woman who believes that she can. On the other hand, if a person believes that gender should confer an ability that is perceived as lacking, the person will experience stress if he or she does not live up to the gender script. Take the case of a man who believes that a man should be able to find his way around a strange city by himself. This man will feel stress if he perceives himself as lost, because being unable to find one's way is not masculine. An additional gender violation of needing help will produce additional stress. A woman under no such gender-based constraints will experience less stress because being lost in a strange city is not a violation of femininity, and because she can easily cope with the situation by asking for help. In this way, learned gender appraisals about what is expected according to one's sex can produce stress beyond the difficulties of the situation itself.

A Consolidated Masculine Gender Role Stress Paradigm

Borrowing from Bem's theory that gender role schema predispose men to view the world through masculine-tinted cognitive lenses, from Pleck's (1995) view that culturally imposed masculinity predisposes men to masculine gender role strain, and from Lazarus and Folkman's (1984) views about the crucial role of cognitive appraisal in stress reactions, we have developed the following propositions that help explain the development of masculine gender role stress and how it may lead to health problems in men.

1. The sociocultural contingencies that reward masculine attitudes and behaviors while punishing nonmasculine attitudes and behaviors result in the development of masculine gender role cognitive schemata in the vast majority of males. These schemata, reinforced by peers and adult role models, eventually operate independently through a self-evaluation process in which a child says to himself, "This is a good (i.e., masculine) way for me to behave."
2. Masculine schemata are then employed by men in varying degrees to appraise threats and challenges from the environment as well as to evaluate and guide their choice of coping strategies. Masculine schemata guide the selection of men's responses from a restricted range of male-sanctioned alternatives. Thus when challenged, for example, men are more likely to display aggression than to employ cooperative responses.
3. Based on their disparate experiences, there are important differences among men as to how committed they are to culturally accepted models of masculinity. At one extreme, men may be so committed to masculinity that they believe that violence against women and children is necessary in various circumstances. At the other end of the scale, some men have relinquished their commit-

ment to masculinity by choosing to stay at home and raise their children.

4. Masculine gender role stress may arise from excessive commitment to and reliance upon culturally approved masculine schemata. Some highly committed men may experience severe loss of self-esteem from losing in a competitive game; others who are less committed to masculine values are able to cope with the loss by feeling that they played well.

5. Masculine gender role stress may also arise from the belief that one is not living up to culturally sanctioned masculine gender role behavior. Men may experience stress if they feel that they have acted in an unmanly fashion.

FACTORS UNDERLYING DIFFERENTIAL HEALTH PROBLEMS IN MEN

The above formulation of masculine gender role stress suggests that men have a higher risk of developing certain kinds of health problems based on masculine lifestyles and behaviors. However, it should be noted that men who exhibit certain "socially desirable" masculine traits are not necessarily at high risk for physical or mental health problems. Instrumental behaviors such as being assertive, decisive, and acting independently may contribute to positive health behaviors for both sexes. Nevertheless, there is growing evidence (e.g., Good & Mintz, 1990; Eisler & Skidmore, 1987; Eisler et al., 1988; Lash, et al., 1990) that some men's adherence to certain aspects of culturally approved masculinity may be unhealthy and stress producing. In this section, we investigate the particular areas of masculine ideology and behaviors that are likely to promote health-related problems in men.

Eisler and Skidmore (1987) conducted a factor analytic study of masculine gender role stress, as measured by the Masculine Gender Role Stress Scale (MGRSS). The results indicate several components of masculinity that can lead to stress. First, many men place tremendous emphasis on being able to prevail in situations that require physical strength and physical fitness. Being perceived as weak or sexually below par is a major threat to self-esteem for many men. Second, men tend to become distressed by women who they perceive to be equal or superior to them in traditional masculine domains such as competitive activities or earning capacities. Third, it is important for men to view themselves as supremely decisive and self-assured. Men value acting in a rational as opposed to an emotional manner because the latter is seen as feminine and ineffective. Fourth, many men are committed to external performances; that is, they wish to be perceived as triumphant in the areas of work achievement and sexual prowess. Finally, many men feel uncomfortable in situations that require expression of tender emotions because doing so is perceived as a major violation of traditional masculine norms.

Masculine Gender Role Stress and Cardiovascular Reactivity

Positive associations found between Masculine Gender Role Stress scores and measures of anger arousal and blood pressure led researchers (e.g., Eisler & Skidmore, 1987; Skidmore, Eisler, Blalock, & Sikkema, 1988; Lash et al., 1990) to hypothesize that a high predisposition to masculine gender role stress, as measured by the MGRSS, may be associated with cardiovascular disease processes. There has been much conjecture that men's greater cardiovascular reactivity to stressors was primarily a function of biological differences between men and women. However, some studies (e.g., Van Egeren, 1979) have shown that when women are placed in certain kinds of stressful situations, they exhibit similar or even greater cardiovascular reactivity than men. Thus researchers have speculated that reactions to particular situations may sometimes be a function of gender differences in men's versus women's cognitive appraisal of these situations as stressful (Jorgenson & Houston, 1981; Polefrone & Manuck, 1987). As discussed below, a number of seminal studies have shed light on the connection between masculine gender role stress and cardiovascular reactivity in men.

In one study (Skidmore et al., 1988), MGRSS scores were compared with physiological measures of subjects' cardiovascular responses to pain via exposure to the cold pressor stress test, a test during which the subject places his hand in ice water for a period long enough to generate acute pain. The magnitude of increases in blood pressure and heart rate response were used as measures of the men's reactivity to this stressor. In addition to the physical stress of the cold pressor test, high-, medium-, and low-scoring MGRSS subjects were subjected to the masculine threat interview, a psychologically stressful interview by a female confederate who frequently challenged the subject's masculinity. Interestingly, results indicated that there was a linear relationship between masculine gender role stress (MGRSS scores) and systolic blood pressure reactivity to both the pain and to the masculine threat interview. There was a progressive increase in blood pressure reactivity associated with higher MGRSS scores. The stress of both physical pain and psychological threat had very similar effects. Thus the nature of the challenge, whether physical or psychological, was less important than the subject's tendency to appraise the situation as a threat to his masculine competence. In this study, both the implied ability to withstand pain and the masculine threat interview could be viewed as masculine relevant challenges. However, it is possible that men who are high in masculine gender role stress (high MGRSS) are simply more highly reactive to all stressors than are men who are low in masculine gender role stress, even if the threats are not relevant to masculinity. Therefore, the researchers looked at the stress responses of high and low MGRSS men to situations that differed in threats to masculinity.

In the follow-up study, Lash et al. (1990) exposed both high-MGRSS and low-MGRSS men to the cold pressor test under different gender-relevant instructions. In the high-masculine challenge condition, subjects were told that the cold pressor was a test of their strength and endurance, and in the low-challenge condition, subjects were told that the investigator was simply interested in looking at their physiological responses to cold water. As expected, results showed no differences in cardiovascular reactivity between high- and low-MGRSS scorers for the low-masculine challenge condition. However, for men in the high-masculine challenge condition, large differences in reactivity emerged, with high-scoring MGRSS men showing much greater blood pressure both prior to and during immersion in the cold water. High-MGRSS men exhibited more stress than low scorers only when confronted with a challenge to their masculinity.

In this context, it appears that MGRSS measures a tendency for some men to appraise environmental challenges in terms of whether or not they threaten the individual's masculine self-image. Outside of the laboratory, however, it remains to be determined what situations are most likely to cause stress in men predisposed to perceive events that reflect on their masculine adequacy or performance.

Masculine Gender Role Stress and Anger

Do men who are highly concerned about masculine adequacy and performance also tend to experience excessive anger? Our research thus far has shown a consistent relationship between masculine gender role stress scores and measures of anger. This is congruent with research on Type A behavior patterns, which have shown that negative emotional states, such as impatience and hostility, are associated with Type A health risk (Price, 1982). Goldfried and Friedman (1982), in discussing Type A behavior patterns, refer to such masculine schemata as "learned invulnerability." In their view, learned invulnerability is a male schema containing beliefs that a man must vigorously cope with any and all obstacles without revealing any of his fears or doubts. Similarly, O'Neil (1981) suggests that anger, hostility, and rage result from men's repression of feminine values, attitudes, and behaviors. The frustrations that result from men's learned inability to reveal or express these feelings may lead to greater levels of anger in men compared with women. In turn, this may explain why men tend to use anger as a response to stress and as a coping device.

Masculine Gender Role Stress and Emotional Inexpressiveness

One of the most powerful masculine mental frameworks influencing men is the strict prohibition against emotional expressiveness. This, we believe, results in men's perceptions that interpersonal situations involving emotional expressiveness, often with women, are stressful. The reluctance of many men to be emotionally expressive restricts the range of their coping strategies and impairs the success of their relationships. Research reported by Eisler (1995) and O'Neil, Good, and Holmes (1995) revealed that men have extraordinary difficulties with the expression of feelings of love, compassion, fear, and hurt. In addition, this research found that men are comparably troubled by having to cope with the emotional expressions of others.

In a related vein, Pennebaker, Hughes, and O'Heeron (1987) developed a theory, with some empirical support, that inhibition of unpleasant emotions may produce chronic nervous system arousal and psychosomatic health problems. To test this hypothesis, Pennebaker et al. (1987) had college undergraduates of both sexes self-disclose traumatic events. Although the data were not analyzed for sex differences, they did show that high self-disclosers had consistently lower arousal (skin conductance) following disclosure than did low self-disclosers. In a follow-up study, Pennebaker, Kiecolt-Glaser, and Glaser (1988) required undergraduates to write about either traumatic experiences or superficial topics over a 4-day period; measures of immune functioning and health center visits served as dependent variables. Interestingly, the results indicated that students in the self-disclosure of traumatic events condition had a higher lymphocyte immune system response and fewer health center visits than did students in the control condition. These studies seem to indicate that the masculine characteristic of inhibiting emotional expressiveness surrounding painful or stressful events may have adverse effects on health.

Emotional Inexpressiveness, Relationship Issues, and Social Support

Lazarus and Folkman (1984) have suggested that the ability to obtain social support is a form of coping competence, and that the availability of social support in time of stress will depend on how well the individual has cultivated his or her social resources prior to the time of crisis. Social support has been hypothesized to buffer the impact of stressors (Enkenrode & Gore, 1981). The degree of perceived social support is positively related to physical and mental health outcomes (Husaini, Neff, Newbrough, & Moore, 1982; Sarason, Shearin, Pierce, & Sarason, 1987).

As might be expected, men's tendency toward emotional inexpressiveness is thought to adversely affect a range of interpersonal relationships. It is axiomatic that the expression of affection, warmth, sympathy, and tenderness are essential to the development of intimate and caring relationships. Research suggests that men find it difficult to be expressive in intimate arrangements, including marriage. Fitzpatrick and Indvick (1982) reported that husbands in couples with both traditional and non-traditional communication styles perceived themselves as generally incapable of discussing or expressing their feelings.

There is also evidence that women must take on the responsibility of expressing emotion in relationships (Rusbult, Johnson, & Morrow, 1986). Relationships between men and women may break down because women have the sole responsibility for the emotionally expressive aspects of the relationship. Because men tend to deny their needs for emotional support from their partners, they may find it difficult to find and utilize emotional support in close relationships.

Studies on gender variation and social support have consistently shown that women have more close friends, perceive that they have more available sources of support, are more likely to request emotional support when they need it, and are more likely to offer emotional support to others (Butler, Giordano, & Neren, 1985; Dunkel-Schetter, Folkman, & Lazarus, 1987). In fact, recent evidence suggests that lack of social support may have more of an impact on the development of stress-related disorders in men than women. Seeman and Syme (1987) found that social network support was significantly related to lesser degrees of coronary atherosclerosis in men, but not women. In addition, level of social support has been found to be inversely related to coronary artery disease in Type A individuals, but not in Type B individuals (Blumenthal et al., 1987).

Differential Health Practices of Men

In addition to differences in physical and mental health issues, there are also substantial differences between men and women in terms of the ways in which each manages health requirements. There is no question that men, like women, need a variety of preventive and therapeutic health care services; however, men tend to utilize such services less than women. For example, researchers (e.g., Verbrugge, 1985) have found that women consistently visit the doctor more than men, even when women's reproductive-related visits are excluded. Further, after analyzing data from the National Medical Care Expenditure Survey, Cafferat, Kasper, and Bernstein (1983) found that women were almost twice as likely as men (15.5% vs. 8.1%) to have obtained psychotropic drugs. This is often interpreted to mean that women experience higher levels of distress. However, an equally valid interpretation is that current gender roles make it less acceptable for men to acknowledge morbidity and ask for help by utilizing health services during early stages of illness. Adding to this, others (e.g., Waldron & Johnson, 1976) have suggested that men also are not sufficiently attuned to their own internal warning signals of illness; that is, men seem to have greater difficulty identifying and processing emotional states (Levant, 1990).

Once aware of illness, men are much more resistant to adopting the "sick role" leading to their seeking health care (Marcus & Seeman, 1981; Woods & Hulka, 1979). Men's resistance to the sick role may be due to their tendency to view the sick role as submissive, dependent, and power-less, and therefore an unmasculine role. To make matters worse, physicians, the majority of whom are men, may foster the traditional masculine gender role health behaviors by their reluctance to identify men as "ill" relative to women. Researchers report that physicians are more likely to label women as "mentally ill" because, in this perspective, women are seen as weaker, more emotional, and less able to manage stress than men (McCauley, Stitt, & Segal, 1980). If this is the case, it would not only perpetuate the traditional masculine gender role but it would also dis-courage men from utilizing health services as means of coping with stress and managing their mental health.

Further supporting this notion, Baffi et al. (1991) report that college males with an androgenous gender role identity engaged in preventive health behaviors significantly more often than did those with more mas-culine gender role identities. In addition, Good, Dell, and Mintz (1989) recently found that traditional attitudes regarding the male role were significantly related to negative attitudes toward seeking and utilizing psychological health services. Men who are strongly committed to a tradi-tional masculine lifestyle appear to be more likely to underutilize avail-able health care systems.

HEALTH-RELATED INTERVENTION STRATEGIES FOR MEN

Based on our previous analysis, we believe that health interventions are misguided if not impossible without viewing individuals within the context of their gender and cultural roles. Men appraise, experience, and cope with stressors differently than women, and they manage stress-related health problems differently. Therefore, health interventions for men must take gender into consideration if they are to be most effective. Traditional helping relationships, regardless of therapeutic orientation, typically require some amount of patient subordination to the mental or physical health "expert," and this subordination is likely to be resisted to varying degrees by most male patients. Based on experience with male patients in a psychological services environment, we would like to suggest a number of alternative tactics and procedures that may ameliorate some of the male gender role related obstacles that seem to prevent men from fully utilizing health-related services.

Consciousness Raising

When working with men either individually or in groups, consciousness raising can be a vital first step in addressing their presenting problems. Thus, it is important to raise questions about the man's wholesale acceptance of traditional masculine values as his own. For instance, most men may have never questioned their socially conditioned assumptions that men must be strong, rational, and responsible under all circumstances. During the intake phase of psychological or medical treatment, when male patients show difficulty discussing their discouragement, fears, or lack of control over events, the tactic of emphasizing the appropriateness and normality of expressing these emotions can be implemented. Many men find it extraordinary that other men have ever experienced similar doubts or fears. This gives testimony to the code of silence most men observe when it comes to sharing their vulnerability with other males.

Often the next stage of consciousness raising, following reassurance that a man's masculinity is not in jeopardy, is to challenge his preconceived notions of what a man should be or what man must do. In one case at our clinic, a middle-aged man presented for sexual counseling after being persuaded to do so by his wife who saw her sexual desires increasing while her husband's desires were waning. This man had labeled his lack of sexual arousal as "impotence" due to aging and had sought medical evidence to support this interpretation. Consciousness raising consisted of pointing out that he, like most men, is not *always* in the mood for sexual opportunities and, in fact, has the right to postpone sexual encounters or suggest alternative ways of expressing affection. This was found to be an effective way of challenging the patient's rigid interpretation of the problem situation. Thus, it is important during consciousness raising to help men evaluate the pros and cons of rigidly adhering to what a man must do.

Modeling Self-Disclosure

Another important part of treating men's health-related problems is helping them feel more comfortable self-disclosing their problems and concerns. Self-disclosure is important because self-revelation provides the helping professional much needed information about the details and context of the patient's problem. Self-disclosure also signals the health worker that the patient is willing and able to accept the needed help in a collaborative fashion. This, in turn, makes the health worker more motivated to extend himself or herself in helping the client. Finally, releasing pent-up feelings has healing properties in itself (e.g., Pennebaker et al., 1988).

One effective way of encouraging men to disclose their concerns is for the health provider to model self-disclosure for the patient. Particularly when both the health provider and patient are male, the health provider's self-disclosure models for the patient the acceptability and potential value of honesty in self-expressive communication. The health provider's self-disclosure also promotes a safe therapeutic environment for the patient by reducing the threat of competition many men feel when attempting to relate to other men. Modeling self-disclosure has also been found effective in a psychoeducational, group therapy context in which men learn and role-play specific interaction skills that they can apply to their own problem environment (Levant, 1990). Support for modeling self-disclosure has been found in a men's anger control group (Eisler, 1994) in which men learn from therapists, and from each other, the acceptability and value of self-disclosure in dealing with issues surrounding their anger problems. By practicing self-disclosure to other males, men gain confidence and security in expressing feelings while also learning to process their problem issues on an emotional rather than strictly intellectual level. Practicing self-disclosure to other men also helps them feel more comfortable revealing personal information to their health providers.

Assignments in "Unmasculinity"

Aside from consciousness raising and increasing men's self-disclosure, it is also critical that men practice health behaviors that run counter to some of the normative masculine behaviors to which they have become so accustomed. Most men are so well practiced at stereotypical masculine behaviors and thoughts that they have difficulty generating alternatives that might be more adaptive in their everyday lives. To counter these masculine habits, we often purposely give patients assignments to behave in ways that are inconsistent with typical masculine values.

In some cases, these prescriptions are geared toward decreasing the highly instrumental nature of many men's activities; other strategies are designed to increase their responsiveness to their own and others' feelings. For example, one assignment involved asking a man to practice a feminine behavior, such as staying at home with his children when they were sick. Another assignment was to ask him to do things he had previously labeled as unimportant. In general, men whose lives are highly structured around being productive and competent at work are encouraged to engage in activities that they might enjoy, but which they might characterize as unmasculine, and thus a threat to self-esteem.

CONCLUSIONS

Although this is a relatively new area of scientific inquiry, meaningful progress has been made toward uncovering lifestyle and socialization factors that contribute to health problems typically experienced by male populations. Undoubtedly there are also important differences between men of diverse cultural and economic backgrounds that would require somewhat different prevention and intervention strategies.

Nevertheless, there appear to be significant gender-related factors that underlie men's distinctive vulnerabilities to health problems. As evidenced by various health statistics (e.g., Cleary, 1987; Harrison et al., 1989; Levant, 1990), men tend to suffer in disproportionate numbers from some mental and physical health disorders. Men are prone to experience mental health problems related to antisocial acts such as anger, violence, and substance abuse, whereas women are more likely to experience anxiety and depression (Cleary, 1987). In terms of physical health, men show a much greater tendency toward type A related illnesses such as coronary artery disease, lung cancer, and cirrhosis of the liver (Cleary, 1987; Harrison et al., 1989).

Commitment to masculine schemata that include displays of physical strength, competitiveness, emotional inexpressiveness, power, and control over the environment severely limit the ways in which men appraise, react to, and cope with life's stressors. We now believe that many of the illnesses to which men are prone may be rooted in commitment to stress-producing aspects of masculine beliefs and values. Thus health providers and researchers must find effective ways to prevent and treat such illnesses through education and modified intervention strategies that take into account gender-role beliefs and behaviors.

REFERENCES

Baffi, C. R., Redican, K. J., Sefchick, M. K., & Impara, J. C., (1991). Gender role identity, gender role stress, and health behaviors: An exploratory study of selected college males. *Health Values, 15,* 9–18.

Bem, S. (1981). Gender schema theory: A cognitive account of sex typing. *Psychological Review, 88,* 354–364.

Blumenthal, J. A., Burg, M. M., Barefoot, J., Williams, R. B., Haney, T., & Zimet, G. (1987). Social support, Type A behavior, and coronary artery disease. *Psychosomatic Medicine, 49,* 331–340.

Butler, T., Giordano, S., & Neren, S. (1985). Gender and sex role attributes as predictors of utilization of natural support systems during personal stress. *Sex Roles, 13,* 515–524.

Cafferat, G. L., Kasper, J., & Bernstein, A. (1983). Family roles, structure, and stressors in relation to sex differences in obtaining psychotropic drugs. *Journal of Health and Social Behavior, 24,* 132– 143.

Calahan, D. (1970). *Problem drinkers.* San Francisco: Jossey-Bass.

Cleary, P. D. (1987). Gender differences in stress related disorders. In R. C. Barnett, L. Biener, & G. K. Baruch (Eds.), *Gender and stress* (pp. 39–72). New York: Free Press.

Dunkel-Schetter, C., Folkman, S., & Lazarus, R. S. (1987). Correlates of social support receipt. *Journal of Personality and Social Psychology, 53,* 71–80.

Eisler, R. M. (1994). *Men's anger control group.* Group therapy program for treating men's anger-related problems. Blacksburg, VA: Virginia Polytechnic Institute and State University.

Eisler, R. M. (1995). The relationship between masculine gender role stress and men's health risk: The validation of a construct. In R. F. Levant & W. S. Pollack (Eds.), *A new psychology of men* (pp. 207–228). New York: Basic Books.

Eisler, R. M., & Blalock, J. A. (1991). Masculine gender role stress: Implications for the assessment of men. *Clinical Psychology Review, 11* 45–60.

Eisler, R. M., & Skidmore, J. R. (1987). Masculine gender role stress: Scale development and component factors in the appraisal of stressful situations. *Behavior Modification, 11*, 123–136.

Eisler, R. M., Skidmore, J. R., & Ward, C. H. (1988). Masculine gender role stress: Predictor of anger, anxiety, and health risk behaviors. *Journal of Personality Assessment, 52*, 133–141.

Enkenrode, J., & Gore, S. (1981). Stressful events and social supports: The significance of context. In B. H. Gottlieb (Ed.), *Social networks and social support* (pp. 43–68). Beverly Hills: Sage.

Fitzpatrick, M. A., & Indvick, J. (1982). The instrumental and expressive domains of marital communication. *Human Communication Research, 8*, 195–213.

Franklin, C. W. (1988) *Men and society.* Chicago: Nelson-Hall.

Franks, V., & Rothblum, E. D. (1983). *The stereotyping of women: Its effects on mental health.* New York: Springer.

Goldberger, L., & Breznitz, S. (1982). *Handbook of stress: Theoretical and clinical aspects.* New York: Free Press.

Goldfried, M. R., & Friedman, J. M. (1982). Clinical behavior therapy and the male sex role. In K. Solomon & N. B. Levy (Eds.), *Men in transition: Theory and therapy* (pp. 309–341). New York: Plenum Press.

Good, G. E., Dell, D. M., & Mintz, L. B. (1989). Male role and gender role conflict: Relations to help seeking in men. *Journal of Counseling Psychology, 36*, 295–300.

Good, G. E., & Mintz, L. M. (1990). Depression and the male gender role: Evidence for compounding risk. *Journal of Counseling and Development and Development, 69*, 17–21.

Good, G. E., & Wood, P. K. (in press). Male gender role conflict, depression, and help seeking: Do college men face double jeopardy? *Journal of Counseling and Development.*

Harrison, J., Chin, J., & Ficarrotto, T. (1989). Warning, masculinity may be dangerous to your health. In M. S. Kimmel & M. A. Messner (Eds.), *Men's lives* (pp. 296–309). New York: Macmillan.

Husaini, B. A., Neff, J. A., Newbrough, J. R., & Moore, M. C. (1982). The stress-buffering role of social support and personal competence among the rural married. *Journal of Community Psychology, 10*, 409–426.

Jorgenson, R. S., & Houston, B. K. (1981). Type A behavior patterns, sex differences, and cardiovascular responses to and recovery from stress. *Motivation and Emotion, 5*, 201– 214.

Lash, S. J., Eisler, R. M., & Schulman, R. S. (1990). Cardiovascular reactivity to stress in men. *Behavior Modification, 14*, 3–20.

Lazarus, R. S. (1991). *Emotion and adaptation.* New York: Oxford University Press.

Lazarus, R. S., & Folkman, S. (1984). *Stress, appraisal and coping.* New York: Springer.

Levant, R. F. (1990). Psychological services designed for men: A psychoeducational approach. *Psychotherapy, 27*, 309–315.

Marcus, A. C., & Seeman, T. E. (1981). Sex differences in reports of illness and disability: A preliminary test of the fixed obligations hypothesis. *Journal of Health and Social Behavior, 22*, 174–182.

McCauley, C., Stitt, C. L., & Segal, M. (1980). Stereotyping: From prejudice to prediction. *Psychological Bulletin, 87*, 195–208.

O'Neil, J. M. (1981). Gender-role conflict and strain in men's lives: Implications for psychiatrists, psychologists, and other human-service providers. In K. Solomon & N. B. Levy (Eds.), *Men in transition: Theory and therapy* (pp. 5–44). New York: Plenum Press.

O'Neil, J. M., Good, G. E., & Holmes, S. (1995). Fifteen years of theory and research on men's gender role conflict: New paradigms for empirical research. In R. F. Levant & W. S. Pollack (Eds.), *A new psychology of men* (pp. 164–206). New York: Basic Books.

Pennebaker, J. W., Hughes, C. F., & O'Heeron, R. C. (1987). The psychophysiology of confession: Linking inhibitory and psychosomatic processes. *Journal of Personality and Social Psychology, 52,* 781–493.

Pennebaker, J. W., Kiecolt-Glaser, J. K., & Glaser, R. (1988). Disclosure of traumas and immune function: Health implications for psychotherapy. *Journal of Consulting and Clinical Psychology, 56,* 239–245.

Pleck, J. (1981). *The myth of masculinity.* Cambridge: MIT Press.

Pleck, J. (1995). The gender-role strain paradigm: An update. In R. F. Levant & W. S. Pollack (Eds.), *A new psychology of men* (pp. 11–32). New York: Basic Books.

Polefrone, J. M., & Manuck, S. B. (1987). Gender differences in cardiovascular and neuroendocrine response to stressors. In R. Barnett, L. Biener, & G. Baruck (Eds.), *Gender and stress* (pp. 13–38). New York: Free Press.

Price, V. A. (1982). *Type A behavior pattern: A model for research and practice.* New York: Academic Press.

Robins, L. N., Helzer, J. E., Weissman, M. M., Orvaschel, H., Gruenberg, E., Burke, J. D., & Regier, D. (1984). Lifetime prevalence of specific psychiatric disorders in three sites. *Archives of General Psychiatry, 41,* 949–958.

Rusbult, C. E., Johnson, D. J., & Morrow, G. D. (1986). Impact of couple patterns of problem solving on distress and nondistress in dating relationships. *Journal of Personality and Social Psychology, 50,* 744–753.

Sarason, B. R., Shearin, E. N., Pierce, G. R., & Sarason, I. G. (1987). Interrelations of social support measures: Theoretical and practical implications. *Journal of Personality and Social Psychology, 52,* 813–832.

Seeman, T. E., & Syme, S. L. (1987). Social networks and coronary artery disease: A comparison of the structure and function of social relations as predicators of disease. *Psychosomatic Medicine, 49,* 341–354.

Skidmore, J. R., Eisler, R. M., Blalock, J. A., & Sikkema, K. J. (1988). *Cardiovascular reactivity in men as a function of masculine gender role stress.* Paper presented at the meeting of the Biofeedback Society of America, Colorado Springs, CO.

Van Egeren, L. F. (1979). Cardiovascular changes during social competition in a mixed motive game. *Journal of Personality and Social Psychology, 37,* 858–864.

Verbrugge, L. M. (1985). Gender and health: An update on hypothesis and evidence. *Journal of Health and Social Behavior, 26,* 156–182.

Waldron, I., & Johnson, S. (1976). Why do women live longer than men? *Journal of Human Stress, 2,* 19–29.

Widom, C. S. (1984). *Sex roles and psychopathology.* New York: Plenum Press.

Woods, N., & Hulka, B. (1979). Symptom reports and illness behavior among employed women and homemakers. *Journal of Community Health, 5,* 36–45.

CHAPTER 13

Psychotherapy with HIV-Infected Gay Men

GARY GROSSMAN

INTRODUCTION: THE PSYCHOLOGICAL IMPACT OF HIV DISEASE

HIV disease has had a profound impact throughout the world. It is a health crisis of tremendous proportions, affecting people of every background, with no foreseeable end in sight. Psychology and related disciplines have devoted substantial attention to the study and exploration of the behavioral and emotional effects of HIV infection. Research has addressed such issues as psychological and behavioral responses to HIV antibody test results (e.g., Jacobsen, Perry, & Hirsh, 1990), coping and psychological functioning (e.g., Folkman, Chesney, Pollack, & Coates, 1993), suicide risks (e.g., Marzuk et al., 1988), and psychological interventions (e.g., Markowitz, Klerman, & Perry, 1992). The psychological impact of HIV infection and disease has been well documented, and the research on effective prevention and intervention strategies continues.

HIV Disease and the Gay Community

Although HIV affects people from all walks of life, it is the gay community that has been hit the hardest in the United States. Estimates of the

GARY GROSSMAN • 2150 Sutter Street, San Francisco, California 94115.

Handbook of Diversity Issues in Health Psychology, edited by Pamela M. Kato and Traci Mann. Plenum Press, New York, 1996.

number of people with HIV infection in the United States have ranged from 1 to 2 million (Curran et al, 1988), and gay men make up the majority. In 1990 the Centers for Disease Control (CDC) estimated that 20% to 30% of gay men in the United States are infected with HIV (CDC, 1990) and as many as 50% of gay men living in large urban areas are infected (Winkelstein et al., 1987). In one way or another, every gay man is confronted with the reality of HIV and AIDS, whether or not he is infected. The psychological ramifications are numerous and complex for the HIV-positive gay man. The impact begins with the initial discovery of antibody status and continues throughout the stages of disease progression to disability and death. The gay community has been ravaged by this disease, suffering such profound loss and devastation that its culture has been irreversibly altered. As members of this community, the impact of HIV on gay men, in contrast to others who are infected, is unique and warrants special attention. To some extent, being a member of the gay community may be an asset, especially if one lives in an urban center. One then has the entire community to turn to for support, assistance, and understanding. In other ways, being gay is an added burden in which men experience multiple losses of friends and lovers, and the specter of AIDS permeates their world.

Psychotherapy and HIV

Many gay men, in response to their emotional and behavioral reactions to having HIV disease, seek assistance from psychotherapists. For some, this is the first time they seek mental health services, because they have had no prior history of emotional difficulties or mental illness. Others have had a history of psychotherapy and return to treatment to deal with the stresses associated with having HIV. In addition, there are gay men who have had a history of mental illness and who experience an exacerbation of their condition in the face of coping with HIV disease.

This chapter will focus on the psychotherapy of gay men with HIV disease, will highlight the issues that frequently arise, and will emphasize some of the unique distinctions and special needs of gay men facing this life-threatening illness.

TERMINAL ILLNESS AND PSYCHOTHERAPY

The extensive literature on death and dying, including Kubler-Ross's (1969) stage model, has contributed significantly to the effective development of self-help and professional psychosocial services for individuals with life-threatening illnesses. The research on psychotherapy with dying patients, however, has been limited. With the onset of the AIDS crisis, more attention has been paid to the process of psychotherapy with dying patients, yielding important discoveries and contributing to our understanding of the psychological impact of terminal illness (e.g., Cadwell, Burnham, & Forstein, 1994).

Over the 15 years that the medical and psychological professions have been working with HIV and AIDS patients, much as been learned about the variable course of this complex disease. The human immunodeficiency virus attacks the immune system, eventually leaving people vulnerable to infections they would otherwise easily fight off. The time between infection and appearance of symptoms can vary greatly from person to person, sometimes taking as long as 15 years. It is because of this broad variability that the psychological impact of HIV disease is unique, and the response to it should be distinguished from the response to other life-threatening illnesses.

The course of HIV disease is less predictable within an individual and more varied from person to person than is typically the case with other life-threatening illnesses. For example, an individual diagnosed with cancer is likely to receive some form of treatment soon after diagnosis. With current advances in medicine and greater attention to the more common forms of cancer, tumor detection is more likely to be early, which increases patients' likelihood of having a positive response to treatment. If patients' symptoms improve, they may then enter a remission for some period of time, often without a recurrence. If the malignancy recurs, patients undergo further rounds of treatment, to which they may or may not respond. If patients don't respond, the disease progresses along a relatively predictable course, with continuous decline. Of course, there is variability in the length of the illness, physical decline, and lifespan, but in general, there is consistency. Once patients fail to respond to treatment and the disease progresses, they do not tend to get better and, instead, gradually or rapidly approach death.

The Roller Coaster of HIV Disease

HIV disease rarely follows the same course across individuals. The manifestations of HIV are so varied that no two individuals with the disease experience the same illness. Because AIDS is a disease that destroys the immune system, people do not die from AIDS but from other opportunistic infections and diseases to which the body has become vulnerable. When cancer patients ask their doctors what to expect, physicians are able to provide them with a reasonable and fixed set of possibilities. When patients with HIV ask their doctors what to expect, there is usually no definitive response. Patients are then left to grapple with the uncertainties of their future. Because of this wide variability and the difficulty predicting the course of illness, someone with HIV may have more difficulty in coming to terms with having a terminal disease. The progression of HIV disease can be like a rollercoaster ride, with many unforeseeable ups and downs.

HIV antibody testing has been available since 1986. Initially, many gay men, the group at highest risk for infection, were reluctant to be tested, even through anonymous test sites. At that point in time, prior to the development of early-intervention strategies, many were concerned that the knowledge of having HIV would be more debilitating emotionally than not knowing and therefore resisted getting tested. In the past several years, since the introduction of antiretroviral agents, such as AZT, and other forms of early intervention, health care professional, as well as AIDS social and political activists, have recommended HIV testing. These recommendations have led to an increased number of gay men who have been tested and who now know their HIV antibody status. If positive, they will probably be in the early stages of the disease process and be symptom free.

A gay man who has discovered his HIV status at a time when he is still asymptomatic feels healthy and does not experience any subjective sense of being sick. This is an awkward time in the life of an HIV infected gay man. He knows he has a deadly virus in his system, yet he has not felt its effects. He has probably known many others in more advanced stages of disease, as well as those who have died, so he knows what lies ahead. As the disease progresses and his immune system begins to deteriorate, he may develop an opportunistic infection and suffer a serious decline in his health, experiencing severe and debilitating illness. He may feel at the brink of death and begin to grapple with the idea of dying, attempting to come to terms with the end of his life. At this point the psychological process may be similar to that of an individual with any other debilitating terminal disease. In the case of a gay male with HIV disease, however, his doctor may discover the source of the infection and treat it. The man begins to improve, to gain weight, to feel stronger, and within a couple of months feels healthy again. He goes out with friends, works out at the gym, and feels energetic and alive. The memory of being at death's door gradually recedes into the background, and he forgets that he thought he was about to die. He no longer thinks about dying, and sometimes even forgets that he has AIDS.

This is a typical scenario for a gay man with HIV and often happens several times during the course of illness. He becomes severely disabled, frail and weak, is in pain, and feels he is near death. Then he responds to treatment and has a dramatic recovery to the point where he feels healthy again and is no longer directly confronted with the possibility of dying. This process of going back and forth between grave illness and relative good health can hinder the acceptance of one's death and interfere with the necessary mourning process. Consider the case of Mr. D:

Mr. D, a 36-year-old gay man, tested positive for HIV antibodies 4 years prior to experiencing any significant symptoms. Because he had been part of a cohort of gay men in a hepatitis study from the late 1970s, he knew that he had been infected for 10 years. Up until his first bout with pneumocystis carinii pneumonia (PCP), he had felt strong, healthy, and unimpaired. He responded quickly to antibiotic treatment, and after a couple of months of infirmity, he felt like his old self again. Over the course of the next 2 years, Mr. D suffered from three more bouts of PCP, each time recovering relatively quickly. He felt reassured that his body was able to recuperate after each illness, which fostered his sense of hope that he could survive. He then began to experience recurring and resistant bronchitis, which although not life-threatening, interfered with his quality of life. Subsequently it was discovered that he had lymphoma in his lungs, and he underwent extensive chemotherapy. Over the course of this treatment, Mr. D became frail and weak, and lost a substantial amount of weight. He felt certain that he was going to die and became increasingly withdrawn and depressed. Gradually, Mr. D began to respond to treatment, developed an appetite, and was able to gain back his lost weight. This period was followed by several months of feeling as if he were healthy again. Mr. D experienced two more episodes of acute illness and physical decline followed by brief periods of health before finally dying.

Each time Mr. D became acutely ill, he came face-to-face with the reality of death and struggled to come to terms with the end of his life, a possibility that he had struggled to deny. As he recovered, however, he returned to his previous state of denial and optimism, submerging any thoughts about his death into the depths of his unconscious. Without conscious access to thoughts about dying, Mr. D was less able to proceed with his mourning process and fought against accepting the loss of his abilities and the inevitability of his death. Because his physical symptoms sometimes changed from day to day, he did not know how to think of his experience. He was not sure whether he was fighting to live or fighting to die. The unpredictable course of HIV disease fostered Mr. D's system of denial and prevented him from sufficiently adjusting to his illness.

The Impact of Age

Although cancer and other life-threatening illnesses can strike at any age, terminal illness is typically associated with older people. In contrast, the majority of people dying from AIDS in the United States are young gay men. Because of his youth the individual who has HIV, as well as his friends and family, are then faced with an additional element that complicates the psychological terrain: the need to come to terms with death and dying in someone who has yet to live a full life. Although coping with death is difficult for anyone, regardless of age, it is, perhaps, somewhat easier to accept if the individual who is dying is elderly and has had the opportunity to live a full life.

Young gay men are forced to confront life circumstances usually associated with old age. Having a lover with AIDS often means that one must care for an adult who is no longer able to attend to his own personal and physical needs. Tending to partners with compromised mental capabilities and making decisions about such things as home health care versus skilled nursing facilities are becoming typical problems for gay men. Surviving multiple losses through the deaths of friends and lovers has become commonplace among gay men in their 30s and 40s. This experience is not expected for most people until more than 30 years later.

Unlike the person facing death late in life, the young gay man with HIV cannot reflect on his long life and console himself with the knowledge that he has lived a rich and full life. He is more likely to feel that he has been cut down in his prime. Kubler-Ross (1969) identifies anger as a typical stage in the mourning process, common in people with terminal disease. When older people are dying, they must come to terms with the loss of life and what was. For younger people who are dying, they must also confront the loss of what might have been. They may feel that they have been robbed of their future. This feeling can lead to a greater sense of rage that may further complicate and impede the mourning process.

PSYCHOTHERAPISTS WORKING WITH HIV

For the past 10 to 13 years, psychotherapists who treat gay men have had to incorporate issues surrounding HIV into their practice. In treating gay men with HIV disease, therapists will be faced with unusual circumstances that may challenge the very structure of the psychotherapy. Decisions will need to be made about what to do if a patient is hospitalized or homebound. Can the psychotherapy continue? Will the patient still gain some benefit from being in therapy? If the patient is unable to come to the therapist, will the therapist go to the patient? What if the patient begins to experience cognitive impairment due to dementia? These are some of the dilemmas that therapists working with HIV patients will face and that require difficult decisions.

When therapists choose to work with gay men, it is important that some thought be given to the reality of HIV disease. Therapists must recognize, accept, and be prepared for the possibility of having patients who are infected. Whether their patients' HIV status is known at the onset of therapy or not, it is important that therapists make informed decisions and recognize the complexities and challenges in the treatment of people with HIV. For therapists who choose to treat gay men with HIV, preparation is essential. Therapists will need to be aware of and attend to their own feelings, attitudes, and values about some emotionally charged issues, such as death, sexual orientation, and AIDS. These are issues that people have strong feelings and opinions about, and therapists will be better able to help their patients if they explore in depth their own attitudes ahead of time. In addition to understanding the emotional component, therapists who choose to do this work also have an obligation to be informed about HIV disease and the resources that are available in their community.

Homophobia and Heterosexual Bias in the Therapist

Each of us has been raised in an environment that is biased against homosexuality and hostile toward homosexuals. Everyone growing up in this culture, whether gay, straight, or bisexual, will internalize some degree of this dominant attitude. Therefore, psychotherapists, regardless of sexual orientation, will have some degree of homophobia (DeCrescenzo, 1984). Although *homophobia* literally means fear of homosexuality, it is a term generally used to describe any bias against homosexuality or attitude rejecting homosexuality as a viable alternative lifestyle. Psychotherapists' biases against homosexuality have been documented in several studies (American Psychological Association [APA], 1991; Garfinkle & Morin, 1978; Morin & Charles, 1983). It is, therefore, essential for therapists who undertake the treatment of gay men to recognize their biases and preconceived notions about homosexuality (Graham, Rawlings, Halpern, & Hermes, 1984). Even therapists who come from liberal backgrounds and are consciously accepting of gay people may still harbor unconscious prejudices against homosexuality. It is only through self-awareness and a willingness toward self-exploration that therapists can recognize their biases and minimize the influence of those biases on the therapy. In an extensive APA study on psychotherapists' biases toward gay and lesbian patients, the Committee on Lesbian and Gay Concerns (CLGC) found numerous occurrences of inappropriate treatment of gay and lesbian patients, including identifying homosexuality as a sickness, discouraging the expression of the patient's sexuality, and minimizing the significance of sexual orientation (APA, 1991). The CLGC concluded that a substantial number of practitioners were in violation of the APA's ethical principles of unbiased treatment and cross-cultural sensitivity and that education and training in gay and lesbian issues was necessary to address this problem (APA).

GENERAL ISSUES FOR PATIENTS IN ALL STAGES OF HIV DISEASE

The progression of HIV disease follows several stages, from early infection without symptoms to the development of illness to end-stage AIDS and death. People with HIV will be faced with a unique set of concerns at each stage of the disease. In addition, there are general issues that therapists and patients will confront regardless of disease progression, including the need for medical monitoring, emotional expression, addressing internalized homophobia, self-destructive behavior, and suicide.

Medical Monitoring

For the individual who is infected with HIV, regular health checkups with a primary care physician are strongly recommended and are extremely valuable in the management of the disease. With advances in HIV medicine, it has become increasingly possible to extend the life span of the infected individual, particularly when prophylactic measures are used. As scientists and doctors have learned more about the disease process, they are able to recognize those points at which an HIV-infected person becomes vulnerable to particular life-threatening infections, and they can begin preventative measures at that time.

Although most patients will have an existing relationship with a primary care physician and are having regular checkups, some patients, for various psychological and emotional reasons, will avoid medical attention when they are feeling healthy. A therapist may need to intervene to help a patient attend to his medical health needs.

> Mr. A, a 26-year-old gay man, had tested positive for HIV 2 years ago but had not yet consulted with his physician. In discussing this situation with his therapist, he insisted that consulting his physician was unnecessary until he began to feel sick. The therapist discovered that Mr. A was poorly informed about HIV disease and unaware of the benefits of early intervention. In addition, both Mr. A and his therapist became more aware of the underlying fear and anxiety that Mr. A had been struggling to avoid. Being able to talk with his therapist about his fears of what the doctor might discover helped Mr. A recognize what he was avoiding. This awareness enabled him to address his anxieties and to seek preventative measures.

Multiple emotional and psychological factors influence the ways an individual will cope with HIV disease. Helping a patient to discover and understand these factors can facilitate the patient in making more informed decisions.

Establishing professional contact with the patient's physician is important for the therapist. Although communication between therapist and physician need not be frequent or extensive, it can be very helpful in making an accurate assessment of the patient and in developing an appropriate treatment plan. For example, if a patient presents with acute psychiatric symptoms such as depression, mania, or psychosis, it is crucial to rule out medical factors. It is also helpful for the therapist to have a general assessment of the patient's current health and the status of his immune system. Knowing a patient's helper T cell count, for example, can provide some degree of prediction for the onset of symptoms[1]. Having an awareness of the patient's stage of HIV infection can also help

[1]The helper T cell is one type of T cell that functions in conjunction with other white blood cells as part of the immune system response. For the purpose of brevity, all references to T cells in this chapter are to helper T cells. The normal helper T-cell range in a healthy individual is from 500 to 1500 (Krowka, 1993). T-cell monitoring provides a useful measurement of immune system functioning. T cells falling below 200 results in a diagnosis of AIDS, and at this level the individual is particularly vulnerable to opportunistic infections.

the therapist assess a patient's response to his illness, including his coping style and the appropriateness of his actions. For example, a patient with a T cell count of 800 who believes he will die within the year and begins to talk about leaving his job to travel can be helped to see the inappropriateness of his reaction. At the other end of the continuum, an asymptomatic patient with less than 100 T cells who has yet to make preparations for disability can be helped to recognize his avoidance of the inevitable. If the therapist is unaware of the patient's stage of disease, assessing the patient's reactions will be difficult.

Therapy as a Place to Express Emotions

Discovering that one is HIV positive and living with that knowledge leads to a full range of emotional reactions, which are often intense and frightening, and, for many, may feel overwhelming and intolerable. Each individual has his own way of coping with such emotions, and many people strive to defend against experiencing their feelings, believing that they must be avoided or kept in check. People will also vary in their ability to manage strong emotions. Some people are better able to tolerate intense feelings and express them in a manner that is contained and modulated. Others are not as well equipped and may experience loss of control over their emotions, responding impulsively, explosively, or becoming immobilized.

Regardless of how an individual manages his emotional reactions to having HIV, therapy becomes a place where the patient can experience and express them. For the patient who is struggling not to feel, who believes he has to avoid his sadness, fear, or rage, the therapist can help the patient discover that he does not have to ignore or deny this part of his experience. The process of warding off the intense affect associated with knowing one has a life-threatening illness may help the individual to cope with the devastating realities of death and dying.

Defense mechanisms are a part of the personality that enable the individual to function by warding off painful emotion. If a defense mechanism is too rigid, however, it can leave the individual cut off from vital aspects of his self and can interfere with effective coping. For example, a patient with low T cells who effectively defends against feeling anxiety might decide to quit a job he has held for 10 years. As a result, he loses his long-term disability benefit and leaves himself vulnerable to financial insecurity. Had he been aware of feeling anxious about becoming disabled, he might have chosen to remain in his current position, or would have made alternate arrangements for financial support. For the person with HIV disease, to be rigidly cut off from his emotional reactions also leaves him at a disadvantage in coping with his grief. The therapist's ability to empathize with the patient's feelings and his or her capacity to tolerate the intensity of the affect can help the patient come to terms with the enormity of his emotional experience. It is not unusual to hear that when a person attempts to share his feelings with a friend or family member, the response is often, "Oh, don't feel that way, everything will be okay." The HIV positive person knows that everything will not be okay, and typically ends up feeling discounted or misunderstood, and may resolve to keep his feelings to himself.

At times, the individual's thoughts and feelings may be of an intensity of content that are confusing and difficult to express to loved ones. In the following two cases, therapy functions as a place that allows feelings of all kinds to be expressed, demonstrating that they can be tolerated.

> Mr. H, a 36-year-old gay man in advanced stages of AIDS, had reached the point of being homebound, too fragile and weak to leave his apartment. His mother, with whom he was very close and generally open, came to take care of him. Over the weeks that his mother was staying with him, Mr. H became increasingly discouraged and despairing, thinking daily about death. He was in significant pain and greatly impaired physically. He revealed to his mother his wish to die, to be out of his misery. His mother responded sharply, saying he shouldn't talk like that, that it wasn't right, and that he would be fine once the doctors find out why he was losing so much weight. Therapy then became the only place where he could talk about his fears and his wishes without being censored or having to worry about the reactions of his family and friends, who were not yet ready to accept his imminent death.
>
> Mr. C, a 33-year-old gay man, tested positive for HIV 2 years ago. He had put off getting tested for many years, believing that he could not cope with knowing he was HIV positive. He had a complete physical at the time that he was tested and his T cell count was hovering around 100. Although he was asymptomatic, at his physician's recommendation he had regular checkups every 6 weeks and began antiviral and prophylactic treatments. He was compliant with all of his doctor's recommendations but insisted that he no longer wanted to know the results of his blood tests or any other medical exams. He would follow his doctor's orders but did not want to know anything, thereby maintaining an illusion that everything was okay. Gradually, Mr. C became severely depressed and withdrawn. He stopped socializing with friends and would, instead, isolate himself in his apartment when not at work. He began missing work, feeling too lethargic to get out of bed some mornings. He eventually sought therapy at the urging of his physician. In therapy, Mr. C expressed his belief that he could not handle knowing about his illness. He could not let himself think about it or experience his feelings associated with having AIDS. It became evident that his depression and withdrawal was a result of his efforts to not know. To keep his thoughts and feeling from himself, Mr. C had to completely shut down and shut out the world. It also became clear that Mr. C was maintaining a state of misery as a means of protecting himself from a deeper sense of grief. To allow himself to enjoy his life while still able would mean there would be more to give up when he became ill and debilitated. If he was miserable, Mr. C realized, then there would be much less to lose in dying. Underlying this position was his belief that he could not cope with the grief he would experience if he was consciously aware of how much he would be giving up.

By approaching patients with the attitude that emotions are acceptable and tolerable, regardless of what they are and whether they are pleasant or painful, the therapist can help to foster an environment in which the patient can begin to experience the full range of affect associated with having HIV.

Internalized Homophobia

When a gay man enters therapy, regardless of the initial reason that he sought treatment, he will eventually address his feeling about being homosexual. For some, this may come in the form of asserting their acceptance of their homosexuality and comfort with their lifestyle. For others, feelings of doubt, negativity, guilt, shame, or regret may emerge. Although many gay men may feel that they have come to terms with their homosexuality in the process of coming out, traces of internalized homophobia often remain (Malyon, 1982). Regardless of the extent to which an individual has confronted his attitudes, beliefs, and feelings about his homosexuality and has consolidated a positive gay identity, there always exists some degree of identification with the dominant culture and its antihomosexual bias. The process of coming to terms with being HIV positive will frequently prompt the resurfacing of unresolved negative feelings about being gay (Isay, 1989). For some men this surfacing may take the form of feelings of guilt and self-blame for becoming infected and may cause strong negative attitudes toward homosexuality to reemerge.

Confronting negative feelings about being gay can complicate the process of adjusting to having HIV. In therapy, it is important to address these feelings and help the patient understand their origin.

> Mr. D, a 32-year-old African-American gay man sought therapy approximately a year after testing positive for HIV. His T cells were above 800, and he was in good general health. Because he was raised Catholic and grew up in the South, he struggled for many years before finally accepting that he was gay and coming out to himself and select friends. Although he was close with his immediate family, his parents and siblings did not know that he was gay, and he stated that he did not have any intention of telling them. He insisted that he was "fine" about being gay, but that he didn't think his family would understand. Mr. D was also very reluctant to reveal to friends that he was HIV positive and was even apprehensive about revealing his HIV status to his therapist. Gradually it emerged in therapy that the shame that Mr. D felt about being infected was very closely tied to his underlying belief that there was something very wrong about being gay. With embarrassment, he disclosed his belief that homosexuality was a sin and a sign of degeneracy. He blamed himself for becoming infected.

It is not unusual to hear a gay man express the thought, "If only I had been straight, this never would have happened to me ...," which can fuel self-blame and feelings of shame and guilt. In order to best facilitate the patient's adjustment to being HIV positive, the therapist must be attuned to the emergence of unresolved conflicts about homosexuality and help the patient to address them.

Self-Destructive Behavior

When working with HIV-positive patients, therapists need to be on the lookout for increased likelihood of self-destructive behaviors. This may be especially true for patients who have had difficulty accepting their homosexuality and who continue to harbor feelings of self-hatred or shame about being gay. Such behaviors are difficult to detect and are not necessarily recognized as dangerous by the patient.

Substance Abuse

A common behavior that is especially harmful in patients with compromised immune systems is substance abuse. Research has pointed to an increased incidence of substance abuse within the gay community (Cabaj, 1990), and substance abuse is frequently an area of attention in psychotherapy with gay men. For a gay man with HIV, even moderate amounts of alcohol or drug use can negatively impact the immune system. Patients who have a problem with substance abuse often do not volunteer this information, and it is not uncommon for substance users to deny the extent to which they are using drugs. Therefore, it is important that therapists actively inquire about patients' drug and alcohol use. Abuse of alcohol or drugs may be a way for the patient to numb himself and thus avoid dealing with having HIV. For others, it might reflect an underlying suicide wish.

> Mr. E sought therapy at the urging of his internist. A 44-year-old gay man, HIV positive for nearly 10 years, Mr. E had been an alcoholic since his late teens. He reported drinking two to three cocktails daily after work, and substantially more on the weekends. He noticed that his drinking had increased over the past several months, with several episodes of blackouts, which he had not often experienced in the past. Although he was concerned about his increased alcohol use and the degree to which it was interfering with his ability to function, Mr. E was reluctant to give it up. He was also increasingly aware of feeling depressed and hopeless. In response to an inquiry by the therapist, Mr. E acknowledged a subtle wish that the alcohol would kill him so that he did not have to die from AIDS the way so many of his friends had.

Active abuse of drugs and alcohol will significantly compromise psychotherapy and limit the benefits a patient might otherwise obtain. Gains made in a session will quickly be undone or impeded by the next episode of substance use. For patients like Mr. E, therefore, it is necessary to treat the substance abuse before the patient can benefit from psychotherapy.

Health Care

A patient who is negligent about his health care may also be acting out unconscious self-destructive wishes. Although it is not as apparent as other overtly dangerous activities, not doing something that is helpful can be extremely harmful. A patient with low T cells who avoids seeing his doctor or who fails to comply with treatment to prevent an opportunistic infection is behaving in a dangerous manner. Helping the patient to recognize the ways in which he sabotages himself or compromises his health is an important role of the therapist. It is the patient's lack of awareness and understanding of his self-destructive actions that enables him to maintain them. Heightening the patient's awareness of how he undermines his health can help him to follow through with his physician's recommendations.

Sexual Behavior

Sex is another area in which gay men frequently act out unconscious self-destructive wishes. For the HIV-infected man, practicing safer sex is extremely important, for the protection of himself as well as his partner. Some HIV-positive men have adopted the attitude that if their partner is also HIV positive, then it is unnecessary to practice safe sex. For some, this attitude may be due to a lack of information or understanding about the virus. For others, it may be due to their denial of danger. Multiple exposure to HIV, even in a person who is already infected, further attacks the immune system and is therefore harmful. For some men, unsafe sex is an expression of a negative attitude toward the self that may be fueled by feelings of guilt and self-blame.

> Mr. P sought therapy to help him make decisions about whether to continue to work or go on disability. In the process of talking about his life, Mr. P described daily alcohol use and frequent casual sexual encounters. When the therapist inquired about the extent of his alcohol use, Mr. P insisted that it was not a problem, that he would only have two or three beers after work, although sometimes more, maybe five or six if he stayed later than usual. When asked about his sexual activity, Mr. P matter of factly stated that if he knew his partner was also HIV positive, he would have passive anal intercourse without a condom. He also responded flatly to his therapist's surprise that he would be willing to engage in such a dangerous behavior, insisting that it was not such a big deal. He believed that his therapist was overreacting to his sexual behavior and alcohol use, asserting that these were not areas of concern. The therapist maintained his stance of treating these as very serious and dangerous behaviors, consistently confronting the patient with his denial of the harm involved. Gradually, Mr. P became increasingly anxious about his behavior, began to wonder about the motivation behind his actions, and for the first time, began to feel uncomfortable with the risks he was taking.

In maintaining a consistent stance that these behaviors are dangerous, the therapist conveys his concern for the patient's well-being, as well as the belief that the patient is worth protecting. This is an important message to be conveyed in therapy, particularly when the patient is struggling internally with feelings of guilt and anger. It is not unusual that when there is no one in the environment that the patient can direct his anger toward, he will unconsciously direct it toward himself.

When treating a patient who engages in any sort of self-destructive behavior, particularly if the patient denies the dangerousness of his actions, it is important that the therapist actively confront the patient's denial and bring the danger to his attention. To not take an active stand against such behaviors is to collude with the patient's belief, conscious or unconscious, that he is not worth protecting.

Suicide

Feelings or thoughts about suicide may emerge at any stage of HIV infection, from the first discovery of being seropositive through end-stage AIDS. The point at which an individual is at greatest risk for suicide is still not well understood. In a study of suicidal ideation among people being tested for HIV infection, researchers found that suicidality does not appear to increase among asymptomatic individuals following a positive test result (Perry et al., 1990). Other studies have suggested that suicidality increases with declining health (Pugh, O'Donnell, & Catalan, 1993; Rabkin, Remien, Katoff, & Williams, 1993). Regardless of the stage of disease, the therapist needs to be alert to the potential for suicidal feelings and wishes in HIV patients.

When a patient introduces thoughts or feelings about suicide, it is important that the therapist respond appropriately. The patient needs to know that he can talk about his suicidal thoughts with his therapist and not feel that he needs to hide them. If the therapist becomes overly anxious, rushing too soon to action or suicide intervention, he may frighten the patient, who may then feel less comfortable bringing up these thoughts. For example, a patient who is still asymptomatic may, in a therapy session, talk about suicide in the context of anticipating severe disability in the future. This may be more likely to emerge in patients who have experienced the decline of a loved one or friend. As one patient has said after caring for his dying lover, "I would kill myself before I would let myself be so helpless, so dependent ... it's humiliating." Another patient, Mr. C, who worked in a medical clinic that had many HIV patients, stated, "Well, I would never let myself get to that point. I would definitely kill myself before that happened ... but then again, I say that now, who knows how I'll actually feel when I'm that sick ... you just never know what you can adjust to until you get there ... "

For some HIV patients, entertaining thoughts of suicide becomes a way of maintaining a sense of control over their life. Knowing that they can chose when their life will end rather than being at the mercy of the disease can help a patient to maintain a sense of power even in the face of feeling helpless. For one patient, the knowledge that he had stored enough medication to overdose, should he ever reach a point of intolerable physical pain and disability, helped him to cope with the stress of his illness.

As patients progress into later stages of HIV infection and begin to experience more agonizing and crippling symptoms, they may express more frequent wishes to die. Even if a patient expresses a suicidal wish, however, it does not necessarily mean that he wants to die. Consider the case of Mr. M.

> Mr. M had survived for nearly 12 years with HIV with relatively few symptoms. In the last months of his life he lost a substantial amount of weight and suffered constant stomach and abdominal pain. He frequently talked about suicide and

sent away for information from the Hemlock Society. He even discussed with
his physician which medication and what amount would be necessary to kill
himself. One of his closest friends was also in end-stage AIDS and in great pain.
Just prior to a therapy session Mr. M learned that his friend had committed
suicide. In the session he talked about envying his friend's courage and wished
that he had the nerve to do the same, wishing he could die and be out of his
misery. All the while, as he talked about death, Mr. M continued to eat his bagel,
slowly and with great difficulty due to the lesions in his throat, and then
carefully took all of his medications and nutritional supplements.

Even in the face of debilitating and painful symptoms, Mr. M's actions
suggest that he had maintained a sense of hope and a desire to survive.
For this patient, suicidal ideation represented more his wish to end his
suffering than an expression of a true wish to die.

In addition to being a symptom of a depressive syndrome, or an
expression of some other wish or anxiety, suicidal ideation may also
emerge as a rational plan to expedite death in the face of pain and suffering at the end stage of a terminal illness. The notion that suicide might be
reasonable and appropriate in certain circumstances continues to be met
with much controversy in this country. The numbers of people suffering
in late-stage AIDS, lingering before death with their quality of life dramatically compromised, has challenged physicians and lay people alike to
reconsider the validity of rational suicide (Slome, Moulton, Huffine, Gorter, & Abrams, 1992).

Many gay men with HIV disease have also gone through the death and
dying process with friends and lovers and know very well what to expect
as their disease progresses. Death from AIDS is often quite horrible, with
a range of debilitating and painful symptoms that leave the individual in a
weak and helpless state. Approximately 10% to 20% of people with HIV
suffer from some degree of dementia, which often renders them completely dependent on care from others (Perry, 1990). Thus, for many
patients, a planned suicide prior to reaching such a painful and debili-
tated state may be a humane and reasonable solution.

ISSUES FOR HIV-POSITIVE ASYMPTOMATIC PATIENTS

The knowledge that one is HIV positive, even in the absence of symptoms, can be highly stressful. For many patients this is even more stressful than having an AIDS diagnosis. The individual is faced with multiple
unknowns and a pervasive sense of uncertainty about the future. "When
will I get sick? What form will my illness take? What can I do to maintain
my health? What's that spot on my leg? How come I'm so tired today?"
These are questions that the HIV-positive gay man may be preoccupied
with. When a person knows that he has HIV, a cold is no longer just a cold.
Any time he feels physically fatigued or slightly under the weather, he
wonders if this is it, the beginning of the decline. He's seen it happen a

dozen times and knows it is inevitable. He just doesn't know when. He's always waiting for the bomb to drop.

Some men are able to lead their lives, not consciously thinking about "when," and not worrying about their health, until something out of the ordinary happens (e.g., a persistent sore throat or a cough). For others, it is frequently on their mind, sometimes to the point of feeling beyond their control.

Stress

Research has found a link between stress and development of illness in patients with cancer and other diseases (Cohen & Williamson, 1991; Rabkin & Struening, 1976.), as well as in people with HIV disease (Rabkin et al., 1991; Temoshok, 1988). The public in general has become much more aware of this connection and people with HIV are often concerned about their levels of stress. For some, the knowledge that experiencing stress might exacerbate their health can, in and of itself, become a source of stress. This feeling may be carried to extremes wherein the individual believes that experiencing any stress, anxiety, or unpleasant emotion will have a negative impact on his health.

Psychotherapy can help the individual to maintain a reasonable perspective on stress as well as help him cope with the stress he inevitably will experience. Certain amounts of stress are expected in all people, and some degree of stress can even be helpful as a source of motivation, stirring people to action. Some people even thrive on stress. Living a life completely free of stress is unrealistic for people in general, and living with HIV is unavoidably stressful. Therapy can help the individual recognize that he need not avoid all stress and that how he copes with his stress is the more important issue. Emphasizing patients' need to develop effective strategies for coping with stress, rather than trying to eliminate it completely, is a more realistic and manageable goal. Learning coping strategies can foster a sense of self-efficacy and can further help to decrease stress (Folkman et al., 1993).

Death and Dying

Regardless of the stage of infection or progression of disease, the HIV-positive person must grapple with issues of death and dying. For the person still early in the process and asymptomatic, these issues may not be as pressing, but they will still be there. For the therapist, it is important to assess the patient's feelings about death. How consciously is he struggling with concerns about dying? What is his attitude about death? Does he expect to die from AIDS or does he believe he'll be one of the survivors? It is helpful for the therapist to know to what degree the patient has accepted the possibility of his death.

The therapist must also be attentive to how realistic the patient's ideas are about his mortality. For example, a patient who recently tested positive for HIV and has high T cells, but who believes his death is imminent, might be so uninformed about HIV disease that he does not realize how extreme his reaction is. John, a 26-year-old gay man with T cells hovering around 500, decided to drop out of school, quit his job, and move to Europe to be "carefree," believing that he would likely die within the year. After spending 9 months in Europe, feeling as good as he did before he left, he returned home to pick up where he left off. Therapy can help the individual become more aware of his beliefs about his life expectancy and more objectively gauge the reasonableness of his expectations.

Denial

Each individual with HIV develops his own unique way of coping with the stress of being infected. Most people will employ denial to varying degrees and at different times during the course of their illness. For many, the use of denial, a common defense mechanism, is adaptive and enables the individual to function. Denying that one is infected can help the individual go about his daily routine without constantly feeling plagued by fear, anxiety, or rage. The psychosocial literature on coping with HIV disease has addressed the importance of "healthy denial" for effective adaptation to the knowledge that one is infected with HIV (Earl, Martindale, & Cohn, 1991; Lackner, Joseph, Ostrow, & Kessler, 1993).

Recognizing when denial has become maladaptive and potentially harmful to the patient may be another important task for the therapist working with HIV-positive gay men (Rosenberger & Wineburgh, 1992). Knowing when to more actively confront the patient's denial often requires a sensitive balancing act and can stir up conflicting emotions within the therapist.

> Mr. M, a 35-year-old gay man, had been asymptomatic and robust since discovering he was HIV positive at age 30. He was very attentive to his health, exercised regularly, ate well, and had regular checkups with his physician. His attention to his health indicated that he was aware of the importance of taking steps to support his immune system. On another level, however, Mr. M behaved as if he would live to a ripe old age, setting long-term personal goals, working 10- to 12-hour days, and looking forward to attending his 3-year-old niece's bat mitzvah (10 years in the future), reflecting a degree of denial about his illness. As his T cells continued to decrease to well below 200, Mr. M still made no mention in therapy of concerns about his ability to work or support himself. He continued working long hours 5 days a week, and had made no plans for future disability. Although aware that this denial was not in Mr. M's best interest, his therapist was reluctant to address it, not wanting to be the one to "burst his bubble." He felt as if this would deprive the patient of hope. After recognizing his own discomfort and becoming more aware of the ways in which he was colluding with the patient's denial, the therapist was eventually able to point out how the patient was avoiding preparing for his disability. Mr. M became intensely

emotional in this session, crying for the first time with his therapist about his
losses, and experiencing fear and sorrow. Gradually, Mr. M began to plan for
the time when he would no longer be able to work. He reduced his work
schedule and developed a very comprehensive support system that included
friends and community services. He began the application process for the
benefits to which he was entitled and had most things in place prior to becoming disabled.

Initially, Mr. M used denial to help him cope with the trauma of being HIV
positive and to maintain a sense of hope. Denial enabled him to go about
his usual daily routine without intrusions of desperation or despair. As
Mr. M's disease progressed and his immune system became more seriously compromised, his defensive style did not adapt to these changes.
His denial then prevented Mr. M from consciously thinking about the
significant changes in his health that required action. His therapist was
also initially not ready to think about the decline in Mr. M's health and
what it represented. It was the therapist's ability to accept and tolerate
the sense of loss and despair that enabled Mr. M to confront and express
these feelings. Once able to experience and accept these painful emotions,
Mr. M was able to plan appropriately for his inevitable disability.

ISSUES FOR AIDS PATIENTS

A diagnosis of AIDS is often a significant milestone for the HIV-
positive person. Up until that point, the individual has had to deal with
the knowledge that he is infected and that his immune system is gradually deteriorating, but he essentially feels healthy. A diagnosis of AIDS
might be due to a T cell count dropping below 200 or an AIDS-related
opportunistic infection.

For those whose diagnosis is a result of T cell count alone, their
experience may be similar to that of an asymptomatic HIV-positive person. Advances in medical management of HIV disease are largely responsible for this similarity. Because of early-intervention strategies and the
increasing number of medications available to prevent the most common
opportunistic infections, people with HIV are enjoying longer periods of
life free from symptoms, even with severely compromised immune systems. Mr. M had been living with a T cell count of 10 for nearly a year
before succumbing to his first opportunistic infection. Mr. C, who discovered that his T cells were at 175 when he tested positive, began immediately on antiviral medications, as well as antibiotics to prevent PCP
infection and cytomegalovirus (CMV), and continues to feel healthy and
robust.

Coping with Losses

For the person with symptomatic AIDS, life becomes a series of coping
with one opportunistic infection after another. Up until this point, the

losses that the individual has had to face may have involved either the deaths of loved ones or the more existential loss associated with the recognition that he will not live a long and prosperous life. Once he has begun to experience symptoms, the person with AIDS must confront and cope with a range of losses affecting him immediately and personally. Initially this may involve the loss of certain physical abilities. Within this physical realm the experience is broad, ranging from the loss of energy, which may be vague and difficult to identify, to problems with walking or loss of bodily function, such as urinary and bowel control. As he experiences greater physical decline and becomes more dependent on others for his care, he must adapt to changes in his self-identity. No longer an independent and competent adult, he must adjust to a state of increasing helplessness.

The inability to enjoy usual and simple pleasures can also represent a substantial loss for someone with AIDS. This may be in the form of no longer being able to participate in social activities with friends, impotence or loss of sexual desire, or not being able to watch television due to blindness from CMV retinitis. Mr. H, who had recuperated from two bouts of PCP and was doing fairly well, had developed lesions in his esophagus from a CMV infection, which made swallowing extremely painful. For him, not being able to enjoy a meal with his family, who had come to spend a religious holiday with him, represented a profound loss. As he described his experience of no longer being able to participate with joy and pleasure in this important family ritual, he could not fight off his tears. He could be there with his family during the meal, but he could not experience the pleasure so evident in everyone else's face. For him each bite was met with excruciating pain. The everyday pleasure of enjoying a good meal was something Mr. H, and many like him, could no longer experience. Eating, although crucial for his survival, became a nightmare.

Death and Dying

As the individual's immune system continues to deteriorate and he is faced with increasing symptoms, the realities of death and dying become more prominent and immediate. At this stage, therapy can facilitate the mourning process, helping the patient to put his life in perspective and come to terms with his accomplishments and successes, as well as his losses and disappointments. The experience of remembering and integrating the good and the bad of his life is an important part of this mourning process. For some, this is not an easy developmental task. Remembering the unpleasant times, the disappointments and failures, can lead to increased feelings of despair if the patient is unable to also maintain an awareness of the happy times.

Mr. R had just begun an exciting new career at 44 years old when he experienced his first opportunistic infection and lost nearly 50% of his body mass. Although he continued to work, he fatigued easily and suffered from frequent bouts of diarrhea. As his physical decline rapidly continued, Mr. R became acutely depressed and withdrew from all social contacts and activities. In therapy he described feeling unable to see his friends, busy and active with their families and careers, because he could not tolerate the envy that he felt. He couldn't even bear to look out his window onto the street below, filled with people bustling about with their daily activities, because of the despair that it would evoke within him. During therapy, his voice was often barely audible, as Mr. R struggled to express himself through his despair. He especially could not bare to talk about his past, to remember any of the joyous times of his life. To remember the happy times felt intolerable in the face of knowing he could not return to them. So accustomed to keeping positive and negative feelings or ideas separate, Mr. R was unable to use his memories of pleasure and happiness to help him cope with his current pain and sorrow. therapy gradually became the arena in which Mr. R could bring his history alive in the moment, no longer afraid that his current agony would destroy the joy of his memories. He was then able to reminisce about his life, his achievements and triumphs, and gradually begin to grieve his losses and accept his pending death.

Finding a balance between the acceptance of death and the maintenance of hope can be difficult to achieve. It requires, in the individual, the ability to hold on to the good and the bad, positive and negative, pleasure and pain, at the same time. Recognizing that one can experience multiple and conflicting thoughts and feelings at the same time enables the individual to both confront, come to terms with, and accept death, and at the same time hope to survive. Maintenance of hope has been found to be associated with lower levels of depression in HIV-infected gay men (Rabkin, Williams, Neugebauer, Remien, & Goetz, 1990) and may also be associated with improved immunological functioning (Jemmot & Locke, 1984). Helping the patient maintain a sense of hope, even at end-stage AIDS, becomes an important function of psychotherapy.

Denial

The use of denial continues to play a role in the coping strategies of gay men in later stages of HIV infection and has the potential to lead to additional difficulties adjusting to illness. A patient whose denial is more fixed and rigid may be unable to appropriately attend to his health care. For example, he may fail to seek treatment when necessary or may not comply with treatments that have been prescribed. He may also be slow to alter his activities and responsibilities to accommodate his physical condition. Mr. D, diagnosed with AIDS for 2 years, had recovered from multiple opportunistic infections including PCP and lymphoma. He had been diagnosed with CMV retinitis, resulting in some visual impairment. When his therapist became aware that Mr. D continued to drive, he wondered with the patient if this was dangerous, given his vision loss. Mr. D assured his therapist that, although his peripheral vision was impaired in his left eye, he could compensate easily for this and saw no reason to stop driving. Not feeling reassured by this, his therapist suggested that Mr. D was trying to put off accepting yet another loss. This helped Mr. D to talk about the significance of the independence that he associated with driving and the helplessness he felt in needing to depend on others for transportation. Given the reliance on the automobile as the primary mode of transportation for so many people in this country, the decision to stop driving is frequently a difficult one for people with AIDS.

> Mr. H had begun experiencing early stages of HIV dementia and had compensated by keeping a notebook to help him remember things. Unbeknownst to his therapist, however, he had continued driving his car. When Mr. H had not arrived for his usually scheduled therapy session, his therapist called him at home. As soon as he heard his therapist's voice on the phone, Mr. H realized how impaired he was. He recounted then to his therapist that he had been on his way to his session, but once he reached the neighborhood of the therapist's office, he could not remember where the office was and ended up driving around for several minutes. Finally, he pulled over and sat on a curb near his car, trying to remember what he was doing. A woman noticed him in his distraught state and sent him home in a cab. He had been reading a magazine when the therapist called, not recalling this ordeal until hearing his therapist's voice. Recognizing that Mr. H was no longer in the position to make completely informed decisions, the therapist told him that he could no longer drive his car and would need to rely on alternative means of transportation to get around. Although he began to cry in response to hearing this, Mr. H was able to accept that he wasn't able to drive safely, no longer needing to deny his impairment.

SUMMARY AND CONCLUSIONS

People with HIV disease seek therapy for a variety of reasons and at various stages of illness. The themes and focus of treatment will be affected by the stage of disease that the patient is in, his premorbid level of psychological functioning, and his existing defensive style. For those patients in early stages of infection, the therapy generally focuses on helping the patient to live with HIV disease. For those at later stages, the therapy focuses more on helping the patient come to terms with his death.

The psychological and emotional impact of HIV is profound for anyone infected, regardless of the route of exposure. Given the devastation within the gay community, the impact on a gay man is unique and warrants special attention. For gay men over 30, AIDS has been part of their life for the last 14 to 15 years, whether they personally are infected or not. Few gay men, particularly those living in urban areas, have been spared the loss of friends and lovers. To have mourned the deaths of dozens of friends by the time one must grapple with his own decline from illness is not at all unusual for an HIV-positive gay man. Many of those men have also been in the role of primary caretaker to a lover or close friend who has died from AIDS and are, therefore, intimately aware of the severity and horror of end-stage disease.

For the gay man with HIV, a core component of his identity—his sexuality—has resulted in his exposure to a deadly virus. Something that was once associated with pleasure, excitement, and love is now connected to loss, disability, and death. All gay men growing up in this society must grapple with homophobia and bias against homosexuality. The degree to which they have become aware of their own internalized homophobia and come to terms with it will vary among gay men and will significantly impact their emotional response to having HIV.

In working with HIV-positive gay men, therapists need to be aware of these distinct experiences in order to understand the complexities of the psychological impact and be in a position to help their patients. Therapists must also be aware of their own attitudes about homosexuality and recognize their biases and misconceptions. Considering homosexuality to be a psychopathology is part of the history of psychology and psychiatry. Many therapists still maintain negative attitudes and beliefs about gay men and lesbians that they may not be fully aware of and that they have not adequately challenged and revised. Even a subtle preference toward heterosexuality can be perceived by a gay patient and interfere with the therapeutic process.

The advantages of providing psychotherapy to patients with HIV disease are multiple. Therapy can help to prevent more serious psychological consequences such as clinical depression and suicide. Psychotherapy can also be a vital resource and support for people with HIV disease. It often becomes the only place where a person with HIV can address his deepest fears and anxieties about becoming sick and dying. In therapy, a patient is able to express the intensity of his emotions without having to censor or protect loved ones. Therapy can facilitate the mourning process, helping the individual to grieve the losses of friends, abilities, identities, and of life.

REFERENCES

Adler, G., & Beckett, A. (1989). Psychotherapy of the patient with HIV infection: Some ethical and therapeutic dilemmas. *Psychosomatics, 30,* 203–208.

American Psychological Association, Committee on Lesbian & Gay Concerns. (1991). *Bias in psychotherapy with lesbians and gay men.* Washington, DC: American Psychological Association.

Bridge, T. P., Mirsky, A., & Goodwin, F. (Eds.). (1988). *Psychological, neuropsychiatric, and substance abuse aspects of AIDS.* New York: Raven Press.

Cabaj, R. (1992). Substance abuse in the gay and lesbian community. In Lowenstein, J., Ruiz, P., & Millman, R. (Eds.). *Substance abuse*: A comprehensive textbook. Baltimore: Williams & Wilkins.

Cadwell, S., Burnham, R., & Forstein, M. (1994). *Therapists on the front line: Psychotherapy with gay men in the age of AIDS.* Washington, DC: American Psychiatric Press.

Centers for Disease Control. (1990). Estimates of HIV prevalence and projected AIDS cases: Summary of a workshop, October 31–November 1, 1989. *Morbidity and Mortality Weekly Report, 39,* 110–119.

Chesney, M., & Folkman, S. (1994). Psychological impact of HIV disease and implications for intervention. *Psychiatric Clinics of North America, 17*, 163–182.

Cohen, M. A. (1990). Biopsychosocial approach to the human immunodeficiency virus epidemic. *General Hospital Psychiatry, 12*, 98–123.

Cohen, S. & Williamson, G. (1991). Stress and infectious disease in humans. *Psychological Bulletin, 109*, 5–24.

Curran, J., Jaffe, H., Hardy, A., Morgan, W., Selik, R., & Dondero, T. (1988). The epidemiology of HIV infection and AIDS in the United States. *Science, 239*, 610–616.

DeCrescenzo, T. (1984). Homophobia: A study of the attitudes of mental health professionals toward homosexuality. *Journal of Social Work and Human Sexuality, 2*, 115–136.

Dilley, J., Pies, C, & Helquist, M. (Eds.). (1993). *Face to face: A guide to AIDS counseling.* San Francisco: AIDS Health Project, University of California.

Earl, W., Martindale, C., & Cohn, D. (1992). Adjustment: Denial in the styles of coping with HIV infection. *Omega: Journal of Death and Dying, 24*, 35–47.

Folkman, S., Chesney, M., Pollack, L., & Coates, T. (1993). Stress, control, coping, and depressive mood in human immunodeficiency virus-positive and -negative gay men in San Francisco. *Journal of Nervous and Mental Disease, 181*, 409–416.

Garfinkle, E., & Morin, S. (1978). Psychotherapists' attitudes toward homosexual psychotherapy clients. *Journal of Social Issues, 34*, 101– 112.

Gorman, J., Kertzner, R., Todak, G., Goetz, R., Williams, J., Rabkin, J., Heino, F., Mayeux, R., Stern, Y., Lange, M., Dobkin, J., Spitzer, R., & Ehrhardt, A. (1991). Multidisciplinary baseline assessment of homosexual men with and without human immunodeficiency virus infection. *Archives of General Psychiatry, 48*, 120–123.

Graham, D., Rawlings, E., Halpern, H., & Hermes, J. (1984). Therapists' needs for training in counseling lesbians and gay men. *Professional Psychology: Research and Practice, 15*, 482–496.

Hays, R., Turner, H., & Coates, T. (1992). Social support, AIDS-related symptoms, and depression among gay men. *Journal of Consulting and Clinical Psychology, 60*, 463–469.

Isay, R. (1989). AIDS: The development of healthy gay men and homophobia. In R. Isay (Ed.), *Being homosexual: Gay men and their development* (pp. 67–81). New York: Farrar, Straus, & Giroux.

Jacobsen, P., Perry, S., & Hirsh, D. (1990). Behavioral and psychological responses to HIV antibody testing. *Journal of Consulting and Clinical Psychology, 58*, 31–37.

Jemmott, J., & Locke, S. (1984). Psychosocial factors, immunologic mediation and human susceptibility to infectious diseases. *Psychological Bulletin, 95*, 78– 108.

Kelly, J., Lawrence, J., & Brasfield, T. (1991). Predictors of vulnerability to AIDS risk behavior relapse. *Journal of Consulting and Clinical Psychology, 59*, 163–166.

Kelly, J., & Murphy, D. (1992). Psychological interventions with AIDS and HIV: Prevention and treatment. *Journal of Consulting and Clinical Psychology, 60*, 576–585.

Kleinman, I. (1991). HIV transmission: Ethical and legal considerations in psychotherapy. *Canadian Journal of Psychiatry, 36*, 121–123.

Krowka, J. (1993). T-cell tests and other laboratory mysteries. In Dilley, Pies, & Helquist (Eds.), *Face to face: A guide to AIDS counseling* (pp. 36–48). San Francisco: AIDS Health Project, University of California.

Kübler-Ross, E. (1969). *On death and dying.* New York: Macmillan.

Lackner, J., Joseph, J., Ostrow, D., & Kessler, R. (1993). A longitudinal study of psychological distress in a cohort of gay men: Effects of social support and coping strategies. *Journal of Nervous and Mental Disease, 181*, 4–12.

Landis, S., Earp, J., & Koch, G. (1992). Impact of HIV testing and counseling on subsequent sexual behavior. *AIDS Education and Prevention, 4*, 61–70.

Malyon, A. K. (1982). Psychotherapeutic implications of internalized homophobia in gay men. In J. Gonsiorek (Ed.), *Homosexuality and psychotherapy* (pp. 59–91). New York: Haworth Press.

Markowitz, J., Klerman, G., & Perry, S. (1992). Interpersonal psychotherapy of depressed HIV-positive outpatients. *Hospital and Community Psychiatry, 43*, 885–890.

Martin, J. (1988). Psychological consequences of AIDS-related bereavement among gay men. *Journal of Consulting and Clinical Psychology, 56*, 856–862.

Martin, J., & Dean L. (1993). Effects of AIDS-related bereavement and HIV-related illness on psychological distress among gay men: A 7-year longitudinal study, 1985–1991. *Journal of Consulting and Clinical Psychology, 61*, 94–103.

Marzuk, P., & Perry, S. (1993). Suicide and HIV: Researchers and clinicians beware. *AIDS Care, 5*, 387–390.

Marzuk, P., Tierney, H., Tardiff, K., Gross, E., Morgan, E., Hsu, M., & Mann, J. (1988). Increased risk of suicide in persons with AIDS. *Journal of the American Medical Association, 259*, 1333–1337.

Morin, S., & Charles, K. (1983). Heterosexual bias in psychotherapy. In J. Murray & P. Abramson (Eds.), *Bias in psychotherapy* (pp. 309–338). New York: Praeger Publishers.

Namir, S., Wolcott, D., Fawzy, F., & Alumbaugh, M. J. (1987). Coping with AIDS: Psychological and health implications. *Journal of Applied Social Psychology, 17*, 309–328.

Ostrow, D., Monjan, A., Joseph, J., VanRaden, M., Fox, R., Kingsley, L., Dudley, J., & Phair, J. (1989). HIV-related symptoms and psychological functioning in a cohort of homosexual men. *American Journal of Psychiatry, 146*, 737–742.

Perry, S. (1990). Organic mental disorders caused by HIV: An update on early diagnosis and treatment. *American Journal of Psychiatry, 147*, 696–710.

Perry, S., Jacobsberg, L., Fishman, B., Weiler, P., Gold, J., & Frances, A. (1990). Psychological responses to serological testing for HIV. *AIDS, 4*, 145–152.

Pugh, K., O'Donnell, I., & Catalan, J. (1993). Suicide and HIV disease. *AIDS Care, 5*, 391–400.

Rabkin, J., Remien, R., Katoff, L., & Williams, J. (1993). Suicidality in AIDS long-term survivors: What is the evidence? *AIDS Care, 5*, 401–411.

Rabkin, J., & Struening, E. (1976). Life events, stress and illness. *Science, 194*, 1013–1020.

Rabkin, J., Williams, J., Neugebauer, R., Remien, R., & Goetz, R. (1990). Maintenance of hope in HIV-spectrum homosexual men. *American Journal of Psychiatry, 147*, 1322–1326.

Rabkin, J., Williams, J., Remien, R., Goetz, R., Kertzner, R., & Gorman, J. (1991). Depression, distress, lymphocyte subsets, and human immunodeficiency virus symptoms on two occasions in HIV-positive homosexual men. *Archives of General Psychiatry, 48*, 111–119.

Rosenberger, J., & Wineburgh, M. (1992). Working with denial: A critical aspect in AIDS risk intervention. *Social Work in Health Care, 17*, 11–26.

Schaffner, B. (1990). Psychotherapy with HIV-infected persons. *New Directions for Mental Health Services, 48*, 5–20.

Schneider, S., Taylor, S., Hammen, C., Kemeny, M., & Dudley, J. (1991). Factors influencing suicide intent in gay and bisexual suicide ideators: Differing models for men with and without human immunodeficiency virus. *Journal of Personality and Social Psychology, 61*, 776–788.

Siegel, K., Raveis, V., & Krauss, B. (1992). Factors associated with urban gay men's treatment initiation decisions for HIV infection. *AIDS Education and Prevention, 4*, 135–142.

Slome, L., Moulton, J., Huffine, C., Gorter, R., & Abrams, D. (1992). Physicians' attitudes toward assisted suicide in AIDS. *Journal of Acquired Immune Deficiency Syndromes, 5*, 712–718.

Temoshok, L. (1988). Psychoimmunology and AIDS. In Bridge, T. P., Mirsky, A., & Goodwin, F. (Eds.), *Psychological, neuropsychiatric and substance abuse aspects of AIDS* (pp. 187–197). New York: Raven Press.

Winkelstein, W., Lyman, D., Padian, N., Grant, R., Samuel, M., Wiley, J., Anderson, R., Lang, W., Riggs, J., & Levy, J. (1987). Sexual practices and risk of infection by the human immunodeficiency virus: The San Francisco Men's Health Study. *Journal of the American Medical Association, 257*, 321–325.

Zegans, L., Gerhard, A., & Coates, T. (1994). Psychotherapies for the person with HIV disease. *Psychiatric Clinics of North America, 17*, 149–162.

CHAPTER 14

Homophobia and the Health Psychology of Lesbians

KATHERINE A. O'HANLAN

INTRODUCTION

American society in the last 30 years has seen an entirely new segment of society coalesce. Sensationalizing media attention has capitalized on Americans' unfamiliarity with gay men and lesbians. The focus on the fringes of homosexual culture has made gay men and lesbians the brunt of multiple levels of prejudice, with negative assumptions about their morality, employability, and integrity. Similar accusations were made against African-Americans, Jews, and other ethnic groups in previous times. Gay men and lesbians have subsequently maintained a hidden subculture, which only recently has become more open and currently weaves through all segments of society. Surveys of the homosexual community suggest that health care providers lack knowledge of the issues salient in the lives of gay men and lesbians and that these health care providers have inadvertently or purposely alienated their patients. The gay and lesbian community needs medical care that recognizes its unique medical demographic profile and that is provided with sensitivity and respect. In this review of lesbian health literature, the medical and psychological effects of heterosexist prejudice from family, educational, religious, and governmental organizations will be discussed, and steps to

KATHERINE A. O'HANLAN • Gynecologic Cancer Section, Stanford University School of Medicine, Stanford, California 94305.

Handbook of Diversity Issues in Health Psychology, edited by Pamela M. Kato and Traci Mann. Plenum Press, New York, 1996.

ameliorate them will be suggested. With greater understanding of who lesbians are and of the psychological effects of societal disdain for them, providers can maintain the highest standard of medical care for all of their patients, including lesbians.

HOMOPHOBIA DEFINED

Homophobia is the "unreasoning fear of or antipathy toward homosexuals and homosexuality" (Random House Dictionary of the English Language, 1987). Homophobia persists when families, friends, teachers, colleagues, religious institutions, government, and the popular media perpetuate the inaccurate perception of gay men and lesbians as child molesters, immoral individuals, or threats to traditional family values or the "natural" order (Fyfe, 1983).

Homophobia operates on dual levels: internally and externally (Isay, 1989; Sophie, 1987). Internal homophobia represents learned biases that all individuals incorporate (internalize) into their belief systems as they grow up in a society biased against homosexuals. External homophobia is the overtly observed or experienced expression of those biases. Such acts range from social avoidance to legal and religious proscription to physical violence.

Various theories of the causes of this prejudice suggest that heterosexuals may express hatred or fear of homosexuals in order to reassure themselves that they are "normal" or "moral" (Ferenczi, 1950). Homophobia has also been described as a variant of sexism, rejecting perceived femininity in men and masculinity in women (Isay, 1989). Although many individuals would not identify themselves as being homophobic, a lack of familiarity with members of the gay and lesbian community can result in acceptance of misinformation and unintentionally biased attitudes toward, or treatment of, members of that community. Knowing one or more gay men or lesbians personally has been associated with less hostility toward homosexuals in general (Ellis & Vasseur, 1993).

Based on extensive review of the psychiatric literature, it can be concluded that there is no scientific basis for homophobic prejudice. There are no differences in levels of maturity, neuroticism, psychological adjustment, goal orientation, or self-actualization between heterosexual and homosexual people (Dancey, 1990; Ferenczi, 1950; Freedman, 1971; Gartrell, 1981; Hart et al., 1978; Hooker, 1969; Peters & Cantrell, 1991; Siegelman, 1979; Thompson, McCandless, & Strickland, 1971). The initial inclusion of homosexuality as a mental disorder in the *Diagnostic and Statistical Manual* (DSM-III) has been reviewed, found to be reflective only of the social mores at the time it was inserted, and rejected. Even the category of ego-dystonic homosexuality appears to reflect only the incorporation of societal homophobia (Suppe, 1984).

Lesbians are not more likely than heterosexual women to have had poor or failed relationships with men or to have been mistreated, molested, or raped by men (Gundlach, 1977). There are no apparent family pathologic variables that have been associated with lesbianism (Shavelson, Biaggio, Cross, & Lehman, 1980). Some studies have revealed slightly higher lifetime rates of depression, attempted suicide, psychological help seeking, and substance abuse (Evans, 1971; Nurius, 1983; Thompson et al., 1971), which most authors attribute to the chronic stress from the endurance of societal hatred (Savin-Williams, 1994) or the designation by society of inferior status (DiPlacido, 1994). Stress from homophobia may have worse mental health implications than other social stressors because of the frequent loss of familial support systems (Brooks, 1981) and the perceived need for concealment and suppression of feelings and thoughts (Larson & Chastain, 1990).

Most lesbians are content with their orientation and function well in society (Bell & Weinberg, 1978). When Ann Landers asked her readership if they were glad to be gay, 75,875 people responded. Only 3% of respondents were not glad, citing victimization by violence, and family, governmental, job, or social discrimination (Landers, 1992).

PSYCHOLOGICAL AND MEDICAL CONSEQUENCES OF HOMOPHOBIA WITHIN THE FAMILY AND SOCIETY

Effects on Girls' Health

A brief description of the developmental steps that lesbians must negotiate helps to explain the psychological injuries to which they become vulnerable (Chapman & Brannock, 1987; Minton & McDonald, 1983; Sophie, 1985; Zera, 1992).

1. Recognition and acceptance of their homosexual orientation despite pervasive familial and societal condemnation.
2. Development of a new identity as a lesbian, a process known as "coming out."
3. Frequent confrontation with ubiquitous homophobia.

Some children as young as 2 to 8 years old experience homosexual feelings and subsequently become isolated and alienated from their family because they perceive that heterosexuality is the only acceptable norm (heterosexism) (Remafedi, Resnick, Blum, & Harris, 1992; Savin-Williams, 1988) Most parents will not inform their children about diversity of affectional or sexual orientation, believing that the information may predispose the children to pursue such behavior and leaving their children's education about this topic to uninformed peers, with the implicit message that homosexuality is unspeakable. Many religions depict homosexuality as an immoral proclivity that must be resisted, telling gay and lesbian children they are "wicked and condemned to hell," unfit to be ministers, and unfit to have their unions blessed (Gibson, 1989; Newman & Muzzonigro, 1993; Swaggart, 1982). Educational institutions do not teach children about diversity of orientation, even though most elementary school children have already begun to notice their orientation (Uribe & Harbeck, 1992). The absence of accurate and positive depictions of gay and lesbian role models in society, with overrepresentation of negative stereotypes of homosexuality in television, theater, and print media, further diminishes the ability of gay and lesbian youth to develop a positive self-identity and to gain respect and understanding from their peers (American Academy of Pediatrics: Committee on Adolescence, 1993). Children also observe the practice of government-enforced military discrimination against its gay and lesbian members, implying that homosexuals are undeserving citizens in American culture, despite the documented absence of security risk or performance inadequacy (Herek, 1990; United States Government Accounting Office, 1992).

The Committee on Adolescence of the American Academy of Pediatrics believes that "[t]he psychosocial problems of gay and lesbian adolescents are primarily the result of societal stigma, hostility, hatred, and isolation. Such rejection may lead to isolation, run-away behavior, homelessness, domestic violence, depression, suicide, substance abuse, and school or job failure" (American Academy of Pediatrics: Committee on Adolescence, 1993). In a 1988 survey of 500 adolescents applying to the Hetrick-Martin Institute, a New York City high school for gay and lesbian teens, 46% of the adolescents reported experiencing physical violence from their family, peers, or strangers because of their orientation (Hunter, 1989).

Psychological Health and Coming Out of the Closet

Learning to live in a society that does not welcome diversity shapes identity development as the child emerges into adolescence (Gibson & Saunders, 1994; Harry, 1989; Remafedi et al., 1992). Conformity, with repression of gay feelings, is encouraged (Kahn, 1991). Children will attempt to conceal their orientation from friends and relatives for fear of reprisals and discrimination, allowing a presumption of their heterosexuality to prevail (Larson & Chastain, 1990). In one study, awareness of sexual orientation occurred at an average age of 10 years, but disclosure to another person did not occur until age 16. From this sample of gay and lesbian youth, 42% acknowledged suicide attempts (D'Augelli & Hershberger, 1993). It is very difficult for these young people to maintain a positive self-image, and they live a double life that is unsatisfactory in both realms (American Academy of Pediatrics: Committee on Adolescence, 1993; Hunter & Schaecter, 1990). Family members and peers tend to view the individual as socially inadequate because of her withdrawn, secretive behavior. For some, this stage of hiding "in the closet" can last well into adulthood.

The dilemma of being out is more acute when multiple oppressive forces are encountered, as is the case among lesbians of color (Greene, 1994; Mays & Cochran, 1988; Phillip, 1993). Disapproval of homosexuality is reported as more intense in the Hispanic and African-American cultures than in European-American culture (Acosta, 1979; Hidalgo, 1984). Christian religiosity, a strong emphasis on family and community commitment, and heterosexual privilege promote bias against homosexuality within the African-American community and can create a conflict of loyalties when African-Americans are confronted with homophobia from their own community (Mays & Cochran). In contrast, Asian-Americans reported more discrimination because of their race than because of their orientation (Chan, 1992). Consistently, Hispanic and black, but not Asian-American youths, are overrepresented victims in studies of gay and lesbian suicide (Phillip, 1993; Rotheram-Borus, Rosario & Koopman, 1991; Schneider, Farberow, & Kruks, 1989).

The decision to come out integrates the separate parts of one's life and results in gradual self-image amelioration. Moreover, coming out, or honestly self-identifying as a gay man or lesbian, has been associated with a significantly higher self-concept (Gartrell, 1981), relationship satisfaction (Berger, 1990), lower social anxiety (Ferguson & Finkler, 1978), trait anxiety and depression (Larson & Chastain 1990; Schmitt & Kurdek, 1987), a greater sense of community, and integration into both family and society (American Academy of Pediatrics: Committee on Adolescence, 1993). Because the color of their skin does not reveal their minority status as homosexuals, most lesbian individuals must remake and renegotiate the decision to come out of the closet in many situations every day of their lives (Stephany, 1992). In two large surveys of lesbians, 15% to 28% of lesbians had disclosed their orientation to everyone in their lives, 29% to 32% remained hidden from their coworkers, and 19% had not disclosed their orientation to their families (Bradford, Ryan, & Rothblum, 1994; Bybee, 1990).

Suicide among Lesbian Youth

A 1989 Report to Louis Sullivan from the Secretary's Task Force on Youth Suicide (Harry, 1989) reported, but provided no data, that homosexual youth account for a disproportionate one-third of youth suicides. Many authors attribute risk for homosexual youth suicide to the youth's experience of familial disapproval and societal hatred (Remafedi, Farrow, & Deisher, 1991; Savin-Williams, 1994; Schneider, Taylor, Hammen, Kemeny, & Dudley, 1991). According to the American Academy of Pediatrics, parental nonacceptance is among the most significant factors in homosexual youth suicide, but because the family typically reflects societal norms, lesbian youth may never get approval or love from this important source of support (American Academy of Pediatrics: Committee on Adolescence, 1993). Of those children surveyed at the Hetrick Martin Institute who were rejected by their families, 44% had suicidal ideation and 41% of young lesbians had attempted suicide (Hunter, 1989). The National Lesbian Health Survey reported that more than 50% of lesbian respondents had suicidal ideation at some time in their lives, and 18% had attempted suicide (Bradford et al., 1994).

In comparison, in the Morbidity and Mortality Weekly Report from the Centers for Disease Control, a random survey of high school students (presumably 90–97% heterosexual) reveals that 8% of teens reported suicide attempts and 2% had required medical attention for their attempt (Centers for Disease Control, 1991). Whether lesbian children are committing suicide at higher rates than heterosexual youth remains unclear and deserves further scientific investigation. However, the importance of parental acceptance in youth self-acceptance has been clearly demonstrated (Savin-Williams, 1989).

Primary Relationships of Lesbians and Their Family Constructs

The prohibition against same-sex marriage denies lesbians the essential ability to form socially legitimate relationships that carry the legal, financial, and psychological perquisites of heterosexual marriage. Though survey data suggests that the majority of lesbians are in long-term relationships (Bradford et al., 1994; Bybee, 1990; Mays, Cochran, & Rhue, 1993), misconceptions persist about the ability of lesbians to form committed and stable involvements. In 1970, researchers from the Kinsey Institute surveyed lesbians from ages 36 to 45 and found that 82% of women were living with a partner (Bell & Weinberg, 1978). More recently, the Michigan Lesbian Survey (Bybee, 1990), the National Lesbian Healthcare Survey (Bradford et al., 1994), and the Black Women's Relationships Project (Mays & Cochran, 1988) report that 60% to 65% of lesbian respondents were in monogamous committed long-term relationships. A 1991 survey of gay and lesbian couples revealed that 75% of lesbian couples shared their income, 88% had held a wedding ceremony or ritual celebrating their union, 91% were monogamous, 7% broke their agreement, and 92% were committed for life (Bryant & Demian, 1990).

Relationship instability in lesbian couples can occur because of the same common relational conflicts of all couples, but it can be compounded by effects of cultural homophobia: coming out issues, self-concept issues, and the absence of wedding traditions and marital role model (Berger, 1990; Cabaj, 1988; Sophie, 1987). Internalized homophobia, with its self-doubt and shame, may make some lesbians feel they cannot develop any relationship at all.

Complications due to isolation from a rejecting family of origin by lesbian individuals can manifest in times of medical crisis. Unless the lesbian couple has specific contracts for mutual medical conservatorship, which are sometimes costly, any blood relative is the legal next of kin. The family of origin can override the role and input of the domestic partner, even though the domestic partner may be the primary caretaker and more knowledgeable of her partner's religious and ethical beliefs. Hospitals may also restrict visitation privileges of "nonrelatives." Although lesbians can circumvent some of these obstacles by designating their medical power of attorney to the person of their choice, unfortunately, only a fraction have taken these sometimes costly legal steps.

Effects on Substance Use, Abuse, and Well-Being

Substance-abuse rates across geographic and class lines for lesbians have previously been reported at 20% to 30% in contrast to 10% for heterosexual women (Cabaj, 1992; Diamond & Wilsnack, 1978; Lesbian & Gay Substance Abuse Planning Group, 1991). Epidemiologists have criticized these studies for using opportunistic sampling techniques, for example, surveys of bar patrons (Paul, Stall, & Bloomfield, 1991). Opportunistic studies are not representative of the lesbian community, as bar patrons are more likely to abuse alcohol and other drugs (Clark, 1981). Recent data regarding lesbian alcohol abuse indicate rates no higher than heterosexual women surveyed in the Chicago or San Francisco areas (Bloomfield, 1993).

Homophobia reduces the success of treatment and recovery for lesbian substance abusers (Hall, 1990). Failure to acknowledge lesbian identity makes recovery more difficult and increases likelihood of relapse (Cabaj, 1992). Lesbian clients are more willing to attend a treatment program that addresses gay issues and provides lesbian counselors (Hall, 1994). Most detoxification and rehabilitation programs show little sensitivity to issues of sexual orientation and generally do not encourage its disclosure (Hellman, Stanton, Lee, Tytun & Vachon, 1989; Morales & Graves, 1983). A questionnaire administered to 98 addiction center treatment providers revealed that 26% scored in the homophobic or marginally homophobic range. Some of the surveyed providers refused to answer the questionnaire, stating that their personal attitudes about homosexuality were not relevant to the quality of care they provided to gay and lesbian patients (Morales & Graves, 1983).

Effects on Rates of Public Violence

In a 1984 random nationwide survey of 2,000 lesbians and gay men by the National Gay and Lesbian Task Force, 19% of respondents had been punched, kicked, or beaten; 27% reported objects thrown at them; 54% had been threatened with physical violence; and 9% had been assaulted with a weapon because of their sexual orientation. Overall, 94% had experienced some type of verbal or physical assault (National Gay and Lesbian Task Force, 1984). The 1992 report from the Philadelphia Lesbian and Gay Task Force documents that 50% of lesbians experienced public verbal abuse and 35% experienced physical violence (Gross & Aurand, 1992). Homicides against gay men and lesbians were recently reviewed and found to be more likely to involve mutilation and torture and more likely to go unsolved, reflecting the intensity of antigay hatred (Dunlap, 1994).

Psychological and emotional injury can also happen to victims of antigay violence. These include posttraumatic stress syndromes, phobias, eating disorders, chronic pain syndromes, and most commonly, depression (Bybee, 1990). A Yale survey revealed that many lesbians and gay male students reported living in secretiveness and feared antigay violence and harassment on campus (Herek, 1993).

The Hate Crime Statistics Act requires the federal government to collect data obtained by police agencies. However, only 12 states include homophobic violence in their definition of hate crimes. Seventeen other states have hate-crime laws that do not count violence based on sexual orientation, and 21 states do not count hate crimes. National documentation of hate crimes would provide valuable information regarding the need to institute specific intervention programs (Herek, 1989). Every episode of antigay violence sends a chilling message of terror and hatred, which, in effect, silences and perpetuates the invisibility of all lesbians, gay men, and bisexuals (National Gay and Lesbian Task Force, 1994). Such violence against any other minority group would be widely viewed as intolerable.

Effects on Earnings and Medical Insurability

Any form of discrimination against homosexuals is legal in all but eight states. The Michigan Lesbian Health Survey reports that the lesbian population surveyed had a median annual income $10,000 lower than that reported by all Michigan women in 1989, even though the lesbian population was more likely to have obtained a college education (Bybee, 1990). An analysis of the 1990 census data, in which gay and lesbian couples could identify themselves as such, found that although 38% of lesbian respondents were college graduates, compared to 34% of male homosexual and 18% of married heterosexuals, lesbian couples had the lowest income of the three groups (Usdansky, 1993). A reduced earning potential may result from actual discrimination (Bradford et al., 1994; Bybee, 1990) or anticipated discrimination (Mays, Jackson, & Coleman, 1991), which inhibits gays and lesbians from seeking higher profile, higher paying jobs. Barriers to insurance for lesbians may keep the lesbian patient from obtaining important yearly screening tests and from seeking health care early in the course of a disease. In fact, in the Michigan study, 58% of lesbians reported not seeking medical care when they felt they needed it because they lacked insurance or financial resources (Bybee, 1990).

EFFECTS OF HOMOPHOBIA IN MEDICINE ON LESBIAN PATIENTS

Effects on the Doctor–Patient Relationship

Homophobia can lead to misrepresentation of facts by patients and misinterpretation of facts by physicians. Numerous studies have revealed a significant prevalence of homophobic attitudes among all types of health care practitioners in the United States. A 1987 questionnaire of midwest bachelor-degree nursing school faculty members revealed that many believed lesbianism was a disease (17%), immoral (23%), disgusting (34%), and unnatural (52%) (Randall, 1989). Fully 17% thought lesbians molest children, and 8% thought them unfit to be registered nurses. More than half said they would never discuss lesbian issues in their classrooms, and more than a quarter said they were uncomfortable providing care to lesbian patients. In another survey, nursing student respondents rated lesbians who preferred nonfeminine garb as even less intelligent, less achievement oriented, less socially desirable, and as having fewer friends than lesbians who wore more feminine garb (Eliason & Randall, 1991). Common opinions about lesbians in the survey were that they "seduced straights" and were a high risk group for AIDS.

A similar bias is observed among physicians. In a 1986 questionnaire returned by 930 physicians of the San Diego County Medical Society, 23% scored as "severely homophobic," with 30% reporting that they would not admit a highly qualified gay or lesbian applicant to medical school or to a pediatric or psychiatric residency, and 40% stated they would stop referring patients to a colleague if they found out that the colleague was gay or lesbian (Matthews, Booth, & Turner, 1986). Fully 40% reported being uncomfortable providing care to gay or lesbian patients. One third of obstetrician/gynecologists and family practice/internists, the primary care providers and gatekeepers in most comprehensive health care plans, self-reported significantly hostile attitudes toward gay and lesbian patients (Matthews et al., 1986).

In a 1994 survey of the 1311 members of the American Association of Physicians for Human Rights, the United States and Canadian gay and lesbian medical association (now called the Gay and Lesbian Medical Association), over one-half of the 711 respondents had specifically observed the denial of care or provision of reduced or suboptimal care to gay or lesbian patients, and 88% had heard their physician colleagues make disparaging remarks about gay or lesbian patients relating to their orientation (Schatz & O'Hanlan, 1994). While 98% of respondents believed that it was medically important for patients to inform their physicians of their orientation, 64% admitted that in so doing, patients risked receiving substandard care, although 14% believed that the quality of patient care would not be jeopardized. Additionally, 17% of practicing physicians reported being refused medical privileges, employment, educational opportunities, and referrals from other physicians because of their orientation. Social ostracism and verbal harassment or insults by their medical colleagues because of their orientation were reported by one-third of physicians and one-half of medical student respondents. Summarizing the survey results, only 12% of respondents felt that "gay, lesbian or bisexual physicians are accepted as equals in the medical profession" (Schatz & O'Hanlan). Medical students have reported frequently hearing overtly hostile comments made about lesbians and gay people by attending physicians during clinical teaching rounds (Tinmouth & Hamwi, 1994). They expressed frustration with the limited information about homosexuality in their curricula and have requested that medical educators present lectures that are updated, inclusive, and deal directly and honestly with gay-related health issues.

Homophobic attitudes of nurses, medical students, and physicians are perceived by patients and negatively affect their experience of and the quality of their medical care. In one study, 72% of lesbians surveyed reported experiencing ostracism, rough treatment, and derogatory comments, as well as disrespect for their partners, by their medical practitioners (Stevens & Hall, 1988). Several studies document extremely negative reactions from health care practitioners commencing after patients revealed their lesbian orientation (Bybee, 1990; Dardick & Grady, 1980; Glascock, 1981; Smith, Johnson, & Guenther, 1985; Stevens & Hall, 1988). Numerous studies also reveal that 67% to 72% of lesbians elected not to reveal their sexual orientation or behavior, fearing sanctions or repercussions if they did (Cochran & Mays, 1988; Glascock; Johnson, Guenther, Laube, & Keettel, 1981). As a result of the broad perception of disrespect for sexual minorities by the medical professions, 84% of surveyed lesbians were hesitant to return to their physicians' offices for new ailments (Stevens & Hall, 1988) and were less likely to return for indicated medical screening tests, for example, Pap smears, blood pressure, cholesterol, stool blood assays, and so on. One respondent answered: "It's like putting your health in the hands of someone who really hates you" (Stevens & Hall, 1990). It is not a surprise that many lesbians employ the services of complementary health care providers who offer more nurturant care in more natural contexts (Bradford et al., 1994). Lesbians also report preferring female, though not necessarily lesbian, health care providers, because women were perceived as less homophobic (Geddes, 1994).

Effects on Public Health

Many physicians have informed their lesbian patients that they do not require Pap smears because they are assumed to be in a low-risk category: having no sex with males. However, most studies reveal that 77% to 91% of lesbians have had at least one prior sexual experience with a male (Bradford et al., 1994; Bybee, 1990), which may be more extensive among black lesbians than white lesbians because of the pressure to participate in the mainstream African-American community (Mays et al., 1993). Sex with men and smoking are both strong risk factors for contracting the human papilloma virus (HPV), the initiating agent for cervical dysplasia and cancer (Holleb, Fink, & Murphy, 1991). The interval between Pap smears for lesbians was reported to be nearly three times that for heterosexual women (Robertson & Schachter, 1981). As many as 5% to 10% of respondents in two large surveys had never had a Pap smear or had one more than 10 years ago (Bradford et al., 1994; Bybee, 1990). There is no prospective data regarding the necessary frequency of Pap smears in women who no longer have sex with men and no advice for lesbians who have HPV regarding the need for safer sex precautions with other women.

Lesbian women, in one study, weighed more, desired a significantly heavier ideal weight, and had less concern for appearance and thinness than heterosexual women (Herzog, Newman, Yeh, & Warshaw, 1992). High body mass index increases one's risk for breast and endometrial cancer, heart disease, diabetes, gall bladder disease, and hypertension (Holleb et al., 1991; Namnoum, 1993). There is no statistically reliable comparison of such data on a large scale because no government sponsored demographic study has yet asked the question of orientation.

The four major lesbian health surveys consistently observed that between 10% and 31% of lesbians have babies during their lifetimes (Bradford et al., 1994; Bybee, 1990; Mays & Cochran, 1988; Warshafsky, 1992). Having a baby is known to reduce by half one's risk for developing endometrial, breast, and ovarian cancers (Holleb et al., 1991). Long duration of oral contraceptive use also significantly reduces the risk for developing endometrial and ovarian carcinoma (Coker, Harlap, & Fortney, 1993). Although no data are available to document lesbian use of oral contraceptives, lesbians are unlikely to have used any contraceptive extensively. Some national studies have suggested that single women, in comparison with married women, have higher rates of cigarette abuse, lower rates of getting mammograms, doing breast self-exams, and getting clinical breast exams (United States Department of Health and Human Services, 1991). Considering all of these factors, lesbians may experience greater morbidity or mortality from multiple cancers and heart disease, especially if they defer seeing a physician until symptoms or signs become extreme or acute.

One-fourth of lesbians over age 40 in the Michigan study had never had a mammogram (Bybee, 1990). In a recent report from the Northern California Cancer Center analysis of local cancer rates and those from the National Cancer Institute's Surveillance, Epidemiology, and End Results (SEER) Program, it was found that white women in the San Francisco–Oakland area have the highest breast cancer rate in the world. The demographic profile was further broken down by race: San Francisco black women have the fourth highest breast cancer rates reported in the world, and Asian and Latina women in San Francisco have the highest reported rates among all Asian and Latina women in California (Greater Bay Area Cancer Registry, 1994). The 1990 census data reveal that San Francisco has the highest concentration of gay and lesbian households in the United States (Krieger, 1993). Unfortunately, no analysis of the impact of orientation can be undertaken in the Cancer Registry Report because the question of orientation was never asked in the survey.

Outside the context of HIV, representative data on health and psychology issues have not been obtained from the gay and lesbian community because researchers have not considered sexual orientation an important question in national probability health surveys (Rothblum, 1994). If reliable demographic information about lesbian health showed a higher incidence, morbidity, or mortality from various cancers or heart disease, then screening or health education programs could be instituted and targeted to the lesbian population. The psychological needs of the lesbian population could also be addressed more effectively, as well as the issues of ethnic minority lesbians.

It appears clear that members of the medical and mental health professions are not immune to the pervasive social stigma against lesbians. Even when research is done, or when homosexuality is discussed in textbooks, the stigma remains apparent. The researchers rarely involved participants beyond the role of providing data, rarely reported feedback, and almost never indicated using data to promote supportive social action (Walsh-Bowers & Parlour, 1992). The photographs employed to portray lesbian individuals presented an inaccurate and unrepresentative view of lesbians (Whatley, 1992). Frequently, even educators who have supportive attitudes hold themselves back from providing lesbian-inclusive and gay-friendly information because they fear that they will also be held in disdain or criticized for their support of immorality (Sears, 1992). These concerns appear to be reflected in the medical profession as well. Currently none of the patient-education brochures created and distributed by the American College of Obstetricians and Gynecologists (ACOG) include information about sexual orientation in their brochures dealing with teenage sexuality, teaching children about sexuality, sexual dysfunction, painful "intercourse" (sic), and sexually transmitted diseases. Numerous requests to the ACOG Patient Education Committee by members of ACOG have been ignored (O'Hanlan, 1991–1993).

CREATING AND IMPLEMENTING SOLUTIONS

It is important to recognize that being lesbian is not inherently (genetically, biologically) hazardous, but that risk factors are conferred through "homophobic fallout." It is the process of homophobia—the socialization of heterosexuals against homosexuals and concomitant conditioning of gays and lesbians against themselves—which must be recognized by health care providers as a legitimate and potent health hazard.

There are many examples of the progress that has already been made: the American Medical Association (AMA) voted in 1993 to include the words "sexual orientation" in its nondiscrimination statement, after having rejected this motion for 4 consecutive years. The AMA just recently passed a policy statement about medical care for gay men and lesbians that reflects the current science that is available regarding sexual orientation. At the 1993 annual meeting, the American Medical Women's Association (AMWA), the 12,000-member association of female physicians, passed, without opposition, a policy statement urging an end to discrimination by sexual orientation. Moreover, AMWA encouraged:

> National, state, and local legislation to end discrimination based on sexual orientation in housing, employment, marriage and tax laws, child custody and adoption laws; to redefine family to encompass the full diversity of all family structures; and to ratify marriage for lesbian, gay and bisexual people ... creation and implementation of educational programs ... in the schools, religious institutions, medical community, and the wider community to teach respect for all humans. (O'Hanlan, 1993, p. 86)

Changes in Medical Education

Recognizing the importance of knowledge about diversity of sexual orientation in clinical practice is an important part of the solution (Davison & Friedman, 1981). Physicians must recognize that as many as 1% to 3% of the patients they currently see, some 1.2 to 3.6 million Americans, are lesbians or bisexual women that are expressing a part of the normal range of human sexuality. Their unique health issues need to be heard, respected, and addressed. A prerequisite is the learned genuine appreciation of the diversity that exists in America today (Wallick, Cambre, & Townsend, 1992). Such information must come from organized curricula in medical school and residency training programs (Gibson & Saunders, 1994; Murphy, 1992). The Temple University School of Medicine provides its medical community with a resource guide that addresses many of the issues described above (Office of Student Affairs, 1992). The American Psychiatric Association has sponsored "A Curriculum for Learning About Homosexuality and Gay Men and Lesbians in Psychiatric Residencies," which describes educational objectives, learning experiences, and implementation strategies for sound clinical practice (Stein, 1994).

Changes in the Provider–Patient Relationship

Health care providers can do much to reduce homophobia within their individual practices. The need for a trusting, supportive, and open relationship is critical in compiling a thorough and accurate medical history of each patient (Erwin, 1993). The AMA policy statement issued December 1994 about gay and lesbian health emphasized the importance of obtaining an accurate, unbiased sexual history from all patients with a focus on behavior, recognizing the alienation of many gay men and lesbians from the medical system, the ubiquity of prejudice against homosexuals, and the psychological effects of the prejudice (O'Neill, 1994). There are numerous ways for physicians to make their practices more welcoming to lesbian patients:

1. Physicians should routinely ask, when discussing sexual behavior (Cass, 1983), whether a woman is sexual with men, women, both, or neither. Physicians should clearly dispel any assumption of heterosexuality by using inclusive language with all patients, inquiring about behavior, not labeling the orientation, and accepting the information of the patient's behavior with neutrality (Meijer, 1993). Simply having a nonjudgmental, nonhomophobic attitude is not enough. The responsible practitioner must convey a nonjudgmental attitude to all patients.

2. Using generic terms such as *partner* or *spouse*, rather than *boyfriend*, for any patient will encourage trust in the physician by removing assumptions. These terms also signify to heterosexual patients the physician's accepting attitude. Comfortable use of language naming sexual behaviors will facilitate the health history by enhancing clarity of communication (Committee on Lesbian and Gay Concerns, 1991).

3. Registration forms and questionnaires that require patients to identify themselves in heterosexual terms such as single, widowed, or divorced should be revised to include "significantly involved" or "domestic partner" in order to avoid making the lesbian patient feel invisible.

4. Informational brochures for patients, especially those dealing with aspects of human sexuality, need to include information about homosexuality. Educational pamphlets in the offices of gynecologists, pediatricians, and family practitioners could provide life-affirming information to youth and provide an educational source for parents, possibly impacting rates of youth suicide as well as public violence and discrimination (American Academy of Pediatrics: Committee on Adolescence, 1993). The American College of Obstetricians and Gynecologists can review the available literature and generate a brochure similar to those that cover so

many salient topics for women. Similarly, the American Academy of Pediatrics should provide information for parents as well as questioning children.

5. If the lesbian patient is partnered, the provider should also welcome her spouse and routinely encourage the couple to consider obtaining a medical power of attorney document—especially prior to any elective surgery or obstetrical delivery. Just as for married individuals, the physician should provide support for the stability of the patient's relationship. The physician should have the skills to counsel for gay-related anxieties and should safeguard against referrals to homophobic colleagues (Randall, 1989).

With this awareness, practitioners can serve as leaders and positive examples in both the medical and the larger community in signaling the need for reduction in societal homophobia (Morrow, 1993).

Inclusion of Orientation in Research Protocols

Efforts are being made to obtain specific morbidity information about lesbians, but obstacles are plentiful. For example, principal investigators of the National Institutes of Health Women's Health Initiative, the largest study ($n = 160,000$) on women's health ever planned, had initially declined to ask participants their sexual orientation out of fear that respondents would quit the study. However, after a review of information on recruitment and retention of lesbians in health trials (O'Hanlan, 1995) and after piloting the question to test groups, the NIH has agreed to include a sexual orientation question. The investigators of the Nurses' Health Study have also decided to stratify their ongoing longitudinal study by sexual orientation to determine morbidity differences (O'Hanlan, 1994). At the Department of Health and Human Services Secretary's Conference for a National Action Plan for Breast Cancer, the Committee for Access to Mammography recommended that all future and ongoing studies be stratified by orientation because of the presence of multiple risk factors for breast cancer within the lesbian community.

Treatment of Young Girls

In order to provide general information as well as specific education for all adolescents, physicians should not reserve their questions about orientation for the gender-atypical individuals, the "sissy" males and the "tomboy" females (Cwayna, Remafedi, & Treadway, 1991). It is impossible to predict which youth are struggling with issues of orientation, and all youth can benefit from the nonbiased demonstration of the health care provider's positive attitude toward issues of orientation. While gender-atypical youth may ultimately develop a homosexual orientation, negative parental attitudes serve only to alienate the parent and isolate the child (McConaghy & Silove, 1992). It is irrational to classify such behavior in youth as abnormal when homosexuality in adults is not considered abnormal (McConaghy & Silove, 1991).

Recognizing homosexuality as a natural sexual expression, the American Academy of Pediatrics (AAP) recommends psychotherapy only for those gay and lesbian youth who are uncertain about their orientation or who need help addressing personal, family, and environmental difficulties that are concomitant with coming out (American Academy of Pediatrics: Committee on Adolescence, 1993). The AAP also understands that families may experience some stress and may need information while supporting a child's newly recognized orientation and recommends that families contact organizations such as Parents, Family, and Friends of Lesbians and Gays (P-FLAG) for information and support or to obtain therapy (Hammersmith, 1987; Neisen, 1987). The AAP further states: "Therapy directed at changing sexual orientation is contraindicated, since it can provoke guilt and anxiety while having little or no potential for achieving changes in orientation" (American Academy of Pediatrics: Committee on Adolescence, 1993, p 633). Conversion therapy has been found to be ineffective, unethical and harmful (Haldeman, 1994). The AMA updated its policy statement regarding the medical treatment of gay men and lesbians in December 1994 (O'Neill, 1994), concurring that aversion therapy, or behavioral therapy to change sexual orientation is no longer recommended, but rather psychotherapy may be necessary to help gay or lesbian individuals to become more comfortable with their orientation and to deal with society's prejudicial response to them.

It is also necessary to establish school-based family counseling programs, develop school and social support programs for gay and lesbian youth, and promote an accurate image of homosexuals through educational programs initially directed toward educators, clergy, and professionals, and later toward the youth themselves and society at large (Griffin, 1992; Harbeck, 1992; Morrow, 1993; Uribe & Harbeck, 1992). Familiarity with issues of orientation as well as openly respectful attitudes of teachers, parents, local organizations, peers, and friends may help frightened youth come to grips with their fears about their sexual identity and begin to confront their own internalized homophobia as their self-concept strengthens (Morrow; Remafedi & Blum, 1986).

Homophobia needs to be addressed within those age ranges in which it is initially recognized: elementary schools (Morrow, 1993; Uribe & Harbeck, 1992). Young girls need access to accurate information in their school libraries and in social studies classes, as well as in sex education curricula (Uribe & Harbeck). Educators are urging that multicultural diversity training programs in elementary schools must include orientation issues in their curricula (Goodman, 1993). To facilitate acculturation of gay and lesbian youth, and the children of gay and lesbian parents, school libraries need to include storybooks of positive role models that resemble their families (Goodman; Phillip, 1993). The state of Massachusetts requires schools to write policies protecting students from harassment, violence, and discrimination because of orientation; train teachers in crisis intervention and violence prevention; create school-based support groups for gay or lesbian as well as heterosexual students; provide information in the school libraries; and write curricula that include gay and lesbian issues (Massachusetts State House, 1993).

Changes in Government

Government-enforced discrimination needs to be addressed. Members of Congress, the courts, and other elected officials must become informed before casting their votes or making decisions about issues of homosexuality and be willing to take a stand on issues based on scientific facts, not popular biases.

It is reasonable to expect lesbians and gay men to desire marriage when their relationships reach a mutual point of intimacy and commitment. The absence of a homosexual's legal right to marry is reminiscent of the case of *Loving v. Virginia*, in 1967, in which the Supreme Court decided that citizens should not be denied the right to marriage on the basis of physical condition or the color of their skin. It would be inconceivable for anti-Semitism or racism to prevail in such a way that Jews or people of color were forbidden from marrying each other, and yet homosexuals are still denied this right.

Some individuals are worried that legal marriage would "endorse homosexuality," making it seem like an acceptable option and resulting in higher numbers of homosexuals. Some are worried about erosion of traditional family values, the concept of the nuclear family, and the effect of having gay or lesbian clergy. Evidence has already been provided showing that there are no conversions to homosexuality, only the natural evolution of the self into an honest and full expression. There is no scientific basis to imagine that gay and lesbian marriage threatens or devalues heterosexual marriage, if such rights were to be extended to all citizens who desired that for which the institution of marriage stands: a monogamous, long-term, mutually supportive, committed relationship. The impact of denial of the institution of marriage, implying that this class of humans does not deserve validation of its highest human function, is deeply corrosive to the self-concept and precludes the natural fulfillment of needs.

Similarly, the practice of military prosecution and discharge of gay and lesbian service members needs to be reviewed by the courts and declared unconstitutional. Based only in bias and prejudice, this practice also perpetuates misinformation among American youth while cutting short the careers of deserving Americans and wasting millions of dollars.

Such situations imposed on any other minority would be considered entirely intolerable.

The APA has concluded that the most effective solution to the problems that result from homophobia is legislation that would make discrimination against gay men and lesbians illegal (Bersoff & Ogden, 1991). Many universities, corporations, cities, and federal agencies now include sexual orientation in their nondiscrimination policy statements and provide domestic partner benefits, including medical insurance, to all registered families. Recently, the United States Departments of Justice, the Interior, Transportation, and Health and Human Services have included sexual orientation in their nondiscrimination policies but do not yet provide benefits. At Stanford University, the first university to offer identical benefits packages to all employees and their families, the 1992 Report of the Subcommittee on Faculty and Staff Benefits regarding domestic partner benefits stated:

> One imagines, for example, that a decision by Stanford 40 years ago to take the lead in eradicating discrimination against blacks, women, or Jews in admissions, hiring, memberships in sororities and fraternities, etc., would have been politically unpopular with many alumni, as well as with the larger political community. One also imagines that had Stanford taken such a leadership role, few in the Stanford community would look back on that decision now with anything but pride. (Fried, 1992, p. 37)

CONCLUSIONS

All individuals, regardless of their orientation, must begin to discard those old views they innocently learned but that science does not validate. All people have a responsibility to examine their attitudes about homosexuality and recognize the views they hold that are not consistent with facts. In our society, health care providers have a unique opportunity to influence others to align their attitudes with objective information. Education of both adults and children about the diversity of orientation will reduce the pervasive, unfounded disdain for homosexuals and maintain lesbian and gay individuals' self-respect. Legislation proscribing discrimination and providing legal recognition for the unions of lesbian and gay families will begin to restore legal, societal, and financial equity to this marginalized population. The resultant increased visibility of lesbians will increase their familiarity in the community and promote more understanding.

Each of these steps will begin to decrease the oppression of lesbians and gay men from society, as well as the learned self-oppression of the individual from within. Improved access to health care, increased integration into family and society, and heightened life satisfaction, will result in better health, especially when homophobia is recognized as a major health hazard to gay and lesbian individuals.

REFERENCES

Acosta, E. (1979, October 11). Affinity for black heritage: Seeking lifestyle within a community. *The Washington Blade*, pp. A–1, 25.

American Academy of Pediatrics: Committee on Adolescence. (1993). Homosexuality and Adolescence. *Pediatrics, 92*(4).

Bell, A., & Weinberg, M. (1978). *Homosexualities: A study of diversity among men and women*. New York: Simon & Schuster.

Berger, R. (1990). Passing: Impact on the quality of same-sex couple relationships. *Social Work, 35*(4), 328–332.

Bersoff, D., & Ogden, D. (1991). APA amicus curiae briefs. Furthering lesbian and gay male civil rights. *American Psychology, 46*(9), 950–956.

Bloomfield, K. (1993). A comparison of alcohol consumption between lesbians and heterosexual women in an urban population. *Drug and Alcohol Dependence 33*(3), 257–269.

Bradford, J., Ryan, C., & Rothblum, E. D. (1994). National lesbian health care survey: implications for mental health care. *Journal of consulting and Clinical Psychology, 62*(2), 228–242.

Brooks, V. (1981). *Minority stress and lesbian women*. Lexington, MA: Heath.

Bryant, S., & Demian. (1990). Summary of results. Partners' national survey of lesbian & gay couples. *Partners*, 2–6.

Bybee, D. (1990). *Michigan lesbian survey* (Report to the Michigan Organization for Human Rights and the Michigan Department of Public Health. Detroit: Michigan Department of Health and Human Services.

Cabaj, R. (1988). Gay and lesbian couples: Lessons on human intimacy. *Psychology Annals, 18*(1), 21–25.

Cabaj, R. (1992). Substance abuse in the gay and lesbian community. In J. Lowinson, P. Ruiz, & R. Millman (Eds.), *Substance abuse: A comprehensive textbook*, (2nd ed., pp. 852–860). Baltimore, MD: Williams and Wilkins.

Cass, V. C. (1983). Homosexual identity: A concept in need of definition. *Journal of Homosexuality, 9*(2–3), 105–126.

Centers for Disease Control. (1991). Attempted suicide among high school students in the United States. *Morbidity and Mortality Weekly Report, 40*(37), 1–8.

Chan, C. (1992). Cultural considerations in counseling Asian American lesbians and gay men. In S. Dworkin & F. Gutierrez (Eds.), *Counseling gay men and lesbians* (pp. 115–124). Alexandria, VA: American Association for Counseling and Development.

Chapman, B. E., & Brannock, J. C. (1987). Proposed model of lesbian identity development: An empirical examination. *Journal of Homosexuality, 14*(3–4), 69–80.

Clark, W. (Ed.). (1981). *The contemporary tavern* (Vol. 6). New York: Plenum Press.

Cochran, S. D., & Mays, V. M. (1988). Disclosure of sexual preference to physicians by black lesbian and bisexual women. *Western Journal of Medicine, 149*(5), 616–619.

Coker, A. L., Harlap, S., & Fortney, J. A. (1993). Oral contraceptives and reproductive cancers: Weighing the risks and benefits. *Family Planning Perspectives, 25*(1), 17–21.

Committee on Lesbian and Gay Concerns. (1991). Avoiding heterosexual bias in language. *American Journal of Psychology, 46*(9), 973–974.

Cwayna, K., Remafedi, G., & Treadway, L. (1991). Caring for gay and lesbian youth. *Medical Aspects of Human Sexuality, 1*, 50–57.

D'Augelli, A. R., & Hershberger, S. L. (1993). Lesbian, gay, and bisexual youth in community settings: Personal challenges and mental health problems. *American Journal of Community Psychology, 21*(4), 421–448.

Dancey, C. (1990). Sexual orientation in women: An investigation of hormonal and personality variables. *Biological Psychology, 30*(3), 251–264.

Dardick, L., & Grady, K. (1980). Openness between gay persons and health professionals. *Annals of Internal Medicine, 93*, 115–119.

Davison, G. C., & Friedman, S. (1981). Sexual orientation stereotypy in the distortion of clinical judgment. *Journal of Homosexuality, 6*(3), 37–44.

Diamond, D. L., & Wilsnack, S. C. (1978). Alcohol abuse among lesbians: A descriptive study. *Journal of Homosexuality, 4*(2), 123–142.

DePlacido, J. (1994). *Stress, behavioral risk factors, and physical and psychological health outcomes in lesbians.* New York: APA Women's Health Conference.

Dunlap, D. (1994, December 21). Survey on slayings of homosexuals finds high violence and low arrest rate. *The New York Times,* p. A10.

Eliason, M. J., & Randall, C. E. (1991). Lesbian phobia in nursing students. *Western Journal of Nursing Research, 13*(3), 363–374.

Ellis, A. L., & Vasseur, R. B. (1993). Prior interpersonal contact with and attitudes towards gays and lesbians in an interviewing context. *Journal of Homosexuality, 25*(4), 31–45.

Erwin, K. (1993). Interpreting the evidence: competing paradigms and the emergence of lesbian and gay suicide as a "social fact." *International Journal of Health Services, 23*(3), 437–453.

Evans, R. (1971). Adjective check list scores of homosexual men. *Journal of Personality Assessment, 35,* 344.

Ferenczi, S. (1950). Sex and psychoanalysis. In E. Jones (Ed.), (pp. 154–184). New York: Basic Books.

Ferguson, K. D., & Finkler, D. C. (1978). An involvement and overtness measure for lesbians: Its development and relation to anxiety and social zeitgeist. *Archives of Sexual Behavior, 7*(3), 211–227.

Freedman, M. (1971). Homosexuality among women and psychological adjustment. *Dissertations Abstracts International, 28,* 347.

Fried, B. (1992). *Report of the subcommittee on domestic partners' benefits.* University Committee for Faculty and Staff Benefits, Leland Stanford Jr. University, Stanford, CA.

Fyfe, B. (1983). "Homophobia" or homosexual bias reconsidered. *Archives of Sexual Behavior, 12*(6), 549–554.

Gartrell, N. (1981). The lesbian as a "single" woman. *American Journal of Psychotherapy, 35*(4), 502–516.

Geddes, V. A. (1994). Lesbian expectations and experiences with family doctors. How much does the physician's sex matter to lesbians? *Canadian Family Physician, 40*(1), 908–920.

Gibson, G., & Saunders, D. E. (1994). Gay patients. Context for care. *Canadian Family Physician, 40*(1), 721–725.

Gibson, P. (1989). Gay male and lesbian youth suicide. *Report of the Secretary's Task Force Report on Youth Suicide, 3*(DHHS Pub. No. [ADM] 89–1622).

Glascock, E. (1981). *Access to the traditional health care system by nontraditional women: Perceptions of a cultural interaction.* Paper presented at the American Public Health Association, Los Angeles.

Goodman, J. M. (1993, April). Lesbian, gay & bisexual issues in education. *Thrust for Educational Leadership,* 24–28.

Greater Bay Area Cancer Registry. (1994). Breast cancer in the greater bay area. *Greater Bay Area Cancer Registry Report, 5*(1), 1–8.

Greene, B. (1994). Ethnic-minority lesbians and gay men: Mental health and treatment issues. *Journal of Consulting and Clinical Psychology, 62*(2), 243–251.

Griffin, P. (1992). From hiding out to coming out: Empowering lesbian and gay educators. *Journal of Homosexuality, 22*(3–4), 167–196.

Gross, L., & Aurand, S. (1992). *Discrimination and violence against lesbian women and gay men in Philadelphia and the Commonwealth of Pennsylvania: A study by the Philadelphia lesbian and gay task force.* Philadelphia: The Philadelphia Lesbian and Gay Task Force.

Gundlach, R. H. (1977). Sexual molestation and rape reported by homosexual and heterosexual women. *Journal of Homosexuality, 2*(4), 367–384.

Haldeman, D. C. (1994). The practice and ethics of sexual orientation conversion therapy. *Journal of Consulting and Clinical Psychology, 62*(2), 221–227.

Hall, J. M. (1990). Alcoholism in lesbians: Developmental, symbolic interactionist, and critical perspectives. *Health Care of Women International, 11*(1), 89–107.

Hall, J. M. (1994). How lesbians recognize and respond to alcohol problems: A theoretical model of problematization. *Answers and Advances in Nursing Science, 16*(3), 46–63.

Hammersmith, S. K. (1987). A sociological approach to counseling homosexual clients and their families. *Journal of Homosexuality, 14*(1–2), 173–190.

Harbeck, K. M. (1992). Gay and lesbian educators: Past history/future prospects. *Journal of Homosexuality, 22*(3–4), 121–140.

Harry, J. (1989). Sexual identity issues. In Department of Health and Human Services (Ed.), *Report to Louis Sullivan from the Secretary's Task Force on Youth Suicide*. Washington, DC: U. S. Department of Health and Human Services.

Hart, M., Roback, H., Tittler, B., Wietz, L., Walston, G., & McKee, E. (1978). Psychological adjustment of non-patient homosexuals: Critical review of the research literature. *Journal of Clinical Psychiatry, 39*, 604–608.

Hellman, R., Stanton, M., Lee, J., Tytun, A., & Vachon, R. (1989). Treatment of homosexual alcoholics in government funded agencies: Provider training and attitudes. *Hospital and Community Psychiatry, 40*(11), 1163–1168.

Herek, G. M. (1989). Hate crimes against lesbians and gay men. Issues for research and policy. *American Psychology, 45*(9), 1035–1042.

Herek, G. M. (1990). Gay people and government security clearances. A social science perspective. *American Psychology, 44*(6), 948–955.

Herek, G. M. (1993). Documenting prejudice against lesbians and gay men on campus: the Yale sexual orientation survey. *Journal of Homosexuality, 25*(4), 15–30.

Herzog, D., Newman, K., Yeh, C., & Warshaw, M. (1992). Body image satisfaction in homosexual and heterosexual women. *International Journal of Eating Disorders, 11*(4), 391.

Hidalgo, H. (1984). *The Puerto Rican lesbian in the United States*. Palo Alto, CA: Mayfield.

Holleb, A., Fink, D., & Murphy, G. (1991). *American cancer society textbook of clinical oncology* Atlanta, GA: American Cancer Society.

Hooker, E. (1969). Parental relations and male homosexuality in patient and nonpatient samples. *Journal of Consulting and Clinical Psychology, 33*(2), 140–142.

Hunter, J. (1989). *Violence against lesbian and gay youth: A report from the Hetrick Martin Institute*. New York: Hetrick Martin Institute.

Hunter, J., & Schaecter, R. (1990). Lesbian and gay youth. In M. Rotheram-Borus, J. Bradley, & N. Obolensky (Eds.), *Planning to live: Evaluating and treating suicidal teens in community settings*, (pp. 297–316). Tulsa: University of Oklahoma Press.

Isay, R. (1989). *Being homosexual: Gay men and their development*. New York: Avon Books.

Johnson, S. R., Guenther, S. M., Laube, D. W., & Keettel, W. C. (1981). Factors influencing lesbian gynecologic care: A preliminary study. *American Journal of Obstetrics and Gynecology, 140*(1), 20–28.

Kahn, M. J. (1991). Factors affecting the coming out process for lesbians. *Journal of Homosexuality, 21*(3), 47–70.

Krieger, L. (1993, September 12). San Francisco remains a mecca for gay couples. *San Francisco Examiner*, pp. A1, A19.

Landers, A. (1992, April 27). Readers answer the poll: Are you happy to be gay? *San Francisco Sunday Examiner and Chronicle*, p. D2.

Larson, D., & Chastain, R. (1990). Self-concealment: Conceptualization, measurement, and health implications. *Journal of Social and Clinical Psychogy, 9*, 439–455.

Lesbian & Gay Substance Abuse Planning Group. (1991). *San Francisco lesbian, gay and bisexual substance abuse needs assessment*. Paper presented at the Lesbian & Gay Substance Abuse, Sacramento, CA.

Massachusetts State House. (1993). Governor's commission on gay and lesbian youth. Boston: Massachusetts State House.

Matthews, W., Booth, M. W., & Turner, J. (1986). Physicians attitudes toward homosexuality: Survey of a California county medical society. *Western Journal of Medicine, 144,* 106.

Mays, V. M., & Cochran, S. D. (1988). The black women's relationships project: A national survey of black lesbians. In M. Shernoff & W. A. Scott (Eds.), *A sourcebook of gay/ lesbian health care* (2nd ed.). Washington, DC: National Gay and Lesbian Health Foundation.

Mays, V. M., Cochran, S. D., & Rhue, S. (1993). The impact of perceived discrimination on the intimate relationships of black lesbians. *Journal of Homosexuality, 25*(4), 1–14.

Mays, V. M., Jackson, J. S., & Coleman, L. S. (1991). *Perceived discrimination, employment status and job stress in a national sample of black women.* Unpublished manuscript.

McConaghy, N., & Silove, D. (1991). Opposite sex behaviors correlate with degree of homosexual feelings in the predominantly heterosexual. *Austalian and New Zealand Journal Psychiatry, 25*(1), 77–83.

McConaghy, N., & Silove, D. (1992). Do sex-linked behaviors in children influence relationships with their parents? *Archives of Sexual Behavior, 21*(5), 469–479.

Meijer, H. (1993). Can seduction make straight men gay? *Journal of Homosexuality, 24*(3–4), 125–136.

Minton, H. L., & McDonald, G. J. (1983). Homosexual identity formation as a developmental process. *Journal of Homosexuality, 9*(2–3), 91–104.

Morales, E., & Graves, M. (1983). *Substance abuse: Patterns and barriers to treatment for gay men and lesbians in San Francisco* (Report to Community Substance Abuse Services). San Francisco: San Francisco Department of Public Health.

Morrow, D. F. (1993). Social work with gay and lesbian adolescents. *Social Work, 38*(6), 655–660.

Murphy, B. C. (1992). Educating mental health professionals about gay and lesbian issues. *Journal of Homosexuality, 22*(3–4), 229–246.

Namnoum, A. (1993). Obesity: a disease worth treating. *The Female Patient, 18*(33), 33–44.

National Gay and Lesbian Task Force. (1984). *Report on anti-gay/lesbian victimization: A study by the national gay and lesbian task force in cooperation with the gay and lesbian organizations in eight U.S. cities.* Washington, DC: National Gay and Lesbian Task Force Policy Institute.

National Gay and Lesbian Task Force. (1994). *Anti-gay/lesbian violence, victimization, & defamation in 1993.* Washington, DC: National Gay and Lesbian Task Force Policy Institute.

Neisen, J. H. (1987). Resources for families with a gay/lesbian member. *Journal of Homosexuality, 14*(1–2), 239–251.

Newman, B. S., & Muzzonigro, P. G. (1993). The effects of traditional family values on the coming out process of gay male adolescents. *Adolescence, 28*(109), 213–226.

Nurius, P. (1983). Mental health implications of sexual orientation. *Journal of Sexual Research, 19,* 119.

O'Hanlan, K. A. (1991–1993). Personal correspondence with members of the ACOG Patient Education Committee.

O'Hanlan, K. A. (1993). Position paper on lesbian health. *Journal of the American Medical Womens' Association, 49*(3), 86.

O'Hanlan, K. A. (1994). Personal communication with Walter Willett, MD and Patricia Case, MPH. Nurses Health Study II, Harvard Medical School and School of Public Health.

O'Hanlan, K. A. (1995). Recruitment and retention of lesbians in health research trials. *Recruitment and retention of women in clinical studies* (NIH Publication #95-3756, 101–104). Washington DC: National Institutes of Health.

O'Neill, J. (1994). *Health care needs of gay men and lesbians in the U.S.* (Report presented by the Council on Scientific Affairs). Chicago: American Medical Association.

Office of Student Affairs. (1992). *A community of equals: a resource guide for the Temple medical community about gay, lesbian and bisexual people.* Philadelphia: Temple University School of Medicine.

Paul, J., Stall, R., & Bloomfield, K. (1991). Gay and alcoholic: Epidemiologic and clinical issues. *Alcohol Health and Research, 5*(2), 151–160.

Peters, D. K., & Cantrell, P. J. (1991). Factors distinguishing samples of lesbian and heterosexual women. *Journal of Homosexuality, 21*(4), 1–15.

Phillip, M. (1993). Gay issues: Out of the closet, into the classroom, racism, fear of reprisals force black gays and lesbians to keep low profile on campus. *Black Issues in Higher Education,* 20–25.

Randall, C. E. (1989). Lesbian phobia among BSN educators: A survey. *Journal of Nursing Education, 28*(7), 302–306.

Random House dictionary of the English language (2nd ed.). (1987). New York: Random House.

Remafedi, G., & Blum, R. (1986). Working with gay and lesbian adolescents. *Pediatric Annals, 15*(11), 773–783.

Remafedi, G., Farrow, J. A., & Deisher, R. W. (1991). Risk factors for attempted suicide in gay and bisexual youth. *Pediatrics, 87*(6), 869–875.

Remafedi, G., Resnick, M., Blum, R., & Harris, L. (1992). Demography of sexual orientation in adolescents. *Pediatrics, 89*(4 Pt 2), 714–721.

Robertson, P., & Schachter, J. (1981). Failure to identify venereal disease in a lesbian population. *Sexually Transmitted Diseases 8*(2), 75–76.

Rothblum, E. D. (1994). Introduction to the special section: Mental health of lesbians and gay men. *Journal of Consulting and Clinical Psychology, 62*(2), 211–212.

Rotheram-Borus, M., Rosario, M., & Koopman, C. (1991). Minority youths at high risk: Gay males and runaways. In M. E. Colten & S. Gore (Eds.), *Adolescent stress: Causes and consequences* (pp. 181–200). New York: Aldine de Gruyter.

Savin-Williams, R. C. (1988). Theoretical perspectives accounting for adolescent homosexuality. *Journal of Adolescent Health Care, 9*(2), 95–104.

Savin-Williams, R. C. (1989). Parental influences on the self-esteem of gay and lesbian youths: A reflected appraisals model. *Journal of Homosexuality, 17*(1–2), 93–109.

Savin-Williams, R. C. (1994). Verbal and physical abuse as stressors in the lives of lesbian, gay male, and bisexual youths: Associations with school problems, running away, substance abuse, prostitution, and suicide. *Journal of Consulting and Clinical Psychology, 62*(2), 261–269.

Schatz, B., & O'Hanlan, K. (1994). *Anti-gay discrimination in medicine: Results of a national survey of lesbian, gay and bisexual physicians.* San Francisco: The Gay and Lesbian Medical Association.

Schmitt, J., & Kurdek, L. (1987). Personality correlates of positive identity and relationship involvement in gay men. *Journal of Homosexuality, 13,* 101–109.

Schneider, S. G., Farberow, N. L., & Kruks, G. N. (1989). Suicidal behavior in adolescent and young adult gay men. *Suicide Life Threatening Behavior, 19*(4), 381–394.

Schneider, S. G., Taylor, S. E., Hammen, C., Kemeny, M. E., & Dudley, J. (1991). Factors influencing suicide intent in gay and bisexual suicide ideators: Differing models for men with and without human immunodeficiency virus. *Journal of Personality and Social Psychology, 61*(5), 776–788.

Sears, J. T. (1992). Educators, homosexuality, and homosexual students: Are personal feelings related to professional beliefs? *Journal of Homosexuality, 22*(3–4), 29–79.

Shavelson, E., Biaggio, M. K., Cross, H. H., & Lehman, R. E. (1980). Lesbian women's perceptions of their parent-child relationships. *Journal of Homosexuality, 5*(3), 205–215.

Siegelman, M. (1979). Adjustment of homosexual and heterosexual women. *British Journal of Psychiatry, 120,* 477.

Smith, E. M., Johnson, S. R., & Guenther, S. M. (1985). Health care attitudes and experiences during gynecologic care among lesbians and bisexuals. *American Journal of Public Health, 75*(9), 1085–1087.

Sophie, J. (1985). A critical examination of stage theories of lesbian identity development. *Journal of Homosexuality, 12*(2), 39–51.

Sophie, J. (1987). Internalized homophobia and lesbian identity. *Journal of Homosexuality,* *14*(1–2), 53–65.

Stein, T. S. (1994). A curriculum for learning in psychiatric residencies about homosexuality, gay men and lesbians. *Academic Psychiatry, 18*(2), 59–70.

Stephany, T. M. (1992). Faculty support for gay and lesbian nursing students. *Nurse Educators, 17*(5), 22–23.

Stevens, P. E., & Hall, J. M. (1988). Stigma, health beliefs and experiences with health care in lesbian women. *Image Journal of Nursing Schools, 20*(2), 69–73.

Stevens, P. E., & Hall, J. M. (1990). Abusive health care interaction experienced by lesbians: A case of institutional violence in the treatment of women. *Response, 13*(3), 23.

Suppe, F. (1984). Classifying sexual disorders: the diagnostic and statistical manual of the American Psychiatric Association. *Journal of Homosexuality, 9*(4), 9–28.

Swaggart, J. (1982). *Homosexuality: Its cause and its cure.* Baton Rouge, LA: Jimmy Swaggart Ministries.

Thompson, N., McCandless, B., & Strickland, B. (1971). Personal adjustment of male and female homosexuals and heterosexuals. *Journal of Abnormal Psychology, 78,* 237.

Tinmouth, J., & Hamwi, G. (1994). The experience of gay and lesbian students in medical school. *Journal of the American Medical Association, 271*(9), 714–715.

United States Department of Health and Human Services. (1991). *Health: United States prevention profile for 1991.* Washington DC: Department of Health and Human Services.

United States Government Accounting Office. (1992). *Report to congress on homosexuality in the military.* Washington, DC: United States Congress.

Uribe, V., & Harbeck, K. M. (1992). Addressing the needs of lesbian, gay, and bisexual youth: The origins of PROJECT 10 and school-based intervention. *Journal of Homosexuality, 22*(3–4), 9–28.

Usdansky, M. (1993, April 12). Gay couples, by the numbers, data suggest they're fewer than believed, but affluent. *USA Today,* pp. 1a, 8a.

Wallick, M. M., Cambre, K. M., & Townsend, M. H. (1992). How the topic of homosexuality is taught at U.S. medical schools. *Academic Medicine, 67*(9), 601–603.

Walsh-Bowers, R. T., & Parlour, S. J. (1992). Researcher-participant relationships in journal reports on gay men and lesbian women. *Journal of Homosexuality, 23*(4), 93–112.

Warshafsky, L. (1992). *Lesbian health needs assessment.* Los Angeles: The Los Angeles Gay and Lesbian Community Services Center.

Whatley, M. H. (1992). Images of gays and lesbians in sexuality and health textbooks. *Journal of Homosexuality, 22*(3–4), 197–211.

Zera, D. (1992). Coming of age in a heterosexist world: The development of gay and lesbian adolescents. *Adolescence, 27*(108), 849–854.

PART IV

ISSUES OF ETHNICITY IN HEALTH PSYCHOLOGY

CHAPTER 15

On Nothing and Everything
The Relationship between Ethnicity and Health

Pamela M. Kato

INTRODUCTION

The use of ethnicity as a grouping variable in health research is disturbing to scientists. It is poorly defined, is not objectively measured, and cannot be studied in a true experiment. Thus, scientific conclusions about the causal relationship between ethnicity and health are difficult to make. To a large extent, ethnic categories are problematic because they are socioculturally constructed categories. Depending on the culture, definitions and criteria for ethnic categories vary. Even within cultures, such as the United States, criteria for membership differs from one context to another. However, ethnicity as a grouping variable should not be discarded because it is not scientific. It deserves careful study because it *is* associated with important health outcomes. It is well known that ethnic groups differ dramatically on many measures of health outcomes (e.g., U.S. Department of Health and Human Services, 1985).

Cancer, the second leading cause of death in the United States, is but one example where interesting patterns of ethnic differences and health outcomes can be found. These ethnic differences in health demonstrate

PAMELA M. KATO • Department of Psychiatry and Behavioral Sciences, Stanford University School of Medicine, Stanford, California 94305.

Handbook of Diversity Issues in Health Psychology, edited by Pamela M. Kato and Traci Mann. Plenum Press, New York, 1996.

the complex nature of the relationship between ethnicity and health. Asians and Pacific Islanders tend to have low rates of cancer compared to nonminorities but have a higher annual average incidence rate of stomach cancer compared to nonminorities (Miller, 1980). African-Americans have extremely high average annual excess cancer deaths compared to whites (DHHS, 1985). The smoking rate for Hispanics is slightly higher than that of non-Hispanic whites (40% vs. 38%), but Hispanics have lower incidence rates of smoking-related cancers than non-Hispanic whites (DHHS, 1985). Similarly, Native Americans experience the *lowest* annual incidence of cancer of all U.S. population groups, but once they are diagnosed with cancer, they are more likely to die of cancer than any other subgroup in the population (DHHS, 1985).

Similar patterns of ethnic differences in health outcomes can be found in other domains of health such as cardiovascular disease, infant mortality, morbidity, and life expectancy. All of the statistics show that ethnic differences in health outcomes exist and are robust. They also suggest that it is not clear why these differences exist. Perhaps biological or genetic factors correlate with this socially constructed factor, but other factors that interact with ethnicity correlate as well and should be carefully evaluated.

If the health of ethnic groups is to improve, the relationship between the sociocultural construction of ethnic categories and health must be carefully scrutinized. In this chapter, we first explore definitions of ethnicity, then examine various factors that may play a role in differences in health outcomes, and finally demonstrate how attention to ethnicity can improve interventions.

DEFINING ETHNICITY

Many purported definitions of ethnicity are vague and misleading. It is often thought that ethnic categories distinguish people who differ in terms of physical characteristics. This categorization is supposed to capture biological differences between groups of people. Hence, the term *ethnicity* is often used interchangeably with race (Zuckerman, 1990). Ethnicity is also commonly ascribed to people in an attempt to capture the ways in which people differ in terms of their national origin (e.g., Mexican-American) or general geographic origin (e.g., Asian-Pacific Islander). These definitions seem to indicate objective distinctions between people, yet careful study reveals that they are neither reliable nor valid indicators of ethnic groupings. More commonly, research scientists are acknowledging that ethnic categories are sociocultural constructions that are derived from systems of rules that groups of individuals within a culture share. There is social agreement on who belongs to which ethnic group. This agreement is not based on objective rules, but on social agreement of what criteria are important for inclusion in a particular ethnic category, what feels like a "natural" category, and what rules matter more than others in deciding upon ethnic categorization.

To understand how ethnicity is associated with health outcomes, we must understand how the dividing lines between ethnic groups are delineated. In this section, racial, geographic, and sociocultural constructions of ethnicity are examined although other constructions of ethnicity do exist (e.g., language and cultural affiliations). None of these alone define ethnic groups. Each purported definition in combination with the others is filtered through a sociocultural rule system to contribute to the ethnic categorization of individuals in different contexts. We begin by outlining purported criteria for creating ethnic categories, starting with race, and end by explaining the sociocultural construction of ethnic categories.

Racial Definitions

Ethnic classifications are often used interchangeably with racial classifications. Race has been defined at various levels with questionable success. Traditional definitions of race are based on attempts to classify people based on differences between various biological systems. At the lowest level of biology, attempts have been made to provide a taxonomy of races based on genetic analyses. This has included attempts to classify race by genetically determined factors, such as blood types. At other levels, race has been defined based on physical characteristics that are assumed to be a good proxy for genetics. Years of scientific inquiry have failed to show evidence of distinct biological differences between the races.

Race was originally a term used as part of a system of biological taxonomy for the classification of plants and animals. Race referred to an "inbreeding, geographically isolated population that differs in distinguishable physical traits from other members of the species" (Zuckerman, 1990). Because racial categories were constructed to inform knowledge in biology, it is not surprising that scientists made attempts to group populations based on studies of genetic systems (Latter, 1980). Their findings, however, pointed to the questionable validity of race as an indicator of genetic differences between groups of people.

Boyd (1950) defined a race as a population that differs significantly from other human populations in the frequency of one or more of the genes it possesses. In his first attempt to classify groups of people, he found six races, similar in many ways to early classifications of race based on physical characteristics. In 1958, Boyd amended his number of different races to 13 after the discovery of a number of new blood-group genes. Other anthropologists have claimed that there are anywhere from 30 to

34 races based on geography, physical characteristics, and genetic analyses (Coon, Garn, & Birdsell, 1950; Dobzhansky, 1962). Modern taxonomists debate the existence of 3 to 60 or more races (Garn, 1971). Still others have claimed that there are hundreds of racial groups, depending on the indicators used (Gottesman, 1968). Current data on the distribution of human genes indicate that there is surprisingly little evidence of any relationship between a deep analysis of genetic traits and stereotypical physical traits that superficially seem to differentiate groups of people (Cavalli-Sforza, Menozzi, & Piazza, 1994).

At yet another level, race is defined on the basis of physical characteristics. For example, scientists might classify an individual's race on the basis of height, skin color, head shape and size, hair type, or facial characteristics (e.g., eye shape, nose shape, nose size). Because races appear to differ in physical characteristics and physical characteristics are handed down genetically, it is thought that differing physical characteristics indicate that races differ in their biology. However, this method of classifying individuals based on physical characteristics is inadequate.

Classifications of race based on physical characteristics are culturally influenced. A particularly salient example of cultural influences in classification occurs when classifying biracial people. For example, an individual with one African-American and one white parent will have physical characteristics of both and will carry 50% of the genes of the African-American parent and 50% of the genes of the white parent. In the culture of the United States, this individual is likely to self-identify as African-American (Poussaint, 1984), is likely to be considered African-American by the larger society, and for the purposes of research, to be classified as African-American. Objectively speaking, this designation is arbitrary. In Brazil, a person with one black and one white parent would receive a racial classification as *mulato*. This classification acknowledges the race of both parents. The difference in racial classifications between the United States and Brazil points to the arbitrary nature of racial classifications and the impact of culture on racial classifications.

Attempts to genetically determine racial groupings and attempts to classify race based on physical characteristics have failed. Racial classification of individuals based on these methods are unreliable and subject to cultural influences. The failure of these past methods has led scholars to acknowledge the sociocultural construction of ethnicity as race. In sum, when we speak of race and racial differences, we are not speaking of groups of people who differ from each other by any distinct biological measures even though certain biological measures may be correlated with certain races (e.g., gene for sickle cell). We are speaking of differences determined socioculturally. This practice suggests that when examining racial differences in health outcomes, care should be taken not to overattribute the differences to biology and to consider the role of sociocultural influences that affect the individual within a particular racial group.

Ethnicity as National or Geographic Origin

Ethnicity is sometimes used to designate national origin. In fact, the word *ethnicity* is derived from the Greek *ethnos* meaning "nation." It is also used to more generally refer to one's geographical origin. Classifications of this type are not strongly representative of the within-group diversity that usually exists.

For example, the label, Mexican-American, is intended to capture a subgroup of the U.S. population with origins in the country of Mexico. This category, however, also includes individuals whose ancestors emigrated from nations in Europe to Mexico, individuals who trace their ancestry from the indigenous people of Mexico, and finally, people who trace their ancestry from a combination of the aforementioned geographical areas. The ethnic category, Mexican-American, can include people whose ancestors have never even lived in present day Mexico. These people may have their roots in areas of the southwest United States that were once Mexico before the United States claimed it as its own. These Mexican-Americans, or Chicanos, culturally and politically assert their ties with both present day Mexico and the Mexico that existed before its land was claimed by the United States. Ethnicity defined by national origin is clearly not consistently a sensitive representative label for within-group diversity.

Ethnicity as national or geographic origin is also not sensitive to the number of generations an individual has been in the United States. First-generation immigrants may be very different from second-generation immigrants. For example, first-generation immigrants from Mexico tend to give birth to infants with low birthweight. Second-generation Mexican-Americans, however, tend to give birth to infants with higher birthweights within the healthy range. The second-generation birthweights are closer to standard birthweights found in the United States (Kleinman, 1990). Simply assessing ethnicity as national origin does not capture generational differences within groups.

Geographical origins may be related to health differences to the extent that certain beliefs and practices of people who have immigrated from certain regions carry on these traditions in the United States. This definition of ethnicity, however, like racial, linguistic, and cultural definitions, is neither an objective, reliable, nor valid measure of what it purports to represent. We turn to the possibility of ethnicity as a sociocultural construction.

Sociocultural Definitions

Ethnic categories are not objectively measured and are not reliably determined. Ethnic groupings are not based on biological, psychological, or social differences between people. Ethnic groupings are perhaps more accurately described as a combination of these differences, which are decided upon by sociocultural rules. These sociocultural rules that guide ethnic groupings are culturally derived frameworks that organize the functioning of individuals within groups. The main characteristics of these sociocultural rules of ethnic categorization are (1) overall agreement, (2) "naturalness", and (3) a hierarchy of rules. On a larger level, the categorization process is based on naive theories about differences between and within ethnic groups. These naive theories that drive ethnic categorizations determine people's identities and the identities people assign to others. The self- and other-assigned identities make up the cultural framework in which people pursue their needs through institutions, function psychologically, and practice "acceptable" behaviors.

Despite the shortcomings of the factors that purportedly define and delineate ethnic groupings, there seems to be an agreement on who belongs to which ethnic group. An individual who has Asian physical features, or "looks" Asian, is classified as Asian, even if this person does not engage in practices consistent with his or her culture. Cultural ties to American Indian tribes counts for an American Indian classification. Ancestry from Mexico counts for a Hispanic classification.

Despite the vagueness of the categories, the boundaries of ethnicities feel natural. People have an intuitive sense that these groupings are natural and even biologically based. This sense persists despite a lack of empirical evidence of a biological structure of ethnic groupings.

In addition to our consensus and naturalness, we use a hierarchy of rules to determine ethnicity. Physical attributes count very heavily in determining ethnic group identity. Physical attributes usually take precedence over national origin and cultural affiliations in determining ethnic groupings. People who look Asian are considered Asian even if they were born in Canada and even if they have few cultural ties with Asia. National origin usually takes precedence over cultural affiliations such as linguistic abilities. A person whose ancestors are from Mexico but who does not speak Spanish is likely to be identified as Hispanic.

The social agreement of ethnic categories, their perceived naturalness, and their hierarchical rules for determining categories are characteristics of what D'Andrade (1984) has called "constitutive rules." *Constitutive rules* are systems of rules that say "X counts as Y in context C" (D'Andrade). For example, in the case of ethnic classifications, constitutive rules may say that a person who comes from Puerto Rico is considered Hispanic by virtue of what is filled out on a form, but this same person may be considered African-American by a doctor or nurse caring for this person who does not inquire about patients' ethnic background. In most instances, we classify people based on constitutive rules.

Recent work in cognitive psychology suggests that the coherence of a concept may exist because the concept fits a person's background knowledge or naive theories about the world (Murphy & Medin, 1985). Interactions with people of the same or differing ethnicities may lead people to form naive theories and implicit assumptions about ethnic groupings that in turn contribute to the agreement, naturalness, and hierarchy of rules that characterize ethnic categorizations. The sociocultural construction of ethnicity suggests that a combination of sociocultural factors may contribute to observed ethnic differences in health outcomes.

FACTORS THAT CONTRIBUTE TO ETHNIC DIFFERENCES IN HEALTH

The health of individuals in ethnic groups can be affected by a number of structural and psychological factors. Structural factors such as resources, environment, institutions, and policies may (or may not) impact the health of ethnic groups depending on levels of both overt and covert discriminatory or racist policies that structure the interactions individuals have with these structural factors. The medical delivery system in the United States is set up by the white middle and upper classes, with white middle- and upper-class assumptions about how to serve people. These assumptions may not be consistent with the beliefs and needs of all ethnic groups. This mismatch of assumptions results in the failure of the institution to serve all patients well while perhaps misplacing blame on certain groups of patients for their ill health because they have failed to abide by the rules of a system that was not set up for them (see Kleinman, 1980, for a more thorough discussion).

Everyday psychological factors including schemas for treatment processes, concepts of health, and beliefs about personal agency impact health through the behaviors and practices that are associated with them. If individuals differ on these factors by ethnic group, health outcomes will differ by ethnic grouping. People who identify with certain ethnic groups may more or less value eating certain foods, engage in culturally approved high-risk health behaviors, and believe in the efficacy of pursuing traditional medical interventions.

Ethnic group members will differ on health outcomes if they have distinct notions about who they are as a member of an ethnic group, what is "right" to do as a member of their ethnic group, and how other people will treat them because of their ethnic group identity. These notions related to ethnic identity can interact with beliefs that health professionals hold. For example, it may feel more right for certain members of ethnic groups to question their doctor's treatment directives and to be very aggressive and controlling in the patient role. Members of other ethnic groups may feel that it is more natural for a patient to give the utmost respect to the doctor, not express doubt, and trust that the doctor has the expertise to know what is best for the patient. In contrast, doctors of certain ethnic identities may be more or less understanding of the meaning and intent of patients who are more or less active in their patient roles, which in turn can impact patient care and health outcomes.

Structural and psychological factors that impact health are numerous and complex. They interact with ethnicity because they seem to be correlated with the ways that ethnic groups are categorized. These factors should be considered along with biology in order to elucidate the relationship between ethnicity and health. We examine these factors and their relation to ethnic differences in health using the example of ethnicity and breast cancer.

The Example of Breast Cancer and Ethnicity

There are ethnic differences in the incidence and survival rates for women with breast cancer. White women in the United States tend to have higher incidence rates of breast cancer than women in ethnic groups. White women have a 20% higher incidence of breast cancer than African-American women (91 compared with 73 per 100,000; National Center for Health Statistics, 1991). (We focus on whites and African-American females because much research has focused on the discrepancy between these two ethnic groups and health outcomes.) Although proportionately more white females are diagnosed with breast cancer than African-American females, white females are more likely to survive breast cancer than African-American females. About 76% of white females have a five-year relative survival rate compared to African-American females who have a 63% relative survival rate (DHHS, 1985). In sum, although more white females than African-American females get breast cancer, African-American females are more likely to die of breast cancer once diagnosed. In the following section, explanations for these ethnic differences in health are explored.

Factors Relating to Ethnic Differences in Incidence of Breast Cancer

There is a great deal of evidence that a number of factors play a strong role in the incidence of breast cancer. Structural and psychological factors that impact ethnic groups differentially are examined.

Structural factors, such as access to resources, may influence ethnic differences in incidence of breast cancer. One study that investigated the role of breast cancer screening through early symptoms and mammographic screening found that mammographic screening contributed to the higher reported incidence of breast cancers among white women compared to African-American women (Liff, Sung, Chow, Greenberg, & Flanders, 1991). This suggests that increased detection through screening may contribute to ethnic differences in the incidence of breast cancer. White females may have greater access to resources because screening facilities are more accessible in their communities.

Psychological factors, such as personal agency, may contribute to differences in screening behaviors. White females may feel more of a sense of personal agency and sense of control over their health to enact behaviors that promote the early detection of breast cancer because a higher proportion of white females are in higher socioeconomic status (SES) groups than African-American females. High perceived self-efficacy is generally related to the practice of health-promoting behaviors and overall better health (Grembowski, Patrick, Diehr, & Durham, 1993). People in lower SES groups often experience a lack of control over their environment. The lack of perceived control in the domain of health has been hypothesized to be a factor in poor health outcomes among lower SES groups (Dutton & Levine, 1989).

Everyday psychological factors such as health-related nutrition beliefs and practices can influence ethnic differences in the incidence of breast cancer. Diet is an important determinant of breast cancer risk. African-American women tend to have diets high in protective agents against breast cancer that may be related to their lower incidence of breast cancer. One study on ethnic differences in nutritional risk factors for breast cancer found that African-American women eat more foods that are protective against cancer, such as fruits and vegetables, than white women eat (Zang, Barrett, & Cohen, 1994). Ethnic variation in beliefs about what is good to eat every day and the consequent nutritional practices can contribute to ethnic variation in the incidence of breast cancer.

In addition to dietary factors, reproductive behaviors contribute to the incidence of breast cancer. Reproductive behaviors are culturally determined psychological factors that reflect beliefs about when it is good, right, or acceptable to start a family or have a child. Finally, sociocultural pressures from families, communities, and institutions among certain ethnic groups may dictate when it is good or right to have a child or to have no children at all. Women who have their first child after the age of 30 or who do not have children at all are at increased risk for breast cancer (Musey, Collins, Musey, Martino-Saltzman, & Preedy, 1987). In one study, black adolescents were more likely to expect early childbearing than other ethnic groups (Trent, 1994). If these beliefs translate to practice, these young women could lower their risk for breast cancer by their early childbearing.

In the realm of biology, scientists have identified genes that predispose women to breast cancer and have examined familial risk factors for breast cancer. It is thought that only a minority of breast cancer cases are genetically determined. The gene for breast cancer, BRCA1, accounts for only about 5% of all cases (Claus, Risch, & Thompson, 1991). Few studies have addressed ethnic differences in genetic risk for breast cancer (for a recent exception, see FitzGerald et al. [1996]). There is also a paucity of studies investigating familial patterns of breast cancer among minority populations. However, one small study found that family history of breast cancer in a first-degree relative was a risk factor to the same degree for both African-American and white patients (Bondy, Spitz, Halabi, Fueger, & Vogel, 1992). Care should be taken in inferring a biological basis in familial patterns of cancer because other psychosocial risk factors for cancer can be shared within families as well.

In sum, counseling that includes not only information about genetic and familial risk factors but also information about other psychosocial risk factors outlined above would likely promote early detection for all ethnic groupings. Attention to culturally determined factors that increase risk within ethnic groups would further promote disease prevention and contribute to the effectiveness of health interventions.

Factors Relating to Ethnic Differences in Survival Rates of Breast Cancer

Ethnic differences in survival rates, like incidence rates, may also be related to factors that impact ethnic groups differently. These differences may reflect ethnic differences in health at diagnosis, structural environments, or psychological factors, to name a few.

White females may have a survival advantage if their cancer is diagnosed at an early stage. In fact, white females in upper education or income levels are more likely to be diagnosed with breast cancer at an early stage (c.f., Jones, Kasl, Curnen, Owens, & Dubrow, 1995; Wells & Horm, 1992). Cancer treatment at early stages is generally associated with improved survival. This difference between ethnic groups in stage at diagnosis may be related to a number of structural and psychological factors.

Differences in survival may reflect structural differences in the communities where most African-American and white women live. White females may simply have better access to better health facilities in their communities. Better access can increase treatment compliance and satisfaction with treatment that may be related to survival. In addition, the medical system in general is set up to serve middle-class patients. Adequate treatment may not be attainable within a system that is not set up to meet the needs of all patients or of patients from other ethnic backgrounds.

White females may have improved survival rates because of their place in the social hierarchy. Socioeconomic status is a composite representation of one's economic status (e.g., income), social status (e.g., education), and work status (e.g., occupation) (Dutton & Levine, 1989). Proportionately more white females are in middle- and upper-socioeconomic status groupings than are African-American women. Recent research has outlined a persistent health gradient from lower to upper classes (Adler, Boyce, Chesney, Cohen et al., 1994; Marmot, Ryff, Bumpass, Shipley, & Marks, 1995) with upper classes showing a reliable health advantage. In one large epidemiological study, the survival differences between black and white women with breast cancer disappeared after adjusting for social class differences (Bassett & Krieger, 1986). This suggests that survival differences are largely associated with socioeconomic factors.

Psychological factors on the part of the patient and doctors may also explain ethnic differences in breast cancer survival. White and African-American females may differ in their attitudes about the usefulness or effectiveness of practicing preventive behaviors such as breast self-examination or mammography. Beliefs that preventive behaviors will be ineffective may lead to a diagnosis of cancer when the patient's cancer is advanced. White and African-American women may also differ in their general beliefs about the effectiveness of health-maintenance and disease-prevention behaviors. These beliefs and practices may differentially affect their overall health and treatment of the cancer once diagnosed.

Doctors may differ in their attitudes toward African-American and white female patients. Differences in survival can arise if patterns of care differ between ethnic groups. Doctors may have certain beliefs about the effectiveness of teaching African-American and white women how to perform preventive behaviors such as breast self-examinations. Doctors may also have certain beliefs about how to care for African-American versus white females that may affect their health care practices. One large study of 7,781 patients with breast cancer found that even after controlling for age and stage of disease, African-American patients experienced significantly different care than white patients experienced (Diehr et al., 1989). African-American patients with breast cancer were less likely to receive certain tests or to be referred for postsurgical rehabilitation. They were also more likely to undergo procedures such as liver scans and radiation therapy in situations where these procedures are deemed "less appropriate." Even after controlling for ethnic differences in health insurance, hospital characteristics, and physician characteristics, ethnic differences in care persisted.

Ethnic differences in survival, like ethnic differences in incidence of breast cancer, are affected by sociocultural factors. These factors include but are not limited to structural factors, status differences, self-efficacy beliefs, and implicit racial discrimination. Acknowledgment of these factors along with socioculturally sensitive interventions can promote improved survival for all ethnic groups.

PAYING ATTENTION TO ETHNICITY IN INTERVENTIONS

General health interventions can be more effective if they are targeted toward ethnic groups. The chapters in this volume illustrate how attention to ethnicity can improve health promotion and treatment interventions.

Three of the chapters in this section specifically focus on ethnicity and disease prevention. Jackson and Sellers (1996, this volume) argue that attention to individual, intermediate, and societal issues that impact African-Americans across the life span should be considered in interventions directed toward African-American health. Castro, Coe, Gutierres, and Saenz (1996, this volume) emphasize cultural issues in creating health-promotion programs that attend to specific Latino issues in health and focus specifically on cancer prevention issues. Schinke (1996, this volume) argues that a behavioral approach to disease prevention that focuses specifically on Native-American health needs, cultural beliefs and practices, collaboration in the community, and an alliance between investigators and Native Americans will provide the most successful disease prevention program.

Two of the chapters in this section emphasize issues of treatment and ethnicity. Chun, Enomoto, and Sue (1996, this volume) maintain that attention to somatization among Asians can ensure more effective health interventions. Smith and Lin (1996, this volume) discuss factors related to ethnic differences in response to various drugs that should be considered when treating patients to improve outcomes. Williams and Rucker (1996) argue that attention to the role of SES when examining ethnic differences in health will clarify the causal mechanisms involved in ethnic differences in health outcomes and will promote the development of effective interventions for all ethnic groups.

CONCLUSION

Ethnic groups show dramatic differences on many measures of health. Because ethnic categories are sociocultural creations, not scientific constructions, the concept of ethnicity is, in general, imprecise and poorly defined. Nevertheless, the sociocultural construction of ethnic grouping may be intrinsically related to the pattern of ethnic differences in health outcomes. The cultural nature of ethnic groupings as a process of categorization and the implications this process has for health should be carefully scrutinized in order to promote the health of all groups. An appreciation of the role of culture in the construction of ethnic groupings may contribute to more effective treatment of all groups of people.

REFERENCES

Adler, N. E., Boyce, T., Chesney, M. A., Cohen, S., Folkman, S., Khan, R. L., & Syme, S. L. (1994). Socioeconomic status and health: The challenge of the gradient. *American Psychologist, 49* 15–24.

Bassett, M. T., & Krieger, N. (1986). Social class and black-white differences in breast cancer survival. *American Journal of Public Health, 76*, 1400–1403.

Bondy, M. L., Spitz, M. R., Halabi, S., Fueger, J. J., & Vogel, V. G. (1992). Low incidence of familial breast cancer among Hispanic women. *Cancer Causes Control, 3*, 377–382.

Boyd, W. C. (1950). *Genetics and the races of man.* Boston: Little, Brown.

Castro, F. G., Coe, K., Gutierres, S., & Saenz, D. (1996). Designing health promotion programs for Latinos. In P. M. Kato & T. Mann (Eds.), *Handbook of diversity issues in health psychology* (pp. 319–345). New York: Plenum Press.

Cavalli-Sforza, L. L., Menozzi, P., & Piazza, A. (1994). *The history and geography of human genes.* Princeton, NJ: Princeton University Press.

Chun, C., Enomoto, K., & Sue, S. (1996). Health care issues among Asian Americans: Implications of somatization. In P. M. Kato & T. Mann (Eds.), *Handbook of diversity issues in health psychology* (pp. 347–365). New York: Plenum Press.

Claus, E. B., Risch, N., & Thompson, W. (1991). Genetic analysis of breast cancer in the cancer and steriod hormone study. *American Journal of Human Genetics, 48,* 232–242.

Coon, C. S., Garn, S. M., & Birdsell, J. B. (1950). *Races.* Springfield, IL: Thomas.

D'Andrade, R. G. (1984). Cultural meaning systems. In R. A. Schweder & R. A. Levine (Eds.), *Culture theory: Essays on mind, self, and emotion* (pp. 88–119). Cambridge, UK: Cambridge University Press.

Diehr, P., Yergan, J., Chu, J., Feigl, P., Glaefke, G., Moe, R., Bergner, M., & Rodenbaugh, J. (1989). Treatment modality and quality differences for black and white breast-cancer patients treated in community hospitals. *Medical Care, 27,* 942–958.

Dobzhansky, T. (1962). *Mankind evolving.* New Haven, CT: Yale University Press.

Dutton, D., & Levine, S. (1989). Overview, methodological critique, and reformulation. In J. P. Bunker, D. S. Gomby, & B. H. Kehrer (Eds.), *Pathways to health* (pp. 29–69). Menlo Park, CA: The Henry J. Kaiser Family Foundation.

FitzGerald, M. G., MacDonald, D. J., Krainer, M., et al. (1996). Germ-line *BRCA1* mutations in Jewish and non-Jewish women with early-onset breast cancer. *The New England Journal of Medicine, 334,* 143–149.

Garn, S. M. (1971). *Human races* (3rd ed.). Springfield, IL: Charles C Thomas.

Gottesman, I. I. (1968). *Biogenetics of race and class* (pp. 1–51). New York: Holt, Rinehart and Winston, Inc.

Grembowski, D., Patrick, D., Diehr, P., & Durham, M. (1993). Self-efficacy and health behavior among older adults. *Journal of Health & Social Behavior, 34,* 89–104.

Jackson, J. S., & Sellers, S. L. (1996). African-American health over the life-course: A multidimensional framework. In P. M. Kato & T. Mann (Eds.), *Handbook of diversity issues in health psychology* (pp. 301–317). New York: Plenum Press.

Johnson, S. D. (1990). Toward clarifying culture, race, and ethnicity in the context of multicultural counseling. *Journal of Multicultural Counseling and Development, 18,* 41–51.

Jones, B. A., Kasl, S. V., Curnen, M. G. M., Owens, P. H., & Dubrow, R. (1995). Can mammography screening explain the race difference in stage at diagnosis of breast cancer? *Cancer (Philadelphia), 75,* 2103–2113.

Kleinman, A. (1980). *Patients and healers in the context of culture: An exploration of the borderland between anthropology, medicine, and psychiatry.* Berkeley, CA: University of California Press.

Kleinman, J. (1990). Infant mortality among racial/ethnic minority groups, 1983–1984. *Morbidity and Mortality Weekly Report, 39,* 31–39.

Latter, B. (1980). Genetic differences within and between populations of the major human subgroups. *The American Naturalist, 116,* 220–237.

Liff, J. M., Sung, J. F. C., Chow, W. H., Greenberg, R. S., & Flanders, W. D. (1991). Does increased detection account for the rising incidence of breast cancer? *American Journal of Public Health, 81,* 462–465.

Marmot, M., Ryff, C., Bumpass, L., Shipley, M., & Marks, N. (1995). *Social inequalities in health: A major public health problem.* London: University College London Medical School.

Miller, A. B. (1980). Nutrition and cancer. *Preventive Medicine, 9,* 189–195.

Murphy, G., & Medin, D. (1985). The role of theories in conceptual coherence. *Psychological Review, 92,* 289–315.

Musey, V. C., Collins, D. C., Musey, I. P., Martino-Saltzman, D., & Preedy, J. R. K. (1987). Long-term effect of a first pregnancy on the secretion of prolactin. *New England Journal of Medicine, 316,* 229–234.

National Center for Health Statistics. (1991). *Health: United States, 1990.* Hyattsville, MD: Public Health Service.

Poussaint, A. F. (1984). *Benefits of being interracial* (Vol. 15). New York: Council on Interracial Books for Children.

Schinke, S. (1996). Behavioral approaches to illness prevention for Native Americans. In P. M. Kato & T. Mann (Eds.), *Handbook of diversity issues in health psychology* (pp. 367–387). New York: Plenum Press.

Smith, M., & Lin, K. (1996). A biological, environmental, and cultural basis for ethnic differences in treatment. In P. M. Kato & T. Mann (Eds.), *Handbook of diversity issues in health psychology* (pp. 389–406). New York: Plenum Press.

Trent, K. (1994). Family context and adolescents' expectations about marriage, fertility, and nonmarital childbearing. *Social Science Quarterly, 75,* 319–339.

U.S. Department of Health and Human Services. (1985). *Report of the secretary's task force on black and minority health.* Washington, DC: U.S. Government Printing Office.

Wells, B. L., & Horm, J. W. (1992). Stage at diagnosis in breast cancer: Race and socioeconomic factors. *American Journal of Public Health, 82,* 1383–1385.

Williams, D. R., & Rucker, T. (1996). Socioeconomic status and the health of racial minority populations. In P. M. Kato & T. Mann (Eds.), *Handbook of diversity issues in health psychology* (pp. 407–424). New York: Plenum Press.

Zang, E. A., Barrett, N. O., & Cohen, L. A. (1994). Differences in nutritional risk factors for breast cancer among New York City white, Hispanic, and black college students. *Ethnicity & Disease, 4,* 28–40.

Zuckerman, M. (1990). Some dubious premises in research and theory on racial differences. *American Psychologist, 45,* 1297–1303.

CHAPTER 16

African-American Health over the Life Course
A Multidimensional Framework

James S. Jackson and Sherrill L. Sellers

INTRODUCTION

This chapter outlines a multidimensional life-course framework to help clarify the psychological mechanisms that may contribute to poor physical and psychological health outcomes among African-Americans. We suggest how the framework clarifies major health issues at each life stage and how it might help in designing programs that promote health among African-Americans.

Race and ethnicity have received considerable scrutiny of late (Williams & Collins, 1995). In our usage of race and ethnicity we refer to the socially constructed meanings attached to both an ethnic and racial classification (Wilkinson & King, 1989). Throughout this chapter, we will use black and African-American interchangeably. Both refer to Americans who share a common ancestral descent from people historically indigenous to Subsaharan Africa. In this sense ethnic and racial categories derive their interpretations from the sociohistorical and current milieu in which groups are embedded, as well as from the self-defining properties of these categories used by members of groups with observable boundary-

JAMES S. JACKSON and SHERRILL L. SELLERS • Institute for Social Research, University of Michigan, Ann Arbor, Michigan 48106.

Handbook of Diversity Issues in Health Psychology, edited by Pamela M. Kato and Traci Mann. Plenum Press, New York, 1996.

defining physical characteristics. While some genetic and biological factors may be related to the categorization of peoples of African descent (e.g., sickle-cell anemia, hypertension, osteopetrosis), we believe that the fundamental power and meaning of being African-American is in its socially constituted and derived meanings for self and other.

Compared to Americans of European descent, at every point of their life span African-Americans have greater morbidity and mortality (Jackson, 1991). Among African-Americans, as with most racial-ethnic groups in the United States, cancer and cardiovascular disease are the two leading causes of death. However, because of hypertension, which afflicts one out of every three African-Americans, blacks have a 60% greater risk of death and disability from stroke and coronary disease than whites. In particular, black women have three times the rate of high blood pressure compared to white women (National Center for Health Statistics, 1989). Similarly, cancer incidence rates for blacks are 6% to 10% higher than whites.

Mortality statistics are equally troubling. The infant mortality rate for blacks is 20 deaths per 1,000, twice the rate that occurs among whites (LaViest, 1992). The average life expectancy for whites is 75.3 years, compared to 69.4 years for blacks (Hale, 1992). Hypertension is particularly deadly. Black women are twice as likely as white women to die of hypertensive cardiovascular disease (National Center for Health Statistics, 1989). African-American cancer mortality rates are 20% to 40% higher than the general population (Baquet, Clayton, & Robinson, 1989).

Summarizing these statistics, African-Americans are at a disproportionate risk for negative health outcomes when compared to European Americans. A number of factors may contribute to this disparity, ranging from biological dispositions (Baquet & Ringen, 1989) to dietary habits (Hargreaves, Baquet, & Gamshadzahi, 1989) to a failure to receive adequate health care (Jones & Rice, 1987). The specific mechanisms, however, that produce these differential outcomes are less clear. Given the complex sociohistorical context of African-Americans, it may be less useful to compare between racial and ethnic group outcomes (e.g., black–white differences) than within groups. Black–white comparisons may be less illuminating than the examination of various intragroup social and cultural factors as possible sources of risk and resilience for African-American men, women, and children (Jackson, 1991).

Factors that mediate risk, promote resilience, and encourage healthy outcomes should be conceptualized along a number of dimensions including the personal, interpersonal, and societal levels. For example, risk factors such as racism and chronic poverty may have particularly pernicious effects on the health of African-Americans across the life course, although other factors such as spirituality, kinship ties, and racial-group identity may buffer these risks factors. To explore how these factors influence and interact with group and personal resources to impede and enhance the health of African-Americans, a multidimensional life-course framework is needed (Jackson, 1993).

A MULTIDIMENSIONAL LIFE-COURSE FRAMEWORK

Figure 1 presents the conceptual framework that guides the chapter. The first dimension of the framework includes individual or micro-level variables, most often examined when studying the relationship between race and health outcomes. The second dimension comprises interpersonal or meso-level factors, such as family and neighborhood. The third

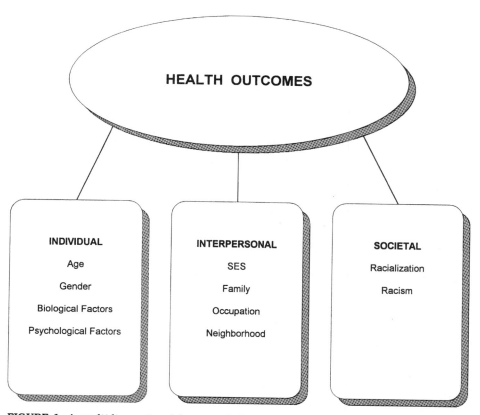

FIGURE 1. A multidimensional framework for examination of health outcomes among African-Americans.

dimension, the societal or macro level, can include a number of societal level factors, such as poverty and racism. Although all the factors noted and impled in this latter dimension are important, in this chapter we will highlight racism as an exemplar of the societal domain. Although not a focus of this paper, it is noted that interactions occur across dimensions, and factors within each dimension influence are influenced by the others.

We speculate that factors within the three dimensions have varying influences on health outcomes and differ in magnitude and importance throughout an individual's life course. The life-course perspective holds that negative environmental, social, and economic conditions early in the life course of African-Americans have deleterious affects on later social, psychological, and biological growth (Jackson, 1981). Such conditions accumulate over the individual life span and may lead to higher levels of morbidity and mortality at earlier periods for African-Americans in comparison to other groups.

A multidimensional, life-course framework places health outcomes within social and structural contexts, producing a more dynamic, less individually focused, sociohistorical model. Such a framework has direct program and policy implications. For example, violence takes its greatest toll on young black men. Furthermore, the deaths and disability of black men early in their life spans have detrimental consequences beyond the individual. These untimely deaths and early disability shape subsequent family structures and processes, including the raising of children and familial access to societal resources (Jackson, 1993). Interestingly, although violence is the single most important cause of death among young black men, even in old age African-American men and women are still more susceptible to violent deaths than are their older white counterparts (Williams & Collins, 1995). Thus although one may postulate lifestyle and culture as major contributory factors in the violence of black youth, this life-course view suggests that other intermediate level factors, such as family and neighborhood, may also be important.

The mortality crossover is another striking example of how a life-course framework is necessary in understanding the factors contributing to the health status of African-Americans. For nearly all diseases, mortality rates for blacks exceed those of whites at every age until late in life. There has been much speculation about the reasons for this crossover, which was at age 73 in 1940 and at age 85 in 1980 (Siegel, 1993). Although a number of explanations have been offered for this phenomena, including age misreporting, recently demographers have concluded that the crossover undoubtedly represents a "survival of the fittest" model in which blacks who survive the health and psychological risks at earlier points in the life course are hardier than their white counterparts at older ages.

Gibson and Jackson (1992) speculated and demonstrated that there may even be successive mortality sweeps among the black population in older ages, successively culling out the less hardy. These mortality sweeps (at 55–64 and 75–85 years of age) result in hardier older blacks over 85 years of age and a "sandwiching" of successive cohorts of relatively morbid and well blacks over the age of 55. We suspect that this survival phenomena begins early in the life course (prenatally) and continues throughout life. This theorizing is consistent with our later speculations regarding the accumulated stress hypothesis, that is, that blacks in the context of relatively meager material resources are continually exposed to environmental stressors and the psychological ravages of second- class citizenship. These resource deficiencies, environmental stressors, and psychological insults are reciprocally related to poor physical and psychological health outcomes over the individual life course. Because of this reciprocal causation over the life course, clear cause-and-effect relationships have been difficult to document empirically. The life course, multifaceted health framework that we are proposing pushes the field toward a conceptual and empirical direction for examining the possible factors and life flows that may help in understanding these admittedly difficult and complex relationships.

Framework Components

We realize that this three-dimension framework does not capture the full complexity and intricacies of the factors that impinge upon considerations of physical and psychological health among blacks. It does, however, provide a useful beginning for moving beyond simplistic individual risk models that are not sensitive to important contextual factors.

In this chapter we will highlight important aspects of these dimensions, rather than providing an encyclopedic treatment of each element. The *individual dimension* includes variables most often examined when studying the relationship between race and health outcomes. These individual-level factors include age, sex, and biological and psychological predispositions, as well as important individual risk factors. A great deal of research has demonstrated gender differences in exposure to such factors as violence (White, 1994), drug and alcohol abuse (Oyemade & Washington, 1990), suicide (Rutledge, 1990), and the health risks of early-teen parenting (Harrison, 1990; Lewis, 1990). Individual social effects (e.g., Reynolds et al., 1994), potential biological factors (Anderson, Myers, Pickering, & Jackson, 1989), and personality factors, for example, John Henryism (James, LaCroix, Kleinbaum, & Strogatz, 1984), have all been shown to contribute to increased risks among blacks for morbidity and mortality.

The *interpersonal dimension* comprises of a range of intermediate-level factors including socioeconomic status, family, occupation, and neighborhood. Since the median income for African-American families is half that of whites and over one-third of all African-Americans are below the poverty threshold, socioeconomic status (SES) holds an important place in examining health outcomes of African-Americans (U.S. Bureau of the Census, 1989). Hence, it is logical to conclude that the connection between race and health is really an issue of class, and considerable research has found that individuals of lower SES have higher rates of morbidity and mortality. Williams (1990) cautions, however, against the uncritical use of SES as a proxy for race. Researchers have found important within-group differences among blacks as well as intriguing between- group (but within class) differences among blacks and nonblacks. Specifically, Kessler and Neighbors (1986) found that most race groups with similar education levels in the upper-income bracket have similar health outcomes, but race groups in the lower-income bracket have disparate health outcomes. Jackson (1993) speculates that perhaps income and other socioeconomic control variables underequate different race groups at lower-income levels and overequate at upper-income levels.

Research on the family's role in producing health outcomes have unduly focused on family instability and risk of poor outcomes for infants and children (Jackson, Chatters, & Taylor, 1993). The family may influence health outcomes in a number of ways. Three of these possible paths are of particular salience from a life-course perspective. First, the family is one of the earliest places an individual receives information and tutoring about health and health behaviors. Norton (1989) suggests, however, that families may teach only what is needed to survive within their environment, an environment that may be unlike that of the wider society. Language, personal style, and interpersonal strategies adaptive within the immediate family environment may be maladaptive in wider society. In addition, the family is a primary transmitter of culture, that is, of attitudes, values, and behavior patterns that communicate the meaning of social experiences. Culture, for African-Americans, may reflect a synthesis of African heritage and American experience. Culture may shape definitions of health and perceptions of illness, as well as health behaviors and health-seeking strategies. In addition, research suggests that family effects may vary in age-specific ways (Wilson & Tolson, 1990). Age-specific patterns, such as increasing influence of peers in the life of the adolescent, suggest the need for varied strategies and models of health promotion and intervention. In summary, research on the family suggests that to be effective, efforts to improve the health outcomes of African-Americans across the life course must be multileveled, culturally sensitive, and linguistically appropriate (Braithwaite, Murphy, & Lythcott, 1989).

Occupation is included in the second dimension. African-Americans have historically been located in lower segments of the occupational structure. These jobs are usually of lower pay; offer less stability; and involve exposure to occupational hazards, waste materials, and toxins (Robinson, 1989). The risks to physical health are coupled with increased mental distress. Recent empirical work suggests that although a majority of black women feel stressed, black women in lower-status occupations were more likely to experience stress and decreased life satisfaction (Rucker, 1994).

A number of scholars have identified *neighborhood* as a factor that may influence a range of life outcomes, including health (Wilson, 1987). The impact of neighborhoods on health outcomes may range from acts of *environmental racism* (e.g., the disproportionate number of cigarette bill-boards and toxic waste dumps in African-American communities) to air-borne dust and dirt that trigger asthma attacks to availability, access, and quality of health care. Empirical research on neighborhood effects are in their nascent stage. Yet this factor may have particular importance for developing an understanding of the relationship between race and health outcomes. Consider, for example, the incidence of lead poisoning in young African-American children. Recent research indicates that not only is there an increased threat of ingesting lead paint but also airborne lead particles threaten the physical and mental health of black children (Reed, 1992).

The third dimension, *societal*, involves the processes of racialization and racism. *Racialization* may be defined as a process of defining a partic-ular group as a race. It is well beyond the scope of this chapter to outline the contemporary debates on race theory (e.g., Omi & Winant, 1986). For our purpose the most salient feature of this debate is the recognition that race is a social construct, not a biological one (Wilkinson & King, 1989; Williams, Lavizzo-Mourey, & Warren, 1994). Consequently, the differen-tials in health outcomes among ostensible racial groups may suggest more about an individual's place in the social structure and perceptions and attributions than about biological factors and genetic dispositions.

Krieger (1990) provides striking evidence to support this claim. In a study of 101 black and white women, Krieger found that perceived gender discrimination was unrelated to hypertension, but among African-American women who reported experiencing unfair treatment, those who kept quiet about the treatment were four times as likely to have high blood pressure than those who talked with others or took some other action in response to the unfair treatment. Krieger also found the black women were six times more likely than white women to report responding passively to unfair treatment. While not definitive, it does suggest that among women who perceive unfair treatment, black women may perceive themselves to have fewer options than white women in actively confronting the problem.

One possible result of racialization is racism. *Racism* encompasses an ideology of superiority of one group over another. It reinforces and justifies individual and institutional discrimination toward the oppressed group. Racism is a pervasive problem for African-Americans across the life course. One need only consider the everyday assaults to an African-American's sense of self, from stereotypical media portrayals to being chronically treated as objects of suspicion and fear, to recognize that

African-Americans are subject to more psychological hazards than their white counterparts. However, the experience of racism may differ in form and meaning as a function of birth cohort, period, and age (Baker, 1987; Cooper, Steinhauer, Schazkin, & Miller, 1981; Dressler, 1991).

The impact of racism on health has received considerable theoretical speculation. Empirical investigations, however, have been difficult for a variety of reasons, including limited samples and difficulty in measuring key concepts such as racism. In one of the few empirical studies, Jackson et al. (1995) uncovered a number of provocative findings on the effects of racism, defined as perceptions and experiences of discrimination, on the physical and mental health of African-Americans. Initial cross-section analysis found that personal experiences of racism and perceptions of discrimination had adverse effects on the physical and mental well-being of African-American adults. Over time, however, those who reported experiencing racism also reported lower numbers of health problems, but also lower levels of subjective well-being and higher levels of psychological distress. The authors speculated that over time a heightened awareness of differential treatment because of race may serve as a buffer (perhaps leading to better health care, greater determination, etc.) against these everyday assaults of racism but at a psychological cost.

The framework we have been describing outlines a multidimensional approach for studying the relationship between racism and health. Biological, psychological, interpersonal, and societal factors are implicated in all stages of health and illness, ranging from behaviors that maintain health to societal factors that may produce severe disease and premature death. This multidimensional perspective can be a guiding model for both research and practice. The essential element of the framework is the life-course perspective. This perspective adds dynamism to an otherwise static approach of relating race and health. Health risk and promoting factors may shift throughout the life course. Racism, for example, may be considered a risk factor and may have a cumulative effect over time on psychological health, which in turn may lead to premature morbidity and mortality. At the same time, however, Neighbors, Jackson, Broman, and Thompson (1995) speculated that, for African-Americans, a psychological orientation of "system blame" may interact with other psychological dispositions to be health protective in the face of stressful environmental factors. These paradoxes and puzzles may, in part, be more fully examined using a multidimensional life-course perspective.

PHYSICAL AND MENTAL HEALTH AND THE AFRICAN-AMERICAN LIFE COURSE

Epidemiologic studies consistently describe the health risks to African-American men, women, and children. This section examines major health issues at each life stage through the lens of a multidimensional life-course perspective. This examination highlights the central premise of the chapter: In order to develop effective health promotion programs, policies, and research agendas, we must conceptualize African-American health outcomes at multiple levels and across the life course.

Infancy and Childhood

Although rarely speculated about in its full life-course implications, we must recognize that African-American children are born with a non-zero probability of being in poverty during a significant portion of their life course. Because of poverty figures that exceed the national average by three and four times and the fact that the largest number of births occur among the poorest segments of the population, some researchers have estimated that upwards of 80% of African-American children born over the next decade will spend the bulk of their childhoods in poverty (Jaynes & Williams, 1989). We need not contemplate a critical-stage theory to understand how and why the increased risk of poverty and single-female-headed households may impact both childhood and later adult development. Early health care, exposure to toxic environments, problematic material resources, and potentially dysfunctional socialization all point to increased risk of poor psychological and physical health outcomes for children born in such circumstances.

Norton (1989) writes, "If we do not understand the tapestry of the early natural experiences of children, if we do not understand what environmental and societal contextual forces shape their world views, ... can we really develop meaningful, relevant and effective services for them and their families?" What we know about the early life of African-American children is troubling. A 1985 Children's Defense Fund investigation found that black infant mortality is twice that of whites and maternal mortality is three times as high. Compared to white children, black children are three times as likely to live in poverty, to die of abuse, to be classified as learning disabled, and are four times as likely to be murdered before their first birthday (White, 1994).

The life trajectory of African-American children is littered with risks. However, health-promoting factors are also evident. Specifically, children and family are of central importance to African-Americans (McAdoo, 1988). Informal within- and fictive-kin adoptions are ready examples. The migration of children from the dangers of northern urban centers to rural southern states is an increasing phenomena within the black community. These strategies for protecting the health and well-being of black children illustrate an intergenerational self-help strategy that black families have implemented across a broad range of health issues, particularly involving the health and well-being of children (Barbarin, 1993; McLoyd, 1990). Research is needed to address the limits to self-help and social support. It is not clear that in an increasingly complicated world of poor material resources and increasing familial demands of single-family households that the traditional intergenerational exchanges among African-Americans can suffice in replacing structured programs and effective family policy (Jackson & Kalavar, 1994).

We are not the first to note that the African-American family and children are very resilient and do well in the face of incredibly negative odds (e.g., McAdoo, 1988). On the other hand, the childhood experiences of a large proportion of black children are not sufficient preparation for the rigors of adolescence. Among boys and girls, lack of educational opportunities, material resources, and poor early health care are already beginning to take a toll. Diets that are insufficient in basic nutrients and high in fat and starches may already be laying the groundwork for later hypertension, heart disease, and cardiovascular problems.

Adolescence and Early Adulthood

For the most part, vast numbers of African-American children are poorly situated to enter the rigors of adolescence in terms of their educational, social, and psychological preparation. Weakened family structures, poor schools, and deteriorated neighborhoods contribute even further to the physical and material ravages. Many of these children will lack the appropriate psychological framework for interpreting their life circumstances and understanding their appropriate roles. Adolescence is not only a period of physical maturation but also a time of dynamic psychosocial maturation. For African-American adolescents, developmental tasks may be further challenged by environmental stressors such as racism. For others, living in largely a nonblack world may produce group identity conflicts, in addition to overt and covert racism, and make the struggle especially difficult (Whaley, 1993).

Adolescents are bombarded with media messages about the "good life" and quickly come to understand that socially acceptable means of accomplishment may not be available. Combined with hormonal and physical changes, the lack of psychological resources and perceived material means to success may take their toll early in the life of many black adolescents. When combined with ready opportunities for advancement though alternative means available in their environments, school dropout, early family development, and criminal behavior become explicable, if no less acceptable.

Two of the most salient health issues for African-American adolescents are pregnancy and violence. Media accounts seem to portray teenage pregnancy as a cause and consequence of the "degenerating" black family. This portrayal is a gross distortion of the reality of growing up in the contemporary United States. Although one out of every four black children is born to a teenage mother, according to the Alan Guttmacher

Institute, class, rather than race, is the strongest determinant of teen pregnancy (Jackson, Chatters, & Taylor, 1993). Class, however, may be understood as an indicator of lack of resources. Hence, the very framing of degeneration is a misdirection. Rather, family structures may be changing while resources to provide for families are dwindling. Even more problematic is the integral relationship between socioeconomic status and race. These are not independent factors. Thus attempts to empirically control for one factor while observing the influence of the other factor is extremely difficult operationally and may be a conceptually flawed approach.

A disproportionate amount of research on adolescent parenting has focused on the teen mother. This single focus is illustrative of a tendency to consider African-Americans in a homogenous manner, even without consideration of the possible differentials in health outcomes between African-American men and women. Although it is beyond the scope of this chapter to address this complex issue formally, a multidimensional life course perspective is particularly sensitive to the impact gender may have on health outcomes. One might consider gender within the third dimension as a social construct that may be an interlocking factor with racism.

Barbarin notes, "the effects of family life on child development are not the same for boys and girls" (Barbarin, 1993, pg. 388). For males, the external environment, one's neighborhood, seems to play a more significant role. For many black males, the neighborhood is a violent one (Akbar, 1980). The homicide rate for black males 15 to 44 years is considerably higher than that of white males in the same age group (Prothrow-Stith & Weissman, 1991).

Thus given poor schooling, early family development, exposure to environmental health risks (including toxins), violence, and a lack of psychological nurturance culminates in an entry into early adulthood without appropriate material resources and poor psychological prospects for achievement in ways that are socially acceptable to the larger society. Early adulthood becomes a period of limited success, constraining both accomplishments and the acquiring of skills and resources appropriate for later development. This lack of individual and family resources is compounded by environmental conditions and economic circumstances that harden into a nonsupportive context (Henly, 1993). For example, in an increasingly sophisticated world, there is a growing need for greater education and highly technical skills. Unlike an earlier era when education was a luxury or the exclusive preserve of upper classes, today education and training is a necessity for acquiring entry-level skills into a profession or career. Jobs in the lower service sector do not provide adequate recompense for the accumulation of the resources necessary for adequate family formation or the material competency to acquire the trappings of a middle-class existence. The physical outcomes are clear. The psychological consequences are no less real, and all too quickly many

African-American young adults find themselves at midlife without adequate resources, no accumulated wealth, and poor prospects for the
future. What for many has been called the command generation, that is
the period of intense accomplishment and the accumulation of material
resources (Neugarten, 1968), turns out to be the generation of regret and
bleak hopes for many African-Americans.

Midlife

Midlife is often envisioned as a period of reflection and consolidation
(Neugarten, 1968). Unfortunately, for many African-Americans their re-
flections are hopeless, and there is little to consolidate. Health care has
been at best sporadic during previous periods of relative good health
(Jackson & Perry, 1989). Thus much preventive health care and healthy
promotive behaviors may not have been practiced. For example, nearly
35% of black women between the ages of 20 and 45 and over 50% of black
women 45 to 55 are overweight. Obesity has potentially dire health consequences. Excess weight places African-American women at higher risk for
heart disease, diabetes, and hypertension, illnesses responsible for disproportionate numbers of deaths within the African-American community (White, 1994).

A second health issue of particular importance for African-Americans
in midlife is alcoholism. Prior to 1950, alcohol-related mortality rates were
higher for whites than for blacks. From 1951 to 1980, deaths due to
cirrhosis tripled among black men, while these alcohol-related deaths
increased only sightly for white men. One puzzle of alcoholism is that the
rates for white males seem to rise sharply during adolescence and then
decline and level off by midlife. For African-American males the pattern is
reversed. A life-course perspective suggests a cumulative effect of the
stress of racism with alcoholism as a possible coping strategy. However,
equally likely explanations involving cohort and period effects are also
viable. More research is needed to examine how stress accumulates and
the strategies African-American use to address these stressors. In addition, research is needed to examine day-to-day hassles of racism as predictors of psychological distress and physical illness over the life course.

Old Age

Black elders are the fastest growing group of African-Americans.
Between 1970 and 1980, the number of African-American elderly increased 34%, whereas the total black population increased by only 16%.
Through approximately age 75, whites can expect to live longer than
blacks. However, after age 75, blacks can expect to live longer than
whites. Researchers have offered several possible explanations for this
phenomenon, which has been labeled the *mortality crossover*. Along the

individual dimension, it has been suggested that blacks who have reached advanced age are biologically stronger (Gibson & Jackson, 1992, Siegel, 1993). Focusing on the intermediate level, Gibson (1986) found that particular help-seeking behaviors may serve as a protective factor. African-American elderly utilized a wider range of informal support helpers and were more willing to substitute helpers than were their white counterparts.

A particular perspective on racism may also serve as a protective factor. Jackson, Antonucci, and Gibson (1990) found that, in large measure, blacks and whites do not differ significantly on various measures of individual aging. However, they do differ in their coping processes (Jackson et al., 1990). In particular, a view of life that emphasizes the existence of structural barriers may be especially important for African-Americans to explain why hard work does not lead to positive outcomes. Jackson (1993) suggests that this fatalistic orientation may be particularly important as one ages. Group identity may also be a protective mechanism, serving as a way of interpreting individual contributions to the entire African-American community.

CONTEXTUAL APPROACH TO AFRICAN-AMERICAN HEALTH SERVICE NEEDS

As the above examples illustrate, a multidimensional life-course framework suggests a movement away from a deficit model of African-American health to one that examines cultural strengths as well as structural barriers to health promotion and illness prevention. Interventions to promote individual health behaviors are in abundance. Unfortunately, few of these efforts move beyond individual change efforts. Thomas (1992) challenges this orientation, suggesting that

> One must be mindful that the ethnicity of an individual is not an independent risk factor. In other words, blacks do not have higher morbidity and mortality rates compared to whites because they are black. The relationship between poor health and socioeconomic status has been well documented. People with the least education, people who live in the least desirable neighborhoods, and people who work at the least prestigious jobs are all more likely to die earlier than people on the other end of these scales. This is why disease prevention policies that assign primary responsibility to individual men and women are unjust. (p. 343)

Efforts to improve the health status of African-American men, women, and children must take a multidimensional focus on the individual, the community, and the wider society. Black men and women do have measurable control over their own health destinies. Risk factors such as smoking, alcohol consumption, lack of exercise, and failure to use appropriate methods to prevent the spread of AIDS are, in large measure, under individual control.

Yet forces such as advertising to promote tobacco and alcohol consumption may be beyond individual change efforts and require action at the interpersonal level. Community-based health promotion and illness prevention programs may be an effective approach to improving health outcomes of African-Americans. This recommendation, however, is not to suggest that communities can solve these health care problems alone. This caution is particularly relevant in the current climate of mounting pressures to contain health care costs. If community-based efforts are to be effective, they must have sufficient resources. Black churches, for example, may be an important site for health care services and health-promotion programs. However, programming, staffing, and promoting these additional efforts may be beyond a congregation's or community's means.

At the societal level, the absence of a single, charismatic national figure or organization does not indicate the lack of efforts to improve the economic, social, political, and health conditions of African-Americans. The National Black Women's Health Project (NBWHP) provides an excellent example of such efforts. NBWHP is a grassroots organization dedicated to the promotion of health, prevention of illness, and improvement of health care system and policy formation for black women (Avery, 1992). Its activities range from individual change efforts, such as the walking-for-health campaign, to lobbying Congress for additional funding for breast cancer research. Similar activities are now underway by the Save Our Children campaign being conducted by the Children's Defense Fund.

SUMMARY

From cradle to grave, African-Americans are at disproportionate risk for physical, social, and psychological harm (Jackson, 1993). We suggest that in order to develop effective health-promotion programs, policies, and research agendas, we must conceptualize and assess African-American health outcomes at multiple levels and across the life course. One central implication of this framework is the need to design programs that address the health of African-Americans comprehensively, across the life cycle, and as members of a racialized group embedded in a particular socio-historical context. Put simply, the framework suggests that health outcomes are a complex interaction of individual, group, and structural factors—factors that must be considered simultaneously if the disparities in health outcomes are to narrow.

In summary, health is an individual, social, economic, and political phenomenon. Consequently, efforts to promote health, prevent and treat illness, and improve the health care system and health policy must be approached from multiple levels. Eliminating the disparities in health outcomes between blacks and whites requires more than individual, psychological change efforts. Eliminating these disparities will require challenging structural barriers as well.

REFERENCES

Akbar, N. (1980). Homicide among black males: Causal factors. *Public Health Reports, 95*(6) 549.

Anderson, N. B., Myers, H. F., Pickering, T., & Jackson, J. S. (1989). Hypertension in blacks: Psychosocial and biological perspectives. *Journal of Hypertension, 7,* 161–172.

Avery, B. (1992). The health status of black women. In R. Braithwaite & S. Taylor (Eds.), *Health issues in the black community* (pp. 35–51). San Francisco, CA: Jossey-Bass.

Baker, F. M. (1987). The Afro-American life cycle: Success, failure, and mental health. *Journal of the National Medical Association, 7,* 625–633.

Barbarin, O. (1993). Emotional and social development of African American children. *Journal of Black Psychology, 19*(4), 381–390.

Baquet, C. R. & Ringen, K. (1985). *Advances in cancer control: Health care financing and research.* New York: Liss.

Baquet, C., Clayton, L., & Robinson, R. (1989). Cancer prevention and control. In L. Jones (Ed.), *Minorities and cancer* (pp. 67–76). New York: Springer-Verlag.

Centers for Disease Control, Division of Debates Translation. (1991). *Diabetes surveillance report.* Atlanta, GA: Centers for Disease Control.

Cooper, R., Steinhaurer, M., Schatzkin, A., & Miller, A. (1981). Improved mortality among U. S. blacks. 1968–1978: The role of the antiracist struggle. *International Journal of Health Services, 11,* 511–522.

Dressler, W. W. (1991). Social class, skin color, and arterial blood pressure in two societies. *Ethnicity and disease, 1,* 60–77.

Gibson, R. (1986). Blacks in an aging society. *Daedalus, 115,* 349–372.

Gibson, R. C., & Jackson, J. S. (1992). The black oldest old: Health, functioning, and informal support. In R. M. Suzman, D. P. Willis, & K. G. Manton (Eds.), *The oldest old* (pp. 321–340). New York: Oxford University Press.

Harrison, A. (1990). High risk sexual behavior among black adolescents. In A. R. Stiffman & L. E. Davis (Eds.), *Ethnic issues in adolescent mental health* (pp. 175–188). Newbury Park, CA: Sage.

Hale, C. (1992). A demographic profile of African Americans. In R. Braithwaite & S. Taylor (Eds.), *Health issues in the black community* (pp. 6–20). San Francisco, CA: Jossey-Bass.

Henly, J. (1993). The significance of social context: The case of adolescent childbearing in the African American community. *The Journal of Black Psychology, 19*(4), 461–477.

Jackson, J. J. (1981). Urban black Americans. In A. Harword (Ed.), *Ethnicity and medical care* (pp. 37–129). Cambridge, MA: Harvard University Press.

Jackson, J. J., & Perry, C. (1989). Physical health conditions of middle-aged and aged blacks. In K. Markides (Ed.), *Aging and health* (pp. 111–176). Newbury Park, CA: Sage.

Jackson, J. S. (Ed.). (1991). *Life in black America.* Newbury Park, CA: Sage.

Jackson, J. S. (1993). Racial influences on adult development and aging. In R. Kastenbaum (Ed.), *The encyclopedia of adult development.* (pp. 18–26) Phoenix, AZ: Oryx Press.

Jackson, J. S., Antonucci, T. C., & Gibson, R. C. (1990). Social relations, productive activities, and coping with stress in later life. In M. A. P. Stephens, J. H. Crowther, S. E. Hobfoll, & D. L. Tennenbaum (Eds.), *Stress and coping in later life families* (pp. 80–97). Washington, DC: Hemisphere.

Jackson, J. S., Brown, T., Williams, D., Torres, M., Sellers, S., & Brown, K. (1996). Perceptions and experiences of racism and the physical and mental health status of African Americans: A thirteen year national panel study. *Ethnicity and Disease 6*(1,2), 132–147.

Jackson, J. S., Chatters, L. M., & Taylor, R. J. (1993). Status and functioning of future cohorts of African-American elderly: Conclusions and speculations. In J. S. Jackson, L. M. Chatters, & R. J. Taylor (Eds.), *Aging in black America* (pp. 301–318). Newbury Park, CA: Sage.

Jackson, J. S., & Kalavar, J. (1994). Equity and distributive justice across age cohorts: A life-course family perspective. In L. Cohen (Ed.), *Justice across generations: What does it mean?* (pp. 175–183). Washington, DC: American Association of Retired Persons.

James, S. J., LaCroix, A., Kleinbaum, D., & Strogatz, D. (1984). John Henryism and blood pressure differences among black men. II: The role of occupational stressors. *Journal of Behavioral Medicine, 7,* 259–275.

Jaynes, G. D., & Williams, R. M. (1989). *A common destiny: Blacks and American society.* Washington, DC: National Academy of Sciences Press.

Jones, W., & Rice, M. (1987). Black health care: An overview. In W. Jones & M. Rice (Eds.), (pp. 3–20). *Health care issues in black america: Policies, problems and prospects* New York: Greenwood Press.

Kessler, R., & Neighbors, H. (1986). A new perspective on the relationship among, race, social class, and psychological distress. *Journal of Health and Social Behavior, 27,* 107–115.

Krieger, N. (1990). Racial and gender discrimination: risk factors for high blood pressure? Social *Science Medicine 30*(12), 1273–1281.

LaViest, T. (1992). The political empowerment and health status of African Americans: Mapping a new territory. *American Journal of Sociology, 97*(4), 1080–1095.

Lewis, S. Y. (1990). Black teens parenting in the inner city. In A. R. Stiffman & L. E. Davis (Eds.), *Ethnic issues in adolescent mental health* (pp. 208–219). Newbury Park, CA: Sage.

McAdoo, H. P. (1988). *Black families.* Newbury Park, CA: Sage.

McLoyd, V. (1990). The impact of economic hardship on black families and children: Psychological distress, parenting, and socioemotional development. *Child Development, 61,* 311–461.

National Center for Health Statistics. (1989). *Health, United States, 1988* (DHHS Publication No. PHS 89-1232). Hyattville, MD: Public Health Service.

Neighbors, H. W., Jackson, J. S., Broman, C., & Thompson, E. (1996) Racism and the mental health of African Americans *Ethnicity and Disease 6*(1,2), 167–175.

Neugarten, B. (1968). The awareness of middle-age. In B. L. Neugarten (Ed.), *Middle Age and Aging* (pp. 93–98). Chicago: University of Chicago Press.

Norton, D. G. (1989). *Research theory and design of relevant culturally and ecologically sensitive interventions.* Paper presented at the Biennial Faculty Training Institute of the National Center for Clinical Infant Programs, Washington, DC.

Omi, M., & Winant, H. (1986). *Racial formations in the United States: From 1960s to the 1980s.* New York: Routledge & Kegan Paul.

Oyemade, U. J., & Washington, V. (1990). The role of family factors in the primary prevention of substance abuse among high risk black youth. In A. R. Stiffman & L. E. Davis (eds.), *Ethnic issues in adolescent mental health* (pp. 267–284). Newbury Park, CA: Sage.

Prothrow-Smith, D., & Weissman, M. (1991). *Deadly consequences.* New York: Harper Collins.

Reed, W. (1992) Lead poisoning: A modern plague among African-American children. In R. Braithwaite & S. Taylor (Eds.), *Health issues in the black community* (pp. 178–192). San Francisco: Jossey-Bass.

Reynolds, P., Boyd, P., Blacklow, R. S., Jackson, J. S., Greenberg, R. S., Austin, D. F., Chen, V. W., & Edwards, B. K. (1994). The relationship between social ties and survival among black and white breast cancer patients. *Cancer Epidemiology Biomarkers and Prevention, 3,* 253–259.

Robinson, J. C. (1989). Trends in racial inequality and exposure to work-related hazards, 1968–1986. In D. P. Willis (Ed.), *Health policies and black Americans* (pp. 404–420). New Brunswick, NJ: Transaction.

Rucker, T. (1994). *Black women, work and life satisfaction.* Paper presented at National Council on Family Relations Annual Conference, Minneapolis, MN.

Rutledge, E. M. (1990). Suicide among black adolescents and young adults: A rising problem. In A. R. Stiffman & L. E. Davis (Eds.), *Ethnic issues in adolescent mental health* (pp. 339–351). Newbury Park, CA: Sage.

Siegel, J. S. (1993). *A generation of change.* New York: Russell Sage.

Thomas, S. (1992). The health of the black community in the twenty-first century: A futuristic perspective. In R. Braithwaite & S. Taylor (eds). *Health Issues in the Black Community* (pp. 338–349). San Francisco: Jossey-Bass.

U.S. Bureau of the Census. (1988). *1989 household and family characteristics, March 1988* (Current Population Reports Series P-20, No, 437). Washington DC: U.S. Government Printing Office.

Whaley, A. (1993). Self-esteem, cultural identity, and psychosocial adjustment in African American children. *Journal of Black Psychology, 19*(4), 406–422.

White, E. (Ed.). (1994). *The black women's health book: Speaking for ourselves.* Washington, DC: Seal Press.

Wilkinson, D. Y., & King, G. (1989). Conceptual and methodological issues in the use of race as a variable: Policy implications. In D. P. Willis (Ed.), *Health policies and black Americans* (pp. 56–71). New Brunswick, NJ: Transaction.

Williams, D. (1990). Socioeconomic differentials in health: A review and redirection. *Social Psychology Quarterly, 53*(2), 81–99.

Williams, D., & Collins, C. (1995). US socioeconomic and racial differences in health: Patterns and explanations. *Annual Review of Sociology, 21,* 349–386.

Williams, D., Lavizzo-Mourey, R., & Warren, R. (1994). The concept of race and health status in America. *Public Health Reports, 189*(1), 26–41.

Wilson, M., & Tolson, T. (1990). Familial support in the black community. *Journal of Clinical Child Psychology, 19*(4), 347–355.

Wilson, W. J. (1987). *The truly disadvantaged: The inner city, the underclass, and public policy.* Chicago: University of Chicago Press.

CHAPTER 17

Designing Health Promotion Programs for Latinos

FELIPE G. CASTRO, KATHRYN COE, SARA GUTIERRES, AND DELIA SAENZ

OVERVIEW OF THE HEALTH STATUS OF LATINOS

In this chapter we examine strategies in program design that include the politics of working with Latino[1] communities. We also examine strategies for reaching hard-to-reach members of this population, for enhancing program effectiveness (effect size), and for maintaining initial gains in healthy behavior change. Our views are based on prior health promotion studies including our recent study, "*Compañeros en la Salud*" (Partners in Health), which is a church-based study of cancer-risk reduction among Latinas, that is, Latino women.[2] Health promotion in Latino populations

---

[1]The literature on Latino health has no consensus regarding the preferred term to use when referring to persons of Latin-American heritage who live in the United States. The terms Hispanic and Latino are both used extensively, although U.S. government documents including U.S. census reports use the term *Hispanic*. Given this mixed usage in the current literature, this chapter will use the terms *Latino* and *Hispanic* interchangeably.

[2]The Spanish-language word for "Latino women" is *Latinas*. We use the terms interchangeably.

FELIPE G. CASTRO and DELIA SAENZ • Department of Psychology and Hispanic Research Center, Arizona State University, Tempe, Arizona 85287.   KATHRYN COE • Hispanic Research Center, Arizona State University, Tempe, Arizona 85287.   SARA GUTIERRES • Social and Behavioral Sciences and Hispanic Research Center, Arizona State University, Tempe, Arizona 85287.

Handbook of Diversity Issues in Health Psychology, edited by Pamela M. Kato and Traci Mann. Plenum Press, New York, 1996.

is challenging, particularly when working with Latinos who live in low-income, disrupted communities where many unhealthy environmental conditions compete with efforts at health promotion. This challenge calls for a deeper understanding of the cultural, social, and psychological factors that must be addressed in designing potent and effective programs that succeed in promoting sound health in various Latino populations.

Principles of Health Promotion

Health promotion has been defined as "prevention plus" (Taylor, Denham, & Ureda, 1982). This definition refers to health promotion's dual goals of preventing disease and also enhancing fitness in people who are currently free of disease. Moreover, the World Health Organization asserts that health promotion is "a process of enabling people to improve their health by synthesizing personal choice and social responsibility" (Glanz, Lewis, & Rimer, 1990, p. 8). Earlier conceptions of health promotion focused on the application of cognitive, behavioral, and social influence methods to promote individual behavior change. More recently, and from a broader systems perspective, community health promotion studies have focused on the application of behavior-change methods in families, in churches, and in entire communities (Fincham, 1992; Glenwick & Jason, 1993).

Generally, health promotion has emphasized three approaches to behavior change: (1) the arrangement of antecedent conditions such as cues that prompt the occurrence of healthy behaviors, (2) the application of operant methods such as contingency management to reward pro-health behavior and discourage unhealthy behavior, and (3) the use of self-control and self-management techniques to help people exert control over their everyday behaviors (Kazdin, 1994). Moreover, social learning constructs such as expectations, self-efficacy, and social reinforcement have also been used to promote healthy behavior change in various populations (Perry, Baranowski, & Parcel, 1990).

Application of Behavior Change Principles to Latinos

The successful application of antecedent, operant, and self-control methods to Latino populations requires a thorough understanding of cultural and environmental factors that create contextual challenges to behavior-change efforts. From a cultural perspective the behavior of Latinos is influenced by several psychological aspects of culture (*subjective culture factors*) that, which include (1) level of knowledge about disease and preventive behaviors, (2) cultural beliefs about the causes of illness, (3) cultural attitudes about one's ability to improve his or her own health, as opposed to relying on doctors and medications, (4) cultural expectations, a person's perceptions about feasible changes that he or she can make relative to that which is "in God's hands," and (5) local community norms, that is, culturally acceptable standards of behavior as related to of weight gain, patterns of alcohol, cigarette and drug use, illness behavior, etc. Efforts to apply behavior change methods without considering these subjective culture factors will likely result in interventions that fail because they lack cultural relevance to members of the target population.

From an environmental perspective, various living conditions can also interfere with efforts at healthy behavior change. These include (1) living in a *large family* in which the actions of other family members can disrupt a focus on efforts at behavior change; (2) *financial pressures* and preoccupations that distract and diminish the relative importance of efforts at healthy behavior change; (3) *environmental stressors* such as crime, noise, and traffic that limit choices for change; and (4) *life emergencies* including marital conflict, family injuries or illnesses, legal problems, home or apartment damages, crime victimization, and the like. While these life events and conditions can and do occur among middle class mainstream Americans, the frequency and severity of these stressful life events among Latinos of lower social class increases their disruptive impact. Efforts at behavior change that do not consider the disruptive impact of these environmental factors are also likely to fail due to a lack of *ecological relevance* of these behavior change strategies in relation to the environmental barriers faced by members of a target population. Thus, these environmental and cultural factors create a different "context," a more difficult and challenging complex of conditions that complicate the task of health promotion (Glenwick & Jason, 1993).

For example, increasing the likelihood that a middle-aged Anglo-American woman will obtain a mammography involves a series of steps that include (1) exposure to the need, (2) inducing motivation, (3) facilitating access with the availability of health insurance or a regular source of medical care, and (4) a strong intention to follow through in obtaining a mammogram. Among low acculturated Latino women, the same steps are necessary, but the process is more complex.

For Latino women, exposure is also a first step. However, in the *Compañeros* study, we have found that for many lower class, low-acculturated Latino women, obtaining a mammography for cancer prevention is a novel idea. Furthermore, paying for a mammography may be regarded as a luxury that has no immediate relevance in daily life. Many low-acculturated, low-income women have no health insurance or regular source of health care, since many work hard in low paying jobs that offer no medical insurance benefits. Other barriers to mammography screening include limited transportation and fear of undergoing medical treatment. The end result is a low probability that these Latino women will obtain a mammogram. This outcome is significant, since the rates of advanced stage breast cancer are higher among Latino women and specifically among lower acculturated, low-income Latino women (Richardson et al., 1987).

Thus in the *Compañeros en la Salud* project, promoting mammography screenings involved designing programmatic interventions that presented health education information in Spanish or in English, prompted motivation, and facilitated access. These intervention approaches included *population segmentation* based on educational and acculturative needs. This population segmentation based on level of acculturation aids in (1) developing targeted health information and educational messages on cancer risk reduction that were congruent with the acculturation–education needs of members of the targeted populations (Balcazar, Castro, & Krull, 1995), (2) mobilizing incentives and social support for participation by having lay health workers, *Promotoras*, encourage women to attend health education classes and health fairs, (3) facilitating access via the availability of low-cost mammograms offered at health fairs conducted at neighborhood churches, and (4) increasing access to lower cost treatment by offering referrals to clinics that had agreed to provide limited follow-up treatment. Despite the apparent costs in planning, the long-term costs are small whether measured in terms of dollars, human suffering, or human lives, when compared with the costs associated with medical treatment if the disease proceeds undetected to an advanced stage.

Latinos in the United States

Table 1 presents a general overview from the 1990 census that summarizes the ambient sociodemographic characteristics for all Latinos nationally as compared with non-Hispanic non-Latino whites (Anglo-Americans). Given the importance of understanding sociodemographic differences among subgroups of Latinos, this table also presents data for the three major Latino subgroups: Mexican-Americans, Puerto Ricans, and Cubans, as well as data for the composite grouping of Central and South Americans (Montgomery, 1994).

As of March 1993, the census counted 22.8 million Latinos, a total that constitutes 8.9% of the total U.S. population. The data in Table 1 show that Mexican-Americans are the largest subgroup of Latinos, 64.3%; followed by Puerto Ricans, 10.6%; and Cubans, 4.7%, although Central and South Americans constitute 13.4% of the total U. S. Latino population within the United States.

In comparisons of all Latinos to non-Hispanic whites, the census data indicate that Latinos are younger; less educated; have a lower mean and median household income; a higher rate of unemployment and higher rates of low-paying labor and service jobs, many of which offer no insurance benefits. Latinos also have lower rates of professional jobs, a larger mean family size, more families with a female head of household, more families who live below the poverty level, and fewer households with access to a telephone. Generally then, Latinos are less well-off as indicated by several of these sociodemographic indicators.

In comparisons that involve the three Latino subgroups and Central and South Americans, these data indicate that Cubans are the oldest and generally the best-off in terms of income, education, employment status, and other indicators. By contrast, Puerto Ricans and Mexican-Americans trade places as the least well-off, depending on the sociodemographic indicator examined. However, overall, most Latino scholars regard Puerto Ricans as the least well-off of the various Latino subgroups. As one example, when measured by the percentage of families who live below poverty level, Puerto Ricans are the least well-off, with 32.5% of Puerto Rican families living below poverty level. This compares with 27.0% for Central and South Americans, 26.4% for Mexican-Americans, 26.2% for all Latinos, 15.4% for Cubans, and only 7.3% for non-Hispanic whites.

Here it must be noted that lower socioeconomic status and low level of acculturation (speaking primarily or only Spanish) are characteristics still observed in native born Latinos who are U.S. citizens. Although there has been a large influx of immigrants from Latin America from 1970 to 1990, in 1990 nearly three-quarters of the Latino population were native born or naturalized citizens (U.S. Department of Commerce, 1993). Thus the large majority of U.S. Latinos are U.S. citizens, and a smaller number are noncitizen legal residents, whereas only a small percentage are undocumented laborers.

In summary, developing a health-promotion program that is responsive to the cultural and economic needs of the targeted Hispanic population depends partly on the subgroup of Hispanics that is being targeted. Furthermore, in the applied setting, a culturally responsive health promotion program must address the local characteristics of the community or *barrio* that is being targeted.

ISSUES IN SEEKING HEALTH CARE

Latinos are expected to become the largest ethnic minority group in the United States shortly after the year 2000, with the largest subgroup within this category being persons of Mexican descent (i.e., Mexican-Americans, Chicanos, Mexicans). Given this demographic trend, a major health care issue concerns access to health care services for Latinos (Marcias, 1977; Trevino & Moss, 1984). Previous work indicates that Mexican-Americans underutilize health services (Anderson, Lewis, & Giachello, 1981; Hough, Karno, & Burnam, 1983). For example, they have been less likely than non-Hispanic whites to use outpatient medical and mental health services (Wells, Golding, Hough, Burnam, & Karno, 1988).

Regarding health service utilization, a lack of health insurance is clearly associated with a lower frequency of health service seeking, partic-

TABLE 1. Selected Characteristics of Hispanics and Non-Hispanic Whites

	Non-Hispanic White	Latinos				
		All Latinos	Mexican Americans	Puerto Ricans	Cubans	Central and South Americans
Population						
Percent of total Hispanic		100	64.3	10.6	4.7	13.4
Male	48.9%	50.1%	50.5%	47.5%	49.1%	51.1%
Female	51.1%	49.9%	49.5%	52.5%	50.9%	48.9%
Age						
Median	33.6	26.7	24.6	26.9	43.6	28.6
Educational attainment						
(Ages 25 and over)						
<5th grade	0.8%	11.8%	15.4%	8.2%	5.3%	7.3%
High school diploma	84.1%	53.1%	46.2%	59.8%	62.1%	62.9%
Bachelor's degree or more	23.8%	9.0%	5.9%	8.0%	16.5%	15.2%
Household income in 1992						
Mean	41,646	29,102	28,448	25,060	35,594	29,682
Median	33,355	22,859	22,938	18,999	25,874	22,812
<$10,000	11.9%	20.4%	18.4%	31.2%	19.8%	18.1%
>$50,000	30.0%	15.5%	14.0%	12.9%	24.5%	16.2%
Below poverty level	9.6%	29.3%	30.1%	36.5%	18.1%	26.7%

Employment					
Unemployment					
Total	6.1%	11.9%	11.7%	14.4%	7.3%	13.2%
Males	7.1%	12.4%	12.1%	17.2%	7.6%	12.4%
Females	5.0%	11.1%	11.1%	11.0%	7.3%	14.4%
Occupation					
Male employed–16 yrs & over					
Laborer/service worker	17.8%	28.4%	29.9%	27.3%	23.3%	28.0%
Professional	29.2%	11.6%	8.7%	15.5%	20.3%	15.3%
Female employed–16 yrs & over					
Laborer/service worker	6.6%	14.8%	15.2%	10.8%	10.6%	19.2%
Professional	30.9%	15.4%	13.6%	18.5%	18.4%	15.7%
Families and households					
Total households	75,735	6,626	3,869	841	405	937
Household size: mean number of persons	2.52	3.41	3.78	2.85	2.65	3.25
Female householder, no husband	8.9%	18.7%	16.1%	31.4%	13.9%	19.8%
Families below poverty level	7.3%	26.2%	26.4%	32.5%	15.4%	27.0%
Availability of telephone					
In household	96.2%	86.0%	85.5%	81.3%	95.1%	85.4%
Available to household	1.0%	2.0%	2.4%	1.5%	0.7%	1.4%
Not available	2.7%	11.9%	12.0%	17.2%	4.1%	13.2%

Source: U.S. Department of Commerce, Bureau of the Census, *Current Population Characteristics* (report No. P20–475), March 1993.

ularly among Mexican-Americans. In an analysis of 1989 Current Population Survey (CPS) data, and in a similar analysis of Hispanic Health and
Nutrition Examination (HHANES) data (1982–1984), Trevino, Moyer, Valdez, and Stroup-Benham (1992) found similar patterns of noncoverage
for the Hispanics who were examined in each survey. These patterns of
insurance noncoverage from CPS data were 10% for non-Hispanic whites,
37% for Mexican-Americans, 16% for Puerto Ricans, and 20% for Cubans.
From HHANES data, these rates were 35% for Mexican Americans, 22%
for Puerto Ricans, and 29% for Cubans. These investigators concluded
that high rates of insurance noncoverage, even among the working poor
who are not insured, have created a potential for a high prevalence of
undiagnosed health needs, as well as low rates of access to preventive
health examinations.

Reasons for Underutilization of Health Services

Numerous reasons have been cited in the literature to explain the
observed disparity in the use of health care services among Latinos as
compared with non-Hispanic whites. These reasons include lack of knowledge regarding available services, as well as pragmatic barriers such as
lack of transportation (Barrera, 1978; Hough, Karno, & Burnam, 1983;
Keefe, 1979; Lopez, 1981; Padilla, Ruiz, & Alvarez, 1975). Another possible
reason cited in the literature is the utilization of alternative health care
systems such as folk healers and religious community leaders (Keefe;
Padilla et al.). Alternatively, a medical systems barrier cited as a cause of
health service underutilization is the lack of staff and facilities that offer
linguistically compatible services for bilingual or monolingual Spanish
speakers (Barrera, 1978). Finally, economic barriers such as low income
or lack of health insurance clearly play a critical role in the underutilization of health services by Hispanics (Wells et al., 1988).

Wells, Hough, Golding, Burnam, and Karno (1987) and Hough and
colleagues (1983) suggest that level of acculturation is an important factor
associated with Mexican-American use of outpatient and health-promotion or preventive services. These investigators found that low-acculturated Latinos (those who speak only or primarily Spanish) sought
health care less often.

Folk Beliefs and Remedies

In the past, several interesting studies examined folk beliefs and the
use of folk practices among Mexican-Americans (Baca, 1969; Clark, 1970;
Currier, 1966; Harwood, 1971; Rubel, 1960). Today, controversy exists
regarding the extent to which Mexican-Americans and other Latinos believe in and use folk healers (*curanderos, santeros*) and folk or herbal
remedies.

Data from the HHANES has revealed that only 4.2% of Mexican-Americans in a sample of 3,623 Mexican-Americans ages 18 years and older indicated that they consulted a *curandero* during the previous 12 months (Higginbothom, Trevino, & Ray, 1990). Those Mexican-Americans who did consult a *curandero*, as compared with those who did not, were persons who preferred taking the HHANES interview in Spanish, expressed dissatisfaction with their health care, had a lower income, had a lower self-perceived health status, and reported having lower perceived control over their health. However, the apparent low rate of help seeking from *curanderos* does not reflect lifetime rates of *curanderos* consultation, and the rates for the past year might operate as underestimates, as many Latinos are not comfortable disclosing that they have consulted a folk healer, and several may have seen a *curandero* sometime in the past.

Beyond the use of *curanderos*, other studies that have examined folk remedies and folk beliefs have noted that Mexican-Americans easily accommodate to the use of two systems of health care: the modern biomedical, and the folk system, where the folk healing system is used to supplement the biomedical system (Mayers, 1989). Some evidence indicates that level of endorsement of folk remedies and endorsement of hot–cold concepts of illness is greater among less acculturated *Latinas*, while endorsement of biomedical beliefs is strong and independent of level of acculturation (Castro, Furth, & Karlow, 1984). Hot–cold concepts include beliefs that relate to health behavior, such as the belief that when a person has a cold, it is unhealthy to drink cold liquids.

The manner in which an acceptance of folk medicine may influence health-related behavior requires further study. Possibly, persons who see themselves as having no personal control over their health may avoid participating in a program of self-change, since they may see no relationship between personal efforts at change and health outcomes. Similarly, persons who invoke God's will as the sole source of health outcomes may eschew efforts at self-directed healthy behavior change. Indeed, among Latinos, particularly those with strong Catholic beliefs, a sense of low or partial control over health and a deference to God's will operate as strong Latino cultural perceptions that influence behavior. Nonetheless, except for extreme cases, these views may not totally discourage most Latinos from selected efforts at healthy behavior change. Accepting a dual system of health concepts allows the belief that despite one's limited control over health, efforts at self-care, *cuidandose* ("taking care of oneself"), are still important and should be pursued.

CULTURALLY RELEVANT MODERATORS OF HEALTH STATUS

The design of culturally relevant health-promotion programs for Latinos should acknowledge four moderators, important factors that describe within-group variability that exists within all Latino populations.

Programs that do not attend to one or more of these factors (level of acculturation, traditionalism, modesty and self-confidence, and family support) may miss important cultural issues that are crucial to program effectiveness for promoting health in Latino populations.

Level of Acculturation

Acculturation is an important factor that has been related to health outcomes in various Latino populations. The general conception of acculturation is that it involves the acquisition of the language, behavioral norms, and values that are characteristic of the host society (Rogler, Cortes, & Malgady, 1991). For Latinos, especially for immigrants, acculturation to U.S. mainstream society involves the process of acquiring new social skills, including English-language skills, that aid in educational and economic upward mobility in the U.S. social system. Acculturation is a process that is more easily conceptualized for immigrants, although native born Hispanics can also undergo a process of acculturation (Castro, Balcazar, & Tafoya-Barraza, 1996).

Although acculturation does not necessarily result in a loss of identity and identification with the home culture, a Behavior Adoption Hypothesis asserts that with acculturation individuals undergo lifestyle changes that mimic the patterns of behavior that are exhibited by members of the host culture. Thus regarding language acquisition, a mark of greater acculturation for immigrating Latinos involves the acquisition of English language skills. In some cases, these Latinos develop bilingual–bicultural skills, whereas in other cases they abandon or suppress their Spanish-speaking skills with the acquisition of English language skills, in part as the result of efforts to evade discrimination from certain members of the host society.

Generally, contemporary acculturation scales for Latinos tend to measure a person's level of cultural involvement and psychological orientation to the Anglo-American and Latino core cultures, as measured along a bidirectional five-point dimension that is evaluated by scale items that examine (1) speaking and reading proficiency in English, Spanish, or both; (2) parental heritage; (3) life experiences in one culture or another; (4) cultural identification; and even (5) cultural pride, depending on the scale used to measure acculturation (Balcazar, Castro, & Krull, 1995; Cuellar, Arnold, & Maldonado, 1995; Cuellar, Harris, & Jasso, 1980; Marin, Sabogal, Marin, Otero-Sabogal, & Perez-Stable, 1987). Given the importance of acculturation issues for most Latinos, a health-promotion theory or model that omits acculturation as a construct and as a moderator–mediating variable is likely to be incomplete (Castro, Harmon, Coe, & Tafoya-Barraza, 1994). Here, the acculturation variable could be regarded as a trait that operates as an antecedent variable, or alternately as a stable mediator of program effects.

Various health-related studies with Latinos have observed a negative health effect for some health outcomes when examined across increasing levels of acculturation. For example, an analysis of data from HHANES (Marks, Garcia, & Solis, 1990) showed that when compared with their less acculturated peers, the more acculturated Latinos exhibited higher levels of alcohol use (frequency and amount) and lower dietary index scores that measured the consumption of balanced, healthy meals. A similar analysis from the HHANES regarding marijuana and cocaine use in relation to level of acculturation also revealed that the more acculturated (English speaking) Mexican-Americans and Puerto Ricans, as compared with their less acculturated (Spanish-speaking) peers were more likely to consume marijuana, cocaine, or both (Amaro, Whitaker, Cofman, & Heeren, 1990). These results support a Behavior Adaptation Hypothesis that indicates that the adoption of the behaviors of members of the host culture population increases with the individual's level of acculturation.

These results, however, are solely suggestive. During the acculturation process, the original social position of an immigrant in the native culture (e.g., being a poor lower class laborer in Mexico) and the immigrant's subsequent social position in the host country (e.g., the United States) may yield very different acculturational experiences and related health practices. For example, in one acculturation pathway, a poor Mexican laborer who immigrates to the United States and sometime thereafter succeeds in upward mobility to a middle-class status and lifestyle might exhibit an overall healthy shift in several health behaviors when emulating the health behaviors of a given health-conscious middle-class American or Latino reference group. By contrast, under a different acculturation pathway, a poor Mexican laborer who migrates to the United States but fails at upward mobility and remains trapped in a U.S. ghetto or barrio may exhibit few healthy shifts in behaviors when emulating the health habits of a lower-class reference group. Further research of a longitudinal nature is needed on the process by which various acculturation pathways may be related to corresponding patterns of change for various health-related behaviors (Castro, Balcazar, & Tafoya-Barraza, 1996).

Traditionalism

Among Mexican-Americans and other Hispanics, traditionalism refers to a set of beliefs, attitudes, and values that reflect conservative and often agrarian life views. Here, within the Latin American/Spanish-speaking cultures, including the cultures of Mexico, the Caribbean, Central America, and South America, Catholicism has been a core aspect of traditional culture practices.

Mexican traditionalism has a strong rural character, and this traditionalism appears to be a core factor within Mexican/Chicano ethnicity

(Castro & Gutierres, in press). Traditions are beliefs and practices about how life should be lived, which are handed down from parents to children. One contrasting force to traditionalism is Western modernization, where new or competing beliefs and practices are introduced and where some of these may operate in conflict with traditionalism. Ramirez has described a traditionalism–modernism dimension that captures variations in life-styles among various groups of Mexican nationals (*Mexicanos*), Mexican Americans, and Chicanos (Ramirez, 1991). The traditional end of this dimension is characterized by traits from nine domains. Here, traditionalism is characterized by (1) distinct gender role definitions (separate male–female role expectations), (2) strong family orientation and loyalty, (3) value of family over individualism, (4) strong sense of community, (5) strong past- and present-time orientation relative to a future-time orientation, (6) reverence for elders, (7) value of traditions and ceremonies, (8) subservience and deference to authority, and (9) spirituality and religiousness.

By contrast with traditionalism, modernism, according to Ramirez, is more prevalent within urban and suburban communities as these are depicted as having a more liberal religious orientation. Modernism emphasizes egalitarianism in child rearing and flexibility in gender role definitions, it emphasizes individualism and competition rather than cooperation, it emphasizes a youth's separation and independence from family early in life, and it emphasizes science rather than religion as the approach toward explaining the "mysteries of life" (Ramirez, 1991).

In the applied setting, elements of both traditionalism and modernism operate concurrently, and individuals within a population will differ in the extent to which they have a preference for traditional or modernistic beliefs and practices. Moreover, there are many individuals who quite comfortably endorse and practice to a high degree both modernistic and traditional practices. As one example, Castro and colleagues (1984) found that many Mexican and Mexican-American women, in a lower-class urban community, concurrently endorsed modernistic biomedical beliefs and practices regarding health and medicine while also endorsing several traditionally oriented folk beliefs about health and illness. Even among Hispanics who were raised or who currently live in a rural setting, the presence of mass media including television signals received via satellite dishes provides an exposure to modernistic health issues and contributes to this dual pattern of health beliefs. More research is needed to evaluate how variations in traditional–modernistic orientation may be related to actual health-related behaviors.

Modesty and *Simpatia*

One aspect of Latino health behavior that is related to traditionalism is modesty in personal health practices, particularly among Latino women who adopt traditional gender roles. This modesty is characterized by (1) caution in observing sexual and social prohibitions, (2) an emphasis on maintaining harmony in family and interpersonal relations (*simpatia*; Marin & Marin, 1991), and (3) deference to the needs and desires of others. For example, regarding the preventive practice of conducting monthly breast self-examinations, it appears that many low-educated, traditional Latino women have not been accustomed to this practice, especially because these women may have been taught that it is improper for a decent woman to engage in self-touching. Thus, promoting breast self-examinations in this population of Latino women requires cultural sensitivity to these traditional views regarding "proper" female conduct.

To date, little work has been conducted on the relationship between traditionalism and various aspects of orientation to health promotion, preparedness for behavior change, and the role of peers as sources of health-related social support. Preliminary analyses from our *Compañeros* projects of the correlation between the traditionalism dimension and level of acculturation among Mexican-American community women suggest that these dimensions are essentially orthogonal, that is, independent, with a correlation that is near zero (Castro & Gutierres, in press). The apparent independence of level of acculturation and level of traditionalism suggests that for Mexican-Americans (and perhaps other Latinos) across levels of acculturation, high traditionalism may be found in high-acculturated and in bilingual–bicultural Mexicans and Mexican-Americans just as often as it is found among low-acculturated Mexican-Americans.

It does appear that with greater acculturation and modernism in their orientation toward Western standards and gender roles, Latino women would exhibit higher levels of personal self-confidence and assertiveness. This assertiveness and self-confidence might promote a stronger orientation towards engaging in self-care. In addition, this more modernistic orientation toward self-care might operate more effectively if it is complemented by support from spouse and family. Such supports would include a message of encouragement that a woman should participate actively in her own health care.

Family Support

The importance of the family as a major source of social support for most Mexican-Americans has been emphasized by many investigators (Keefe, Padilla, & Carlos, 1978; Murillo, 1971; Valle & Vega, 1980). The concept of *familism* or *la familia* (a strong emphasis on reciprocity and strong emotional ties among family members) is a powerful factor in most Mexican-American families (Vega, Hough, & Romero, 1983). However, researchers differ in their evaluation of the effect that social support from the family has on alleviating stress. Several studies have shown that family social support reduces stress for Mexican-Americans (Hoppe &

Heller, 1975; Salgado de Snyder, 1987; Vega & Kolody, 1985), whereas other investigators have questioned the overall effects of strong family bonds when they serve as the sole source of social support (Raymond, Rhoads, & Raymond, 1980). These researchers have concluded that strong family bonds may aid in stress reduction, but they could also interfere with the individual's ability to seek needed help from outside sources. In developing health-promotion programs that work, our *Promotoras* (lay health workers) have advised us that the inclusion of spouse and other influential family members is a critical feature in promoting a woman's full participation in a health program. Given the role of the family among Latinos, efforts to incorporate the spouse and the family should be pursued, although the complexity of this approach must also be acknowledged. The alternative, however, is quite negative; without family support, for many Latinos, efforts at healthy behavior change are likely to fail.

DESIGNING CULTURALLY RESPONSIVE HEALTH PROMOTION PROGRAMS FOR LATINO COMMUNITIES

Cultural Proficiency and Competence

For designing effective health promotion programs, program planners must themselves be culturally competent. That is, they must have a thorough understanding of the cultural health beliefs and practices of various members within a targeted population. Understanding these beliefs and behaviors adds conceptual depth to the program planner's understanding of the cultural nuances that govern family, group, and community dynamics. Program planners must be familiar with general Latino cultural dynamics; yet they must also be familiar with local community dynamics in order to design culturally relevant health promotion programs for various members of a specific Latino population.

Moreover, developing *cultural proficiency* for work with Latino populations involves developing a deeper and ever more intimate understanding of the characteristics and the within-group variability that exists among members of a specific Latino population. Thus, cultural proficiency for developing optimal health promotion programs for members of a given population is an ideal, a high-level capacity. By contrast, a less advanced, yet substantive level of understanding of the culture of a given population is *cultural competence*. Cultural competence has been defined as "a set of academic and interpersonal skills that allow individuals to increase their understanding and appreciation of cultural differences and similarities within, among, and between groups. This requires a willingness and ability to draw on community-based values, traditions, and customs and to work with knowledgeable persons of and from the community in developing focused interventions, communications, and other supports" (Orlandi, Weston, & Epstein, 1992, p. vi).

Political Issues in Working with Latino Communities

In the 1990s, promoting health in Latino populations requires that the health promotion team or program establishes a sincere partnership with community leaders and organizations. In the past, researchers and program developers have given limited aid and resources to communities that have agreed to participate in the proposed research or program. As a consequence, many communities have felt exploited and now resist participating in newly proposed activities or programs (Marin & Marin, 1991).

Today, many Latino community leaders insist on having an equal and reciprocal relationship, a true partnership between themselves and the principal investigator or program director. Accordingly, program planning must include the views of community needs as these are emphasized by community leaders. These views must be considered early in program planning and design. While some community leaders may not understand the technical issues in research or program design and evaluation, they do understand community politics. Thus obtaining their support is crucial to gaining access to various members of a targeted population, especially the hard to reach.

Generally, an attitude of respect and sincerity on the part of the health promotion team is crucial for the establishment of this health partnership. This approach helps to establish trust (*confianza*), which cannot be rushed or approached in a cavalier manner. Community leaders and organizations aim to protect their constituents and thus will avoid compromising their own credibility by endorsing untrustworthy people. Investigators or programs that compromise and therefore lose community trust will experience a withdrawal of support from community leaders and a loss of access to targeted members of that community. Even more important, as community leaders and elders discuss among themselves a betrayal of trust, the investigator or program and its sponsors will lose credibility and develop a negative reputation that can persist for many years. In this regard, most ethnic communities, especially small, traditional communities, have a strong institutional–historical memory and will not be easily persuaded to participate in the near future.

By contrast, given the right attitude on the part of "outsiders," the research or program team can initiate a partnership by the successful implementation of at least five activities: (1) becoming familiar with the community, (2) establishing legitimacy, (3) consulting with community leaders and groups, (4) obtaining the sponsorship of various community leaders and organizations, and (5) providing clear and understandable information about the study or the program to prospective participants (Marin & Marin, 1991). These activities were undertaken by staff of the

Compañeros en la Salud project and ultimately led to the development of our program in 14 local churches (Castro, Elder, Coe, et al., 1995).

Reaching the Hard to Reach

Reaching hard-to-reach members of a community is a challenging task even for experienced investigators who are members of the local community. Often, the "sickest," those with the most severe health problems or those who are the highest risk of contracting disease or illness are also those who are the hardest to reach. In the *Compañeros* project, the channel for access that we chose was churches, miniature communities in which we conducted health education classes and community health fairs.

In partnership with our university's School of Nursing, the *Compañeros* project conducted community health fairs where free screening exams were offered (e.g., vision, hearing, blood pressure, immunizations). At the health fair registration desk we collected some demographic and health-needs data for the purpose of program evaluation and client follow-up. In this data gathering, however, the inclusion of a question on immigration and documented status should be considered carefully and perhaps not asked at all, as such a question can raise suspicion among documented as well as undocumented members of the community and compromise access to the hard to reach.

Additionally, Latino men are typically harder to reach than Latino women, perhaps because many Latino men engage in greater denial about their health and take a less active role in attending to family health issues relative to the role taken by *Latinas*. Accordingly, health promotion programs for Latinos need to include activities that appeal to Latino men and that will attract their participation and support. In this regard, future health promotion programs with Latinos should also emphasize family involvement, including the active participation of the Latino husband in support of the health of his wife.

Promotora Programs

A *Promotora* is a lay health educator who ideally lives within the same community as members of the target population, speaks the same language as the people she is serving as well as the language of the dominant culture, and understands and is intrinsically involved in the host community. In many ways, effective *Promotoras* bridge the gap between two cultures. When she is working with indigenous and ethnic groups, a crucial function of the *Promotora* is to educate while reinforcing the common identity shared by community residents. This task involves understanding and endorsing the shared traditional language, attitudes, values, and beliefs (Harwood, 1981). In most projects that use the *Promotora* model, the peer health worker is selected from within the community and is trained (1) to conduct health education classes in the community and (2) to bridge the gap between the community and health care resources by providing referrals and, in some cases, basic services to hard-to-reach populations in rural or urban settings.

Culturally relevant community health promotion programs that recruit *Promotoras* as staff members, whether paid or unpaid, should prepare these lay health workers to perform a variety of general tasks that fall into five skills areas: education, organization, publicity, outreach, and referral. Promotional development in the area of education, which is generally the most time-consuming task, involves fostering each *Promotora's* commitment to learning important aspects of health and health promotion. Under this skills area, a *Promotora* would attend a series of health education classes followed by additional enrichment classes that may be held once every 6 weeks.

Skills training in organization involves learning about scheduling and planning community activities such as educational classes and health fairs, maintaining attendance records, scheduling appointments for well-women examinations at health fairs that are led by the *Promotora*, and overseeing registration at health fairs. Skills training in the area of publicity involves showing the *Promotora* how to prepare and circulate (via community or church bulletin, bulletin board, or newsletter) announcements about the project and its activities, as well as how to make formal announcements about these activities during church services and at other church-based activities.

Skills training in the area of outreach involves maintaining contact with the organizational leadership (e.g., church hierarchy) and with the cohort of participating church members while informing them about project activities and encouraging their participation. Skills training in making referrals involves providing participants with lists of referral sources, offering follow-up services by aiding women in scheduling appointments, and ensuring that women get to their appointments. One aspect of this skills training in making and completing referrals involves a mastery of relevant medical terminology that allows *Promotoras* to serve as medical interpreters.

Enhancing Program Effect

A major issue in designing community intervention programs involves the efficiency with which the intervention is delivered and, conversely, the effectiveness of the intervention in prompting specific behavior change. From a design standpoint, most community-based health promotion programs have a small-effect size, which means that the level of behavior change in standardized units is typically small ($\delta = .1$ to $.3$). In other words, the amount (level or frequency) of observable change in a targeted behavior is small (e.g., a decrease in scores on a scale of dietary fat consumed per week). Or as measured in another manner, the proportion of cases in a sample that benefit from the intervention is small (e.g., the increase in the percentage of women who participate in mammography screening).

Power is the ability to detect a program effect if the effect is present (Cohen, 1988). Power is defined as $(1 - \beta)$, where beta is the probability of making a type II error, that is, 1 minus the probability of not detecting an effect that is present. Conventional research studies accept a power value of $P > .80$, meaning an 80% capacity to detect an effect that is actually there.

Here the effect size is particularly important, where a stronger program effect will require fewer units to detect that effect at .80 power, while, by contrast, a weaker program effect will require more units. Given that the recruitment and retention of even one additional unit, such as a church, is a major effort-laden task that requires much investment of personnel time and project resources; the minimum number of units needed for adequate power is a major consideration in program design and intervention.

Regarding this issue, Table 2 presents pretest to posttest change scores from the *Compañeros* project. These change scores are presented for the "cancer prevention" (the intervention group) churches and for the "family mental health" (the comparison group) churches. These data are presented for three targeted behaviors that are important in cancer-risk reduction. The sample consists of Latino women who attend their local church although in these analyses, the church is the unit of analysis. These behavioral variables are pretest–posttest changes in (1) frequency of breast self-examinations, (2) mammography examinations obtained during the past year, and (3) scores on a high-fat food scale. The program intervention goals were (1) to increase the frequency of breast self-exams from "none" to "once per month," (2) to increase the proportion of women in the sample who received a mammography this year from a "lower percentage" to a "higher percentage," and (3) to lower the frequency of high-fat foods consumed from a "higher fatty foods scale score" value to a

TABLE 2. Parameters for Power Calculation

Variable	Cancer prevention churches$_c$		Family mental health churches$_f$			Effect size
	M_c	SD_c	M_f	SD_f	D	(ES)
Breast self-exam (BSE)	0.39	0.65	0.19	0.38	.20	.31
Mammography (Mamm)	0.25	0.50	0.10	0.25	.15	.30
High-fat foods (Hical)	−0.44	0.38	0.00	0.80	−.44	.55

$D = M_c - M_f$. (ES) $= M_P - M_F/SD_K$. Here SD. is the *larger* of the two standard deviation values (SD_c or SD_f) in order to yield a more conservative test of effect size.

"lower scale score." For ease of presentation, we are eliminating here the technical details involved in the measurement of these variables.

In a preliminary analysis of the cancer prevention churches (c) (the intervention group), as compared with our family mental health, churches (f) (the comparison group) we observed changes in the appropriate direction from pretest–posttest as presented in Table 2. Across all churches, the church mean scores for the cancer prevention churches (M_c) and the mean scores for the family mental health churches (M_f) are shown in Table 2. Variable (D) in Table 2 refers to the difference in church-level mean scores (i.e., $M_c - M_f$). For the three outcome variables, these difference scores were for breast self-examination (BSE) = .20, for mammography (Mamm) = .15, and for high-fat foods (Hical) = −44. The respective effect sizes (ES) are for breast self-examination = .31, for mammography = .30, and for high-fat foods = .55, respectively. Thus, the church-level behavior change effects for breast self-examinations and for mammography are classifiable as small, and for high-fat foods consumption the effect size is moderate.

Based on the aforementioned data, Table 3 shows the number of churches needed to attain a given level of power, based on the observed mean differences (D). Note that with minor changes in mean scores (D), there is a remarkable change in the numbers of churches (N) needed to attain .80 power in relation to program effect sizes. For example, for the variable of *breast self-exam*, by increasing the program's effect size (i.e.,

TABLE 3. Treatment Effect against Churches Needed

Target behavior	Difference: D	SD_c	SD_f	N	Power
Breast self-exam					
	.20	.65	.38	42	.53
	.30	.65	.38	39	.80
	.40	.65	.38	22	.80
	.50	.65	.38	15	.82
Mammography					
	.15	.50	.25	42	.54
	.20	.50	.25	42	.75
	.30	.50	.25	22	.81
	.40	.50	.25	13	.83
High-fat food					
	.30	.38	.80	42	.71
	.40	.38	.80	31	.81
	.50	.38	.80	20	.81
	.60	.38	.80	14	.81

Note: SD_c is the difference in church means as shown in Table 2. SD_c is the standard deviation for cancer control prevention churches, and SD_f is the standard deviation for the family mental health churches. N is the number of churches needed per group for the indicated power level.

increasing the strength of our intervention and thus effecting larger changes in the outcome variable within intervention group) from .30 to .40, one reduces the number of churches needed from 39 to 22 for the same power level! These results indicate that *design efficiency* for health-promotion programs can be greatly improved simply by making small but significant increases in the strength of the intervention as measured by its capacity to produce a somewhat greater increment in behavior change. This is a very important issue in the design and implementation of future health promotion programs that will make a difference in our communities.

Regarding this issue, Hansen and Collins have identified seven ways to increase the power of a prevention intervention without increasing sample size (Hansen & Collins, 1994). From among these seven approaches, two approaches that directly enhance program effects are (1) maintaining program integrity, that is, fidelity in program implementation and (2) targeting appropriate mediators, that is, identifying and targeting the specific factors (such as attitudes or behavioral skills) that are believed to produce the intended change on the targeted outcome measures. The design of effective programs can benefit from the use of a well-conceived program model, a model that charts the effects of program activities, mediators, and outcomes as these effects are believed to occur. Such conceptual models may help to clarify the anticipated effects of key mediators and how the intervention might be structured to influence the mediators that in turn effect sustained changes in the targeted behaviors.

Potentiating the Intervention

Magnitude of effect on the targeted outcome measures can be increased by focusing staff and program efforts toward changing the outcome measures or changing the mediators that produce healthy changes in behavior (MacKinnon, 1994). Identifying relevant mediators—attitudes, skills, environmental barriers, and the like—requires a clear and culturally relevant model of the factors believed to produce healthy behavior change in members of the targeted population. For work with Latinos, this includes the contribution of the four cultural moderators: level of acculturation, traditionalism, *simpatía*, and family support.

ISSUES AND DIRECTION IN PROGRAM PLANNING

The Challenge of Maintaining Healthy Behavior Changes

One of the biggest health-promotion challenges in all populations, but particularly in ethnic minority populations, involves maintenance of healthy behavior change once it has been initiated. Particularly for low-income minorities who live in unstable, disrupted environments, staying on track with a program of healthy behavior change is indeed difficult.

For example, a 40-year-old Latino woman may initiate a personal exercise program that involves walking 2 miles, three times per week, for the purpose of weight management and to reduce her risk of diabetes, high blood pressure, and to promote cardiovascular fitness. Despite a commitment to this program, various disruptive conditions can compete with her efforts. A nonsupportive husband criticizes her for taking time and attention away from him and their three children. Her 4-year-old son gets the measles, and his illness forces her to postpone her walking program for more than a week. A recent gang shooting near her home makes her wonder whether it is safe to walk, even at the local park. The family car breaks down, and she needs to take it to the repair shop because her husband cannot take time off from work.

These and other environmental constraints can discourage even the most committed efforts at healthy behavior change. The more oppressive, unstable, and nonsupportive the person's environment and family system, the greater the likelihood that a person will abandon efforts at behavior change. Designing viable health promotion programs for Latinos, programs that encourage and support long-term behavior change, must take into account the unique environmental constraints and challenges that face various Latinos, particularly those who live in low-income, disrupted neighborhoods.

Some Guidelines for Program Development with Latino Populations

Program Planning

Given the effects of environmental constraints on lifestyle changes, a first step in the planning stage involves studying the local environment (the neighborhood, family systems) for naturally occurring opportunities and constraints. In connection with this, the program planner should speak with members of the target group to understand them in terms of their level of education and literacy, acculturation, and level of traditionalism, as well as in terms of their preferences and preparedness for participation in a program of healthy behavior change. In understanding the community and its residents, it is also useful to form a partnership with community leaders and organizations that can offer culturally relevant advice and can sanction the proposed program. In the *Compañeros* project, we conducted a series of focus groups with church-going women who served as key informants about the needs and preferences of members of their church. Finally, it is advisable that program planners develop a conceptual model, a "picture" of what factors may facilitate or impede the targeted behavior change as depicted in graphic form, and that shows the anticipated program effects. This model should include the expected influence of the culturally relevant moderators: level of acculturation, traditionalism, *simpatía*, and family support.

Program Participation

In this preparation stage, it is important to make the program activities simple and meaningful to members of the target population. It is also important to include an educational component that offers a clear rationale and clear instructions and to incorporate a simple self-monitoring or self-report system of consumer feedback. However, many Latinos who are low in education and literacy are not accustomed to written communications, such that a system of verbal self- and program monitoring may be needed. In the *Compañeros* project, our team of *Promotoras* served as local experts that provided feedback on the applicability and appropriateness of the health education materials and interventions that we developed, thus allowing for ongoing revisions and refinements of these materials and activities. Besides content and activity development, it is essential to set a formal system for program evaluation in place from the beginning. This system should incorporate outcome and process evaluation components, including formative evaluation (Windsor, Baranowski, Clark, & Cutter, 1994). In this program evaluation it is also important to examine the fidelity of program implementation as well as the level of participant exposure (sessions attended, etc.) to program activities as an indication of program "dose" received by each participant.

Program Implementation

As noted previously, maintaining participation in any ongoing program is a major challenge in working with low-income, ethnic minority populations. Latinos who live in impoverished, disrupted communities will miss several program sessions for a variety of reasons including family emergencies, dwindling commitment, inexperience in sustaining regular attendance in a health program, and transportation problems.

Focus-group feedback from our *Promotoras* at the end of our project yielded useful advice on ways to enhance program implementation and effects. The *Promotoras* recommended a greater effort to involve spouses and other family members as sources of support. Thus one important strategy for increasing participation is to build in social support from spouse, family, friend, or *Promotora*. A buddy-system approach will help sustain participation and active behavior change. In this regard, it is important not only to inform or educate members of the target audience about the benefits of a given behavior change, but also to build commitment by a self-analysis of the advantages and disadvantages of changing a targeted behavior and by anticipating the likely barriers to change that should be avoided or overcome (Watson & Tharp, 1981). Important here as well is building in culturally relevant incentives and rewards for progress in behavior change. Feedback from families or buddies regarding the activities or items that constitute culturally relevant rewards for members of the participating group will help to identify meaningful incentives.

Maintenance

Ideally, a targeted health behavior, when practiced regularly, becomes a habit, one that is incorporated into the person's daily routine or lifestyle. When this occurs, the health behavior acquires naturally reinforcing properties that eliminate the need for external incentives or rewards. Often a targeted health behavior fails to develop into a health habit when it competes with an incompatible unhealthy behavior. In low-income environments many external prompts promote unhealthy behaviors that compete with healthy ones. Given this, Latinos should be helped to restructure their home environments while also enlisting the aid of family members to prompt healthy behavior change. And, they should be helped to identify competing unhealthy behaviors and to work toward eliminating these.

Finally, in any behavior-change effort, relapse to the old, unhealthy ways is a frequent occurrence (Marlatt & Gordon, 1985). Program participants can be advised about the risks of relapse and offered relapse-prevention training that includes family members as aids to relapse avoidance. This training includes an understanding that a slip or lapse does not constitute a failure, but rather a temporary setback that can be remedied if addressed immediately and actively. Along these lines, the participant can be reminded that persistence is the key to success and that success at personal behavior change involves discovering the pathway to change that is comfortable and that works for the individual. This process of discovery involves supportive mentorship from a *Promotora*, from program staff, and from a family member or a peer who is familiar with the person's commitment to change. Allowing for this process of discovery and mentorship also requires flexibility in the manner in which a program of behavior change is designed, presented, and implemented within a given subpopulation of Latino participants.

CONCLUSION

Designing a program for healthy behavior change in Latino populations, especially for low-income populations, is challenging. More research is needed on ways in which standard behavior-change approaches should be modified to lend cultural relevance to these efforts. A partnership among community health leaders, organizations, researchers, and providers will foster a deeper cultural understanding of how behavior-change programs can be tailored to operate effectively in meeting the unique needs of various subpopulations of Latinos.

REFERENCES

Amaro, H., Whitaker, R., Coffman, G., & Heeren. T. (1990). Acculturation and marijuana and cocaine use: Findings from HHANES 1982-84. *American Journal of Public Health*, *80*(Suppl.), 54–60.

Anderson, R., Lewis, S. Z., & Giachello, A. L. (1981). Access to medical care among the Hispanic population of the southwestern United States. *Journal of Health and Social Behavior*, *22*, 78.

Baca, J. (1969). Some health beliefs of the Spanish speaking. *American Journal of Nursing*, *69*, 2172–2176.

Balcazar, H., Castro, F. G., & Krull, J. L. (1995). Cancer risk reduction in Mexican American women: The role of acculturation, education, and health risk factors. *Health Education Quarterly*, *22*, 61–84.

Barrera, M. (1978). Mexican-American mental health service utilization: A critical examination of some proposed variables. *Community Mental Health Journal*, *14*, 35–45.

Castro, F. G., Elder, J., Coe, K., Tafoya-Barraza, H. M., Morrato, S., Campbell, N., & Talavera, G. (1995). Mobilizing churches for health promotion in Latino communities: *Compañeros en la Salud*. *Journal of the National Cancer Institute Monographs*, *18*, 127–135.

Castro, F. G., Balcazar, H., & Tafoya-Barraza, H. M. (1996). Towards measuring acculturation process: Changes in acculturation status across stages of development. Unpublished monograph.

Castro, F. G., Furth, P., & Karlow, H. (1984). The health beliefs of Mexican, Mexican American, and Anglo American women. *Hispanic Journal of Behavioral Sciences*, *6*, 363–383.

Castro, F. G., & Gutierres, S. E. (in press). Drug and alcohol use among rural Mexican Americans. *NIDA Research Monograph*. Rockville, MD: National Institute on Drug Abuse.

Castro, F. G., Harmon, M. P., Coe, K., & Tafoya-Barraza, H. (1994). Drug prevention research with Hispanic populations: Theoretical and methodological issues and a generic structural model. In A. Cazares & L. A. Beatty (Eds.), *Scientific methods for prevention intervention research* (NIDA Monograph No. 139, DHHS Publication No. ADM 94-3631 pp. 203–233). Washington, DC: U.S. Government Printing Office.

Clark, M. (1970). *Health in the Mexican American culture*. Berkeley: University of California Press.

Cohen, J. (1988). *Statistical power analysis for the behavioral sciences* (2nd ed.). Hillsdale, NJ: Erlbaum.

Council on Scientific Affairs. (1991). Hispanic health in the United States. *Journal of the American Medical Association*, *265*, 248–252.

Cuellar, I., Arnold, B., & Maldonado, R. (1995). Acculturation rating scale for Mexican-Americans II: A revision of the original ARSMA scale. *Hispanic Journal of Behavioral Sciences*, *17*, 275–304.

Cuellar, I., Harris, L. C., & Jasso, R. (1980). An acculturation rating scale for Mexican American normal and clinical populations. *Hispanic Journal of Behavioral Sciences*, *2*, 199–217.

Currier, R. L. (1966). The hot-cold syndrome and symbolic balance in Mexican and Spanish-American folk medicine. *Ethnology*, *5*, 251–263.

Fincham, S. (1992). Community health promotion programs. *Social Science and Medicine,* *35,* 239–249.

Ginzberg, E. (1991). Access to health care for Hispanics. *Journal of the American Medical Association, 265,* 238–241.

Glanz, K., Lewis, F. M., & River, B. K. (1990). *Health behavior and health education.* San Francisco: Jossey-Bass Publishers.

Glenwick, D. S., & Jason, L. A. (1993). *Promoting health and mental health in children, youth, and families.* New York: Springer.

Hansen, W. B., & Collins, L. M. (1994). Seven ways to increase power without increasing N. In L. M. Collins & L. A. Seitz (Eds.), *Advances in data analysis for prevention intervention research* (NIDA Monograph No. 142, NIH Publication No. ADM 94-3599 pp. 184–195). Rockville, MD: National Institute on Drug Abuse.

Harwood, A. (1971). The hot-cold theory of disease: Implications for treatment of Puerto Rican patients. *The Journal of the American Medical Association, 216*(7), 1153–1158.

Harwood, A. (1981). *Ethnicity and medical care.* Cambridge, MA: Harvard University Press.

Higginbothom, J. C., Trevino, F. M., & Ray, L. A. (1990). Utilization of curanderos by Mexican Americans: Prevalence and predictors. Findings from HHANES 1982-84. *American Journal of Public Health, 80*(Suppl.), 32–35.

Hoppe, S. K. & Heller, P. L. (1975). Alienation, familism, and the utilization of health services by Mexican Americans. *Journal of Health and Social Behavior, 16*(3), 304–314.

Hough, R. L., Karno, M., & Burnam, M. A. (1983). The Los Angeles Epidemiological Catchment Area research program and the epidemiology of psychiatric disorders among Mexican-Americans. *Journal of Operational Psychiatry, 14,* 42.

Kazdin, A. (1994). *Behavior modification in applied settings* (5th ed.). Pacific Grove, CA: Brooks/Cole.

Keefe, S. E. (1979). Mexican American's underutilization of mental health clinics: An evaluation of suggested explanations. *Hispanic Journal of Behavioral Sciences, 1,* 90.

Keefe, S. E., Padilla, A. M., & Carlos, M. L. (1978). *Emotional support systems in two cultures: A comparison of Mexican American and Anglo Americans* (Occasional Paper No. 7). Los Angeles: University of California, Spanish Speaking Mental Health Research Center.

Lopez, S. (1981). Mexican American usage of mental health facilities: Under-utilization considered. In A. Baron (Ed.), *Explorations in Chicano psychology.* New York: Praeger.

Macias, R. F. (1977). Hispanics in 2000 A.D.—Projecting the number. *Agenda, 7,* 16–20.

MacKinnon, D. P. (1994). Analysis of mediating variables in prevention intervention research. In A. Cazares & L. A. Beatty (Eds.), *Scientific methods for prevention intervention research* (NIDA Monograph No. 139. DHHS Publication No. ADM 94-3631 pp. 127–154). Washington, DC: U.S. Government Printing Office.

Marin, G., & Marin, B. V. (1991). *Research with Hispanic populations.* Newbury Park, CA: Sage.

Marin, G., Sabogal, F., Marin, B. V., Oters-Sabogal, R., & Perez-Stable, E. J. (1987). Development of a short acculturation scale for Hispanics. *Hispanic Journal of Behavioral Sciences, 9,* 183–205.

Marks, G., Garcia, M., & Solis, J. M. (1990). Health risk behaviors of Hispanics in the United States: Findings from the HHANES, 1982–84. *American Journal of Public Health, 80*(Suppl.), 20–26.

Marlatt, G. A., & Gordon, J. R. (1985). *Relapse prevention: Maintenance strategies in the treatment of addictive behaviors.* New York: Guilford.

Mayers, R. S. (1989). Use of folk medicine by elderly Mexican American women. *The Journal of Drug Issues, 19,* 283–295.

Montgomery, P. A. (1994). *The Hispanic population in the United States: March 1993* (Publication No. P20-475, U.S. Department of Commerce, Bureau of the Census). Washington, DC: U.S. Government Printing Office.

Murillo, N. (1971). The Mexican American family. In N. N. Wagner & M. J. Huag (Eds.),

Chicanos: Social and psychological perspectives (pp. 97–108). St. Louis: C. V. Mosby.

Orlandi, M. A., Weston, R., & Epstein, L. G. (1992). *Cultural competence for evaluators.* Rockville, MD: Office of Substance Abuse Prevention.

Padilla, A. M., Ruiz, R. A., & Alvarez, R. (1975). Community mental health services for the Spanish-speaking surnamed population. *American Psychologist, 30,* 82.

Perry, C. L., Baranowski, T., & Parcel, G. S. (1990). How individuals, environments, and health behavior interact: Social learning theory. In K. Glanz, J. M. Lewis, and B. K. Rimer (Eds.), *Health behavior and health education* (pp. 161–186. San Francisco: Jossey-Boss.

Ramirez, M. (1991). *Psychotherapy and counseling with minorities: A cognitive approach to individual and cultural differences.* New York: Pergamon.

Raymond, J. S., Rhoads, D. L., & Raymond, R. I. (1980). The relative impact of family and social involvement on Chicano mental health. *American Journal of Community Psychology, 8*(5), 557–569.

Richardson, J., Marks, G., Solis, J., Collins, L., Berba, L., & Hisserich, J. (1987). Frequency and adequacy of breast cancer screening among elderly Hispanic women. *Preventive Medicine, 16,* 761–774.

Rogler, L. H., Cortes, D. E., & Malgady, R. G. (1991). Acculturation and mental health status among Hispanics. *American Psychologist, 46,* 585–597.

Rubel, A. (1960). Concepts of disease in Mexican American culture. *American Anthropologist, 62,* 795–814.

Salgado de Snyder, N. (1987). *Mexican American women: The relationship of ethnic loyalty and social support to acculturative stress and depressive symptomatology.* Occasional Paper No. 22. Spanish Speaking Mental Health Center. University of California, Los Angeles.

Taylor, R. B., Denham, J. W., & Ureda, J. R. (1982). Health promotion: A perspective. In R. B. Taylor, J. R., Ureda, & J. W. Denham (Eds.), *Health promotion: Principles and clinical applications* (pp. 1–18). Norwalk, CT: Appleton-Century Crofts.

Trevino, F. M., & Moss, A. J. (1984). Health insurance coverage and physician visits among Hispanic and non-Hispanic people in the U.S. *Health—United States, 1983.* Washington, DC: U.S. Government Printing Office.

Trevino, F. M., Moyer, M. E., Valdez, R. B., & Stroup-Benham, C. A. (1992). Health insurance coverage and utilization of health services by Mexican Americans, Puerto Ricans, and Cuban Americans. In A. Furino (Ed.), *Health policy and the Hispanic* (pp. 158–170). Boulder, CO: Westview Press.

U.S. Department of Commerce. (1993). *We the American ... Hispanics.* Washington, DC: U.S. Government Printing Office.

U.S. Department of Health and Human Services. (1994). *Healthy people 2000: National health promotion and disease prevention objectives - midcourse revisions.* Washington, DC: U.S. Government Printing Office.

Valle, R., & Vega, W. (1980). *Hispanic natural support systems: Mental health promotion perspective.* Sacramento, CA: State of California, Department of Mental Health.

Vega, W. A., Hough, R. L., & Romero, A. (1983). Family life patterns of Mexican Americans. In G. J. Powell, J. Yamamoto, A. L. Romero, & A. Morales (Eds.), *The psychosocial development of minority group children* (pp. 194–215). New York: Brunner/Mazel.

Vega, W. A., & Kolody, B. (1985). The meaning of social support and the mediation of stress across cultures. In W. A. Vega & M. W. Miranda (Eds.), *Stress and Hispanic mental health: Relating research to service delivery* (DHHS Publication No. ADM 85-1410). Rockville, MD: National Institute on Drug Abuse.

Watson, D. L., & Tharp, R. G. (1981). *Self-directed behavior: Self-modification for personal adjustment* (3rd ed.). Monterey, CA: Brook/Cole.

Wells, K. B., Golding, J. M., Hough, R. L., Burnam, M. A., & Karno, M. (1988). Factors affecting the probability of use of general and medical health and social/community services for Mexican Americans and Non-Hispanic Whites. *Medical Care, 26,* 441–451.

Wells, K. B., Hough, R. L., Golding, J. M., Burnam, M. A., & Karno, M. (1987). Which Mexican Americans underutilize health services? *American Journal of Psychiatry, 144,* 918–922.

Windsor, R., Baranowski, T., Clark, N., & Cutter, G. (1994). *Evaluation of health promotion, health education, and disease prevention programs* (2nd ed.). Mountain View, CA: Mayfield.

CHAPTER 18

Health Care Issues among Asian Americans

Implications of Somatization

CHI-AH CHUN, KANA ENOMOTO, AND STANLEY SUE

INTRODUCTION

Asian Americans (including Pacific Islander Americans) represent a significant part of the population. They are, in terms of percentage increase, the fastest growing ethnic group in the United States. In 1980, the population of Asian Americans exceeded 3.7 million, easily doubling the 1.5 million figure in 1970 (U. S. Bureau of the Census, 1988). The 1990 population of Asian Americans is about 7.3 million, nearly double that of 1980. Projections are that by the year 2020, the population will be 20 million (Ong & Hee, 1993). The Asian-American population is not only the fastest growing but also the most diverse ethnic group in terms of cultural backgrounds, countries of origin, and circumstances for coming to the United States. For example, the broad Asian-American category includes more than 50 different subgroups, which may primarily speak one of more than 30 different languages. The three largest subgroups in the Asian-American category are Chinese, Japanese, and Filipinos; significant numbers of Asian Indians, Koreans, Southeast Asians (e.g., Viet-

CHI-AH CHUN, KANA ENOMOTO, and STANLEY SUE • Department of Psychology, University of California at Los Angeles, Los Angeles, California 90095.

Handbook of Diversity Issues in Health Psychology, edited by Pamela M. Kato and Traci Mann. Plenum Press, New York, 1996.

namese, Cambodians, Laotians, and Hmong), and Pacific Islanders are also included in the Asian-American category.

Although research on the health status of Asian Americans has not been well developed, Asian Americans have been found to exhibit differences from other groups in terms of health status. For example, mortality rates for Asian-American adults (age-adjusted rates) and infants are lower than those of other ethnic groups including whites (Gardner, 1994). The incidence of all types of cancers combined are lower among Chinese, Japanese, and Filipinos than among whites, although higher rates have been found for certain anatomical sites such as the liver (Jenkins & Kagawa-Singer, 1994). The prevalence of chronic carriers of Hepatitis B is 8% to 15% among Asian Americans, while the prevalence is only a fraction of 1% for the U.S. population as a whole (H. Hann, 1994). Many differences exist among the various Asian-American groups. For example, obesity is much higher among Samoans and Hawaiians than among other Asian-American groups (R. Hann, 1994), and refugees from Southeast Asia have high-prevalence rates for tuberculosis compared to other Americans.

Although some of the findings on health status can be criticized because of methodological and conceptual weaknesses that often plague Asian-American research (e.g., inability to obtain large and representative numbers of respondents, cultural biases in assessment), ethnic differences on health status are not surprising. In fact, we expect the genetic–biological, cultural, dietary, environmental, and behavioral variations found among distinct racial, ethnic, or social groups to be reflected in health-status indicators. Indeed, the most interesting and significant questions are, What accounts for health status differences among ethnic groups? And how can our understanding of ethnic differences assist in the development of research, theory, and intervention (prevention and treatment) strategies that promote human welfare?

In this chapter, we discuss somatization among Asian-Americans as a means of raising some important health psychology issues. *Somatization* refers to complaints about, or the appearance of, physical symptoms such as headaches, stomach pains, inability to concentrate, chronic fatigue, sleep difficulties, loss of sensory functioning, and so on that have a strong psychological basis.[1]

Examining somatization is important for several reasons. First, somatic symptoms may have psychological as well as physical determinants; the interactions of these determinants are clearly germane to health psychology. Second, a controversy exists over the prevalence of somatization. Considerable impressionistic evidence suggests that somatization is more prevalent among Asian-Americans than among West-

---

[1]The definition used here is not confined to somatization disorder, which is a psychiatric condition manifested by multiple physical complaints that have no physical basis.

erners (Kleinman, 1977; Tseng, 1975). Analysis of the prevalence of somatization may be instructive in gaining insight to the complexities of ethnic comparisons in health status. Third, the role of culture in health and in the expression of symptoms is particularly salient in the analysis of somatization. Finally, implications for health practices (prevention, assessment, and treatment) can be drawn.

In this chapter, we argue that little empirical evidence exists to support the notion that Asian Americans have a higher prevalence of somatization; that theoretical formulations attempting to explain the phenomenon of somatization, especially among Asian Americans, have failed to distinguish between disease and illness behavior; and that understanding illness behavior and cultural values can aid in the delivery of effective health interventions.

SOMATIZATION IN THE WEST

Somatization is a common phenomenon in Western societies. Lipowski (1988) defines it as "the tendency to experience and communicate somatic distress and symptoms unaccounted for by pathological findings, to attribute them to physical illness, and to seek medical help for them" (p. 1359). Somatization also exists in the form of amplified symptom expression among people with real medical problems that are often chronic, such as cancer or arthritis. Epidemiological studies in the United States and Europe have estimated the prevalence rate of somatization to be between 12% and 28% (Birdes & Goldberg, 1985; Schepank, 1988; Shepherd, Cooper, Brown, & Katton, 1966). In the past 2 decades, somatization has been the focus of much research because the medical community began to recognize it as a costly phenomenon (Engel, 1977; Katon, Ries, & Kleinman, 1984). More than 50% of primary care visits are made by somatizers who often undergo unnecessary medical exams, surgeries, and procedures, which are not only costly but also damaging to their health (Katon et al., 1982). Thus somatization is an important health care issue with significant fiscal, medical, and psychological relevance.

Researchers have offered many explanations of why people manifest somatic symptoms without medical cause (Katon, 1982; Kellner, 1990; Kirmayer, 1984; Mechanic, 1979). According to Simon (1991), the numerous etiological explanations can be summarized into four basic models. The first model, based on traditional Freudian theory, proposes that somatization is a *psychological defense*. Physical-symptom reporting and health-care seeking are viewed as altered presentations of psychiatric disorder, usually affective or anxious in nature. Therefore, somatization is a "masked" presentation of psychopathology. The second model conceptualizes somatization as a *nonspecific amplification of distress*. Manifestation of both physical and psychological symptoms is viewed as the consequence of nonspecific underlying distress. This model predicts that patients who tend to perceive and report unpleasant sensations will endorse higher levels of all types of symptoms. The third model conceptualizes somatization as a *tendency to seek care for common symptoms* (Simon, 1991). This model assumes that unpleasant physical symptoms are ubiquitous and that negative affective states cause people to seek health care for symptoms they might otherwise ignore. Mechanic (1972) found that psychological distress caused somatizing patients to interpret common bodily sensations as evidence of disease. Mechanic viewed this tendency as a learned pattern of coping with emotional distress by focusing on bodily symptoms and seeking health care. The final model presented by Simon (1991) suggests that somatization is a by-product of the medical care system and other social institutions that selectively attend to physical symptoms. Such *selective attention* often contribute to iatrogenic damages, which are medical damages induced by unnecessary or exessive medical treatments.

SOMATIZATION IN ETHNIC ASIANS[1]

Research in cross-cultural psychiatry suggests that somatization is a more common phenomenon in non-Western cultures, including ethnic Asians living in Asia and in the United States (Kirmayer, 1984). While explanatory hypotheses concerning somatization among ethnic Asians are not inconsistent with the conceptions of somatization in Western societies, researchers have emphasized different cultural values or practices that encourage somatization. In general, these cultural hypotheses propose that certain aspects of Asian cultures facilitate the development of somatization. Ethnic Asians, especially the ethnic Chinese,[2] are thought to deny the experience and expression of emotions, either consciously or unconsciously (Cheung, in press; Kleinman, 1977; Nguyen, 1982; Tseng, 1975). Open displays of emotions are discouraged in order to maintain social harmony or avoid exposing personal weakness. Also, because of the heavy social stigma of mental illness, psychological distress is more readily expressed through the body rather than through the mind (Kleinman, 1977; Nguyen, 1982; Tseng, 1975). Somatic expressions of psychological distress thus constitute the socially recognized and accepted signals of illness. This cultural hypothesis is, in essence, very similar to the psychological defense model of somatization.

[1]Ethnic Asians refer to all those of Asian descent living both in and outside of Asia. Ethnic Asians include Asians living in the United States (i.e., Asian Americans).
[2]Ethnic Chinese refer to all those of Chinese descent living both in and outside of China, Hong Kong, and Taiwan.

Alternatively, because most Asian cultures traditionally hold a holistic view of mind and body, a clear differentiation between the psychological and somatic systems does not exist among many ethnic Asians (Tseng, 1975). Many of the indigenous expressions of psychological states metaphorically describe the states of various bodily organs. Furthermore, Chinese medicine, which has dominated traditional medicine in most of Asia for centuries, emphasizes the balance of two energy forces, yin and yang, as the key to good bodily and mental health. According to Chinese medicine, human problems can disturb the balance of yin and yang. Once an imbalance between yin and yang is created, it should be treated through both mind and body. The philosophy of mind and body of traditional Chinese medicine has had a tremendous influence on ethnic Asian patients' knowledge and conceptualization of their problems. Lastly, Leff (1981) made a controversial reference to the stages of ontogenic development of cultures. He explains that somatization commonly occurs in cultures that are still "primitive" such as those of Asia and Africa, whereas in the more "civilized" Western cultures psychological distress is expressed through psychological symptoms.

Prevalence of Somatization among Ethnic Asians

What do empirical findings suggest about the prevalence of somatization among ethnic Asians? Is somatization really as common as these cultural hypotheses suggest? Considerable research has been done with ethnic Chinese psychiatric patients (Kleinman, 1977; Lin, 1953, 1982; Rin, Schooler, & Caudill, 1973; Tseng, 1975; Tseng & Hsu, 1970). Tseng found that nearly 70% of the psychiatric outpatients at a psychiatric clinic in Taiwan presented with exclusively or predominantly somatic complaints on their initial visit. Similar observations were made across age and socioeconomic status in Chinese Americans living in Boston's Chinatown area (Gaw, 1976). Kleinman (1977) compared symptom presentations of 25 Chinese and 25 American psychiatric patients with depressive syndromes. He found that 88% of the Chinese patients initially reported somatic complaints but no affective complaints, compared with only 20% of the American patients. Somatic complaints were also much more common among Thai depressive patients and Vietnamese soldiers than among European depressive patients residing in Thailand and American soldiers in Vietnam, respectively (Bourne & Nguyen, 1967; Tongyonk, 1972). These findings suggest that somatization is more prevalent in ethnic Asians than in people with European ancestry.

Further evidence of greater somatization among ethnic Asians comes from cross-cultural research on neurasthenia. In China, *shenjing shuairuo*, or neurasthenia, is the most commonly diagnosed psychiatric disorder (Kleinman, 1980, 1982; Ware & Kleinman, 1992; T. Y. Lin, 1982). It is also a widely recognized and used psychiatric lay term in China, Hong

Kong, and Taiwan (T. Y. Lin, 1989) and implies "an ailment with vague, protean signs and symptoms due to weakness of the nervous system, the brain, and the body generally, in which bodily weakness, fatigue, tiredness, headaches, dizziness, and a range of gastrointestinal and other complaints are to be found" (Kleinman, 1982, p. 82). Kleinman found that of the 100 Chinese psychiatric patients diagnosed with neurasthenia he interviewed in China, 93% suffered from various forms of clinical depression and 71% from anxiety disorders (although actual diagnosis of depression was very rare). These neurasthenic patients reported the somatic symptoms of depression and anxiety but suppressed most of the affective symptoms. Kleinman thus argues that, in China, neurasthenia is a culturally sanctioned expression of psychiatric disorder, mainly depression and anxiety. Once again, the implication is that ethnic Chinese tend to somatize their psychiatric disorders.

Research in cross-cultural psychiatry has also "discovered" culture-bound syndromes that are primarily somatic in nature. *Hwabyung* is a somatic disorder found among ethnic Koreans (K. M. Lin, 1983; K. M. Lin et al., 1992). Literally, *hwabyung* means "anger sickness" or "fire sickness" and consists of "a multitude of somatic and psychological symptoms, including constricted, oppressed, or 'pushing-up' sensations in the chest, palpitations, 'heat sensation,' flushing, headache, 'epigastric mass,' dysphoria, anxiety, irritability, and difficulty in concentration" (K. M. Lin et al., 1992, p. 386). Based on the investigation of the symptomology of *hwabyung* and the psychiatric history of Korean Americans who have experienced *hwabyung*, K. M. Lin and his colleagues concluded that *hwabyung* may be a culturally bound somatic expression of major depression.

Koro is a culture-bound syndrome found primarily in Chinese and Southeast Asian cultures. It is conceptualized as a nervous disease because it causes certain nerves to contract. The contraction of the nerves results in shrinkage of the genitals. *Koro* occurs more commonly in men, although *koro* in women has been reported. Men who suffer from *koro* complain about their penis shrinking and fear impending death (Edwards, 1984). *Koro* attacks are said to be random but usually occur after a shock treatment to the patient that causes fear or anxiety or as a result of physical overexhaustion. Other symptoms of a *koro* attack are very similar to those of a panic attack. They include sudden increase in heart rate, palpitations, numbness in the extremities and limbs, fainting, and fear of dying (American Psychiatric Association, 1994). Therefore, *koro* may be viewed as a culturally bound somatic expression of anxiety, fear, or both, in ethnic Chinese and Southeast Asians.

In sum, much of the early cross-cultural research on somatization and the more recent research on neurasthenia and culture-bound syndromes suggest that somatization is quite prevalent among ethnic Asians and possibly more prevalent than among Euro-Americans.

Problems with Cross-Cultural Research in Somatization

While the findings of these early studies provide some support for a higher prevalence of somatization among Asians, there have been conceptual and methodological problems with the cross-cultural research in somatization. First, the definition of somatization is not clear. Somatization has been operationally defined in such various terms as somatic complaints, endorsement of somatic symptoms, initial reporting of somatic symptoms, diagnosis with a somatic disorder such as neurasthenia, and so on (Gaw, 1976; Kleinman, 1977, 1982; T. Y. Lin, 1982; Tseng, 1975). Recently, there have been efforts to refine the definition of somatization (Cheung, 1985 cited in Cheung, in press; Kleinman & Kleinman, 1985). Cheung (1985, cited in Cheung, in press) defined somatization as "the presentation, complaint, or manifestation of somatic symptoms that relate to psychological or emotional problems." This revised definition of somatization may appear to be tautological with the psychological defense model of somatization that conceptualizes somatization as a masked expression of underlying psychological distress. However, it should be noted that Cheung's revised definition does not imply how or why such masking occurs, whereas the psychological defense model states that the masking of underlying psychological distress occurs as a result of internal psychological defenses such as denial, repression, or suppression of emotions.

Kleinman and Kleinman (1985) expanded their definition of somatization by adding the medical-help-seeking component of the phenomenon. Furthermore, they made the distinction between acute, subacute, and chronic somatization. *Acute somatization* refers to temporary somatic complaints and medical help seeking caused by acute life stressors. *Subacute somatization* is a more serious condition that lasts several months and is caused by either persistent stressful life circumstances or a psychiatric disorder such as depression or anxiety. *Chronic somatization*, on the other hand, often consists of physical symptoms of a psychiatric disorder or amplified expression of a chronic medical disease such as arthritis or heart disease. Lipowski (1988) argues that acute somatization is a common and normal response to stress and that only chronic somatization should be considered as a clinical disorder. With the exception of studies on neurasthenia and depression in ethnic Chinese (Kleinman & Kleinman, 1985; Ware & Kleinman, 1992), investigations on somatization in ethnic Asians often failed to distinguish the various types of somatization.

Second, related to the problems of definition, early studies failed to make a distinction between symptom reporting and symptom manifestation (Cheung, in press). Many of them relied solely on patient self-report. One major drawback of self-report is that ethnic-Asian participants tend to hold back information or not report symptoms that may cause themselves or their families shame (e.g., marital conflict, psychotic symptoms, academic or job failure; Uba, 1994). Because of the shame that psychological disorders carry in Asian cultures, subjects in the early studies who were asked to report symptoms may have selectively reported only the somatic symptoms that appeared to have a physical cause. Such selective reporting could certainly give researchers the impression that ethnic-Asian psychiatric patients somatize. In fact, recent studies have found that many of the ethnic-Asian patients who initially reported only somatic complaints also report psychological symptoms when directly probed (Cheung, 1982; Cheung, Lau, & Waldman, 1980; Lin, Masuda, & Tazuma, 1982; Nguyen, 1982; Zheng, Xu, & Shen, 1986). Thus initial reporting of somatic symptoms should not be taken automatically as evidence for a lack of psychological insight or awareness.

Third, most of the early findings on ethnic Asians are descriptive and anecdotal (Kirmayer, 1984). Some reports were based on the clinical experience of the authors (T. Y. Lin, 1982) and some on clinical case analyses (Kleinman, 1977; Nguyen, 1982; Ware & Kleinman, 1992). Others simply reported frequency counts and percentages of people with somatic complaints or number of people who endorsed a particular symptom (Kleinman, 1977, 1982; Nguyen, 1982; Tseng, 1975) Although good descriptive information, impressionistic data, or both can help us develop critical hypotheses, there must be empirical testing of the cultural hypotheses that have been put forth.

Fourth, conclusions drawn from these early findings may be misleading because these studies included only psychiatric patients. As a result, there may have been some selection biases in the samples. For example, Asian psychiatric patients compared to other ethnic patients tend to avoid mental health services, fearing stigmatization. Consequently, they are likely to be more seriously disturbed than other patients. Or individuals with somatic problems may seek medical treatment, whereas those with psychological problems may seek help from other providers such as acupuncturists and herbalists, from nonprofessionals (e.g., spiritual/religious leaders, friends, family), or not seek help at all. If these self-selection and sampling problems are not controlled, comparisons of the prevalence of somatization among different groups cannot be adequately performed.

In fact, recent studies investigating somatization in nonclinical community samples of Asians and Asian-Americans found that somatization is not more prevalent in Asians and Asian-Americans than in ethnic Europeans (Beiser & Fleming, 1986; Cheng, 1989). Kagawa-Singer and her colleagues (under review) interviewed Asian- and Euro-American women with breast cancer using several structured interview measures and found that the number and the type of somatic symptoms not attributable to their medical condition did not differ between the two groups of women. In an epidemiological study in Taiwan, Cheng measured the prevalence rates of somatization to be 19.6% for males and 27.1% for females. Cheng compared these rates to those in the British survey by Jenkins (1985) and from other Western surveys (Woodruff, Murphy, & Herjanic, 1967; Mathew, Weinman, & Mirabi, 1981) and found that they were not different from one another. Raskin, Chien, and K. M. Lin (1992) found that contrary to their hypothesis, which predicted more reporting of somatic complaints in elderly Chinese Americans compared to elderly European Americans, elderly Chinese Americans actually reported less somatic complaints than their Caucasian counterparts. In a later paper, even Kleinman and Kleinman (1985), who originally claimed that somatization was more common among ethnic Chinese, acknowledged that somatization was also very common in the West.

In conclusion, there is insufficient evidence to support the claim that ethnic Asians somatize more than ethnic Europeans (Cheung, in press; Kirmayer, 1984; Singer, 1975). In fact, more recent research evidence suggests that what we saw in the early reports of somatization in ethnic Asians were artifacts of methodology (e.g., poor and inconsistent operational definition of somatization, inadequate sampling strategy, and insufficient probing for psychological symptoms). As mentioned above, many of the early reports did not distinguish between discomfort reporting (or illness behavior) and symptom manifestation. Cheng (1989) warned that the term *somatization* should be used only when primary psychological symptoms are not found in spite of adequate clinical assessment. When reporting bias is controlled for by conducting structured interviews, nonpsychiatric populations are studied, and the prevalence rates of ethnic Asians and ethnic Europeans are directly compared, at least in terms of prevalence, then the phenomenon of somatization in ethnic Asians is not exceptional. What appears to be exceptional in ethnic Asians is the highly common physical symptom-reporting and medical-help-seeking behaviors.

UNDERSTANDING SOMATIZATION IN ETHNIC ASIANS

Despite revealing new evidence, some of which has been mentioned above, it is interesting to note that the myth of greater somatization in ethnic Asians persists. The persistence of the myth is partly due to inadequate dissemination of the new evidence. However, the main fuel for its perpetration appears to be what caused the emergence of the myth in the first place. That is, regardless of their awareness of the psychological nature of their problems, ethnic Asians initially tend to report more somatic complaints and seek medical help for their somatic problems more frequently than do ethnic Europeans.

The clinical implication of this phenomenon is that there is a greater burden on health care providers seeing Asian-American patients to identify patients who may be presenting psychogenic somatic symptoms. This task requires health care providers to understand the meaning of somatic complaints in the Asian-American population. Such understanding should be based on knowledge accumulated not only from clinical experience but also from systematic and well-defined research. Fortunately, the recent studies of somatization in ethnic Asians have gone beyond estimating prevalence rates and have begun to systematically investigate the phenomenon, ultimately searching for etiological factors that may be influenced by culture. The following discussion is our attempt to provide a brief overview of these studies within a common theoretical framework and shed some light on the phenomenon of somatization in ethnic Asians.

Somatization as an Illness Experience

The distinction of illness experience/behaviors from disease has helped recent efforts to improve research on the phenomenon of somatization, especially in ethnic Asians. The disease/illness distinction originally began in the medical field in order to understand symptoms and behaviors of chronically ill patients that are not directly caused by the biological disease (McHugh & Vallis, 1986). *Disease* simply refers to physical ailments or conditions that require medical attention such as cancer, arthritis, and hepatitis. *Illness*, however, refers to one's reaction to, interpretation of, and coping with the disease. Illness can also be described as the psychosocial experience of the disease. Recognizing the limitations of the biomedical model of disease that attributes physical conditions and ailments only to "disordered biology," McHugh and Vallis proposed a biopsychosocial model—the illness behavior model—which integrates both the disease and illness experiences of an individual. It has been proposed that somatization phenomena observed in ethnic Asians may be better explained as illness behaviors (Cheung, in press; Kleinman, 1982; Kleinman & Kleinman, 1985; Ware & Kleinman, 1992).

According to the biomedical model, a disease shares a universal etiology and manifestation (McHugh & Vallis, 1986). Thus, the conceptualization of somatization as a disease would be relatively *culture free*. That is, somatization in the United States is caused by the same factors and is manifested in the same way as somatization in Indonesia. This is the model under which health and mental health care providers commonly operate (Kleinman, 1980). In the fourth edition of the *Diagnostics and Statistical Manual of Mental Disorders* (DSM-IV; American Psychiatric Association, 1994), somatization appears to be conceptualized more as a disease, and the manual lists the criteria of various somatoform disorders. Although the DSM-IV acknowledges some cultural variations of the disorders, the main assumption is that these criteria will be relatively universal.

The illness behavior model, on the other hand, pertains to the experience of disease and acknowledges the influence of the ethnocultural context on the individual (McHugh & Vallis, 1986). According to the illness behavior model, diseases may be universal, but the illness experience accompanying each disease varies from person to person. Illness experience is a set of cognitions and behaviors occurring in reaction to a disease. The illness experience begins with cognitive appraisals of a problem situation (e.g., depression, anxiety, or interpersonal conflict). These cognitive appraisals are influenced by both internal and external factors, such as past learning experience related to illness and social support. Once the situation is considered distressing, coping responses that broadly consist of self-care and help seeking will follow. Sociocultural factors, such as attitudes toward experience of distress and the socially normative treatment of distress, comprise the ethnocultural context that influences the components of the illness experience.

Somatization as an illness occurs in reaction to the underlying disease that can be either life stressors (e.g., unemployment and marital conflict) or psychopathology (e.g. depression and anxiety) (Cadoret, Widmer, & Troughton, 1980; Katon, 1982; Katon, Kleinman, & Rosen, 1982; Kleinman, 1982; Kleinman & Kleinman, 1985). Illness behaviors often take the form of medical help seeking and somatic-symptom presentation. Such illness behaviors are fairly common and even adaptive in both ethnic Asians and ethnic Europeans. However, in some individuals these behaviors persist beyond the negative results of thorough medical examinations and thus become maladaptive. In China, somatization is implicitly understood as an expression of underlying psychological distress or pathology but labeled as a disease (i.e., neurasthenia; T. Y. Lin, 1982; Kleinman & Kleinman, 1985). Kleinman and Kleinman concluded that neurasthenia is a cultural label of somatization, which, in turn, is an illness behavior of "masked depression."

It has been demonstrated that the illness model lends itself to investigations of the ethnocultural influences on somatization, whereas the biomedical disease model places its emphasis on the universal aspects of somatization. The reconceptualizion of the phenomenon of somatization in ethnic Asians as an illness enabled the examination of the specific illness aspects of the phenomenon (Cheung, Lee, & Chen, 1983; Cheung, 1987; Cheung & Lau, 1982; Kleinman, 1982; Kleinman & Kleinman, 1985; Ware & Kleinman, 1992). This approach has advanced our understanding of the ethnocultural influences on somatization by shedding light on how ethnic Asians conceptualize their problems and how these conceptualizations guide the expression of distress, coping, and help-seeking behaviors.

Problem Conceptualization and Symptom Presentation

In the past, the cultural hypotheses stated that ethnic Asians tend to conceptualize their problems mainly in somatic terms and that their conceptualization contributes to their somatic experience and reporting of psychological distress (Kleinman, 1977; Tseng, 1975). However, recent research indicates that somatic symptoms are not necessarily alternative channels for expressions of distress because psychiatric symptoms and somatic symptoms were often found to co-occur (Cheung, Lau, & Waldmann, 1980-81; Lin, Masuda, & Tazuma, 1982; Nguyen, 1982). In fact, exclusive manifestation of somatic symptoms is quite rare. Most patients acknowledge the presence of both somatic and psychological symptoms, but often do not see the link between their physical complaints and psychological distress (Lin, Masuda, & Tazuma). Furthermore, studies investigating problem conceptualization in ethnic Chinese revealed that ethnic Chinese have a multitude of different conceptualizations of their problems that can be broadly categorized as psychological, somatic, and situational (Cheung, 1987; Cheung, Lee, & Chen, 1983).

If ethnic Asians conceptualize their problems in various ways including somatic and psychological, why do researchers repeatedly observe ethnic Asians in psychiatric settings presenting with somatic complaints? Researchers have found that the symptom-reporting behaviors of ethnic Asians may be context-dependent. Ethnic-Chinese patients reported only somatic symptoms to their primary care physicians despite their awareness of psychological symptoms (Cheng & Lau, 1982). Even when they were seen by a psychiatrist, these patients limited their reporting to somatic symptoms because they thought psychiatry treated only problems related to the brain such as headaches and dizziness (Tseng, 1975). In fact, Tseng explained that until recently psychiatry was called "neuropsychiatry" in both China and Japan. In Korea, the term is still being used. Thus, as Kirmayer (1984) suggested, patients' knowledge of psychiatric medicine also contributes to their selection of which symptoms to report.

Coping and Help Seeking

In addition to symptom-reporting behaviors, problem conceptualization also appears to influence the coping and help-seeking behaviors of ethnic Asians. In an investigation of illness behaviors of Chinese college students, Cheung and her colleagues (1983) found that problem conceptualization is related to coping and help-seeking behaviors when the problem is not serious. That is, if the problem was conceptualized mainly in somatic terms, then the student subjects indicated that they would change their somatic states by modifying their diet or doing more exercise. On the other hand, if the problem was conceptualized in both somatic and psychological terms, then the subjects offered both psychological and somatic solutions such as relaxing, changing social and physical lifestyle, and so on. For serious problems, however, the solution was unanimously "seeking medical care" regardless of the subjects' initial problem conceptualizations. Ethnic-Chinese college students reported that for serious problems they would seek professional help from primary care physicians and occasionally from traditional Chinese medicine (Cheung et al.). Even for mild problems, a substantial minority answered that they would consult primary care physicians. Cheung and her colleagues thus concluded that primary care physicians are regarded by ethnic Chinese as professionals to whom they may turn for many different problems.

In contrast, psychiatric care is seldom sought by ethnic Chinese. In the same study by Cheung and her colleagues (1983), even individuals who conceptualized their problems psychologically rarely indicated that they would seek or had sought help from mental health care providers. In fact, they preferred self-care coping strategies that included relaxing, ignoring the problems, or changing their social lifestyle and seeking social support from families and friends (Cheung, 1987; Cheung et al., 1983). Despite the psychological nature of the problems, when these strategies fail to alleviate distress, medical help is sought. One hundred percent of the ethnic Chinese psychiatric patients interviewed in a retrospective study (Cheung) indicated that they had been referred to psychiatric care by their primary care physicians.

This fact does not imply that all individuals seeking medical care for their psychological problems will eventually be referred to psychiatric care. In fact, many of the psychiatric patients, especially those who primarily conceptualized their problems somatically, had frequently changed their physicians because of lack of improvement in their somatic problems (Cheung, 1987; Kleinman, 1985). This "doctor shopping" caused long delays before these individuals consulted psychiatric care. From these findings we can deduce that some patients may never get referred to psychiatric care if their physicians fail to detect the psychosocial nature of their problems. Unfortunately, we know very little about these individuals.

In conclusion, the early impression that ethnic Asians somatize more than ethnic Europeans seems to be associated with particular coping and help-seeking behaviors of ethnic Asians rather than to a tendency to conceptualize problems somatically. In fact, as demonstrated by Cheung and her colleagues (Cheung, 1987; Cheung et al., 1983), ethnic Asians do not limit their conceptualization to somatic terms. By understanding the disease–illness distinction and the cultural conceptions of illness, we can gain insight into the means of devising effective treatment and intervention programs and into the important directions for future research.

IMPLICATIONS FOR CLINICAL PRACTICE

Reconceptualizing somatization as an illness has important clinical implications for health care providers because ethnic Asians tend to seek medical help for problems that are not only somatic in nature but also psychological and social (Cheung, 1987; Cheung, Lee, & Chan, 1983). The clinical implications can be divided into three general areas: assessment, treatment, and prevention of somatizing illness behaviors of ethnic Asians.

Assessment

Because research findings show that ethnic Asians tend to present only somatic symptoms to primary care physicians and psychiatrists for problems that are actually psychogenic, health care providers need to exercise care when assessing the physical health of Asian-American patients. Given the research findings, it would be tempting to conclude that the Asian-American patient is exhibiting somatization illness behaviors when the medical cause of the presented problem is not obvious. A comprehensive interview can prevent health care providers from making diagnostic errors that are based on stereotypical assumptions and can help them assess whether the patient's symptoms are truly due to organic causes only or are illness behaviors of psychological distress or psychopathology other than somatization disorder.

Nevertheless, health care providers need to be sure to probe for possible psychological symptoms related to memory, concentration, and affect that Asian-American patients may not report since studies have found that many of the so-called "somatizers" do admit having psychological symptoms when asked. A structured and comprehensive interview that covers both somatic and psychological symptoms can ensure that such psychological symptoms, if present, do not go unnoticed by practitioners.

The interview may also contain questions regarding the patient's medical treatment history and presence of life stressors. The medical treatment history might reveal the patient's utilization pattern of the health care system. This information can help health care providers identify possible somatizers whose medical treatment history would reveal a pattern of "doctor shopping." Inquiry into past and present life stressors can provide information about what factors precipitated health care utilization. In the cases of patients with real medical problems, the deterioration in their physical condition or appearance of new physical symptoms may have caused them to seek medical care. On the other hand, patients with somatic symptoms that are psychogenic will have experienced some kind of stressful life event or circumstance immediately before the onset of the somatic symptoms or seeking of medical care.

Treatment

Research on somatization in ethnic Asians also has important implications for treatment of Asian-Americans. The evidence demonstrates that ethnic Asians, including Asian-Americans, often hold conceptualizations of their problems that differ from mainstream Western medicine and psychiatry. Unfortunately, for effective, culturally responsive health care services, it is critical that the patient and the health care practitioner share, or at least understand, each other's conceptualizations of the patient's problem. Meichenbaum (1976) notes that when there is incongruity in problem conceptualization between the patient and health care provider, patients are less likely to engage in treatment. If, for example, Asian-American patients believe that their somatic symptoms are caused by an imbalance in hot and cold energy, the patients may resist referrals to mental health care providers. Therefore, in order to facilitate treatment compliance and efficacy, the treatment should initially accommodate the patient's conceptualization of the somatic symptoms (Simon, 1991).

If the patient's problem is identified as somatization illness behavior, the treatment should target the underlying psychological distress or psychiatric disorder. However, the somatizing patient should be "eased" into the psychological treatment by implementing the treatment in primary health care settings, in conjunction with medical services. This process will help reduce the resistance of somatizing patients to psychological interventions. Thus, an ideal treatment for somatization would entail interdisciplinary work between health and mental health professionals.

One such treatment program that has been implemented in primary health care settings is a group treatment program designed by Barsky, Geringer, and Wool (1988). This treatment program has a psychoeducational (i.e., behavioral and cognitive) and supportive orientation. The behavioral component consists of distraction and relaxation techniques that assist patients to reduce sensitivity to bodily sensations. The cognitive component consists of teaching somatizers to reattribute physical sensations to benign causes such as cold and fever. Supportive discussions of life stress and situational factors have repeatedly been found to be helpful, especially to relieve the overall psychological distress. This component may be very important because Kleinman and Kleinman (1985) reported that almost all of the neurasthenic patients they interviewed in the study had experienced stressful life events in the 6 months prior to the onset of their symptoms. Treatment of this nature considers somatic symptoms to be genuine expressions of distress and deals with somatic symptoms not as a defense against the real problem but rather as a real problem (Simon, 1991).

Prevention

Preventive efforts should focus on educating the Asian-American community about the psychogenic nature of some somatic problems. Although somatic expressions of distress are not necessarily abnormal or dysfunctional (Kleinman & Kleinman, 1985), awareness of the dangers of developing maladaptive somatization behaviors that can lead to chronic dependence on health care and iatrogenic damages should be raised in the Asian-American community. Such awareness can minimize unnecessary medical treatment and reduce the delay to appropriate mental health care. Because studies have shown that regardless of how problems are conceptualized ethnic Asians seek professional help from primary care physicians for serious problems, education about available mental health services and the nature of mental health services and psychiatric care are necessary to reduce delay to appropriate care

IMPLICATIONS FOR RESEARCH

Our discussion points to a need for greater understanding of somatization among Asian Americans. First, we need more detailed descriptions of the illness phenomenon in Asian Americans, for example, the nature of somatic complaints, frequency or intensity of somatic symptoms, underlying disease, and the course of the illness. Because findings have largely been derived from the Chinese and some from Southeast Asian refugees, the generalizability of results is thus open to question. Therefore, we need more descriptive data on other groups of Asian Americans.

Second, more sophisticated research designs involving tests of specific hypotheses are needed to identify the specific cultural factors that influence the medical help-seeking behaviors in Asian Americans. Various cultural factors such as collectivistic values (e.g., shame/loss of face), attitudes toward mental illness, and culturally transmitted coping behaviors have been proposed in the past, and some work has begun with the Chinese population in Hong Kong, but not with Asian Americans who are distinctly different because of their biculturality.

Third, research indicates that most ethnic Chinese who seek psychiatric care go through the primary health care system at some point in their attempts to cope with their problems. Investigations into this particular phase of the illness can provide valuable information for designing and implementing prevention and treatment programs.

Fourth, we need to find out what happens when Asian Americans seek nonprofessional help. For example, we know very little about how they seek help from family and friends or mobilize social support. And we know even less about what kinds of help Asian Americans seek from the nonprofessionals and how effective nonprofessional help is.

Finally, we need research on the culturally sensitive assessment, treatment, and prevention of somatization illness behaviors for Asian Americans. This reserach should look at both the innovation and efficacy of new procedures and programs.

REFERENCES

American Psychiatric Association. (1987). *Diagnostic and statistical manual of mental disorders* 3rd ed., Rev. ed. Washington, DC: American Psychiatric Association.

Barsky, A. J., Geringer, E., & Wool, C. A. (1988). A cognitive-educational treatment for hypochondriasis. *General Hospital Psychiatry, 10*, 322–327.

Beiser, M., & Fleming, J. A. E. (1986). Measuring psychiatric disorder among southeast Asian refugees. *Psychological Medicine, 16*, 627–639.

Bourne, P. G., & Nguyen, D. S. (1967). A comparative study of neuropsychiatric caualties in the United States army and the army of the republic of Vietnam. *Military Medicine, 132*, 904–909.

Bridges, K., & Goldberg, D. P. (1985). Somatic presentation of DSM III psychiatric disorders in primary care. *Journal of Psychosomatic Research, 29*, 563–569.

Cadoret, R., Widmer, R. B., & Troughton, E. P. (1980). Somatic complaints: Harbinger of depression in primary care. *Journal of Affective Disorder, 2*, 61–70.

Cheng, T. A. (1989). Symptomatology of minor psychiatric morbidity: A crosscultural comparison. *Psychological Medicine, 19*, 697–708.

Cheung, F. M. (1982). Psychological symptoms among Chinese in urban Hong Kong. *Social Science and Medicine, 16*, 1339–1344.

Cheung, F. M. (1984). Preferences in help-seeking among Chinese students. *Culture, Medicine and Psychiatry, 8*, 371–380.

Cheung, F. M. (1987). Conceptualization of psychiatric illness and help-seeking behavior among Chinese. *Culture, Medicine and Psychiatry, 11*, 97–106.

Cheung, F. M. (in press). Facts and myths about somatization among the Chinese. In T. Y. Lin, W. S. Tseng, & E. K. Yeh (Eds.), *Culture and mental health: Chinese experiences.* Hong Kong: Oxford University Press.

Cheung, F. M., & Lau, B. W. K. (1982). Situational variations of help-seeking behavior among Chinese patients. *Comprehensive Psychiatry, 23*(3), 252–262.

Cheung, F. M., Lau, B. W. K., & Waldmann, E. (1980–81). Somatization among Chinese depressives in general practice. *International Journal of Psychiatry in Medicine, 10*, 361–374.

Cheung, F. M., Lee, S., & Chan, Y. Y. (1983). Variations in problem conceptualizations and intended solutions among Hong Kong students. *Culture, Medicine and Psychiatry, 7*, 263–278.

Edwards, J. W. (1984). Indigenous koro, a genital retraction syndrome of insular Southeast Asia: A critical review. *Culture, Medicine and Psychiatry, 8*, 1–24.

Engel, G. L. (1977). The need for a new medical model: A challenge for biomedicine. *Science, 196*, 129–136.

Gardner, R. (1994). Mortality. In N. W. S. Zane, D. T. Takeuchi, & K. N. J. Young (Eds.), *Confronting critical health issues of Asian and Pacific islander Americans* (pp. 53–104). Thousand Oaks, CA: Sage.

Gaw, A. C. (1976). An integrated approach in the delivery of health care to a Chinese community in America: The Boston experience. In A. Kleinman, P. Kunstadter, E. R. Alexander, & J. L. Gale (Eds.), *Medicine in Chinese cultures: Comparative studies of health care in Chinese and other societies.* Bethesda, MD: Fogarty International Center, National Institute of Health.

Hann, R. S. (1994). Hepatitis B. In N. W. S. Zane, D. T. Takeuchi, & K. N. J. Young (Eds.), *Confronting critical health issues of Asian and Pacific islander Americans* (pp. 148–173). Thousand Oaks, CA: Sage.

Hann, H. W. L. (1994). Tuberculosis. In N. W. S. Zane, D. T. Takeuchi, & K. N. J. Young (Eds.), *Confronting critical health issues of Asian and Pacific islander Americans* (pp. 302–315). Thousand Oaks, CA: Sage Publications.

Jenkins, C. N. H., & Kagawa-Singer, M. (1994). Cancer. In N. W. S. Zane, D. T. Takeuchi, & K.

N. J. Young (Eds.), *Confronting critical health issues of Asian and Pacific islander Americans*. Thousand Oaks, CA: Sage.

Jenkins, R. (1985). *Sex difference in minor psychiatric morbidity*. Psychological Medicine Monograph (Suppl. 7). Cambridge, UK: Cambridge University Press.

Katon, W. (1982). Depression: Somatic symptoms and medical disorders in primary care. *Comprehensive Psychiatry, 23,* 274–287.

Katon, W., Kleinman, A., & Rosen, G. (1982). Depression and somatization: A review, part I. *American Journal of Medicine, 72,* 127–135.

Katon, W., Ries, R. K., & Kleinman, A. (1984). The prevalence of somatization in primary care. *Comprehensive Psychiatry, 25,* 208–215.

Kellner, R. (1990). Somatization: Theories and research. *Journal of Nervous and Mental Disease, 178,* 150–160.

Kirmayer, L. J. (1984). Culture, affect and somatization. *Transcultural Psychiatric Research Review, 21,* 159–217.

Kleinman, A. (1977). Depression, somatization and the "new cross-cultural psychiatry." *Social Science & Medicine, 11,* 3–10.

Kleinman, A. (1980). *Patients and healers in the context of culture*. Berkeley: University of California Press.

Kleinman, A. (1982). Neurasthenia and depression: A study of somatization and culture in China. *Culture, Medicine and Psychiatry, 6,* 117–190.

Kleinman, A., & Kleinman, J. (1985). Somatization: The interconnections in Chinese society among culture, depressive experiences, and the meanings of pain. In A. Kleinman & B. Good (Eds.), *Culture and Depression* (pp. 429–490). Berkeley: University of California Press.

Leff, J. P. (1981). *Psychiatry around the globe: A transcultural view*. New York: Marcel Dekker.

Lin, K. M. (1983). Hwa-byung: A culture-bound syndrome? *American Journal of Psychiatry, 140,* 105–107.

Lin, K. M., Lau, J. K. C., Yamamoto, J., Zheng, Y. P., Kim, H. S., Cho, K. H., & Nagasaki, G. (1992). Hwa-byung: A community study of Korean Americans. *Journal of Nervous and Mental Disease, 180,* 386–391.

Lin, K. M., Masuda, M, & Tazuma, L. (1982). Adaptational problems of Vietnamese refugees: Part III. Case studies in clinic and field: Adaptive and maladaptive. *Psychiatric Journal of the University of Ottawa, 7,* 173–183.

Lin, T. Y. (1953). A study of the incidence of mental disorder in Chinese and other cultures. *Psychiatry, 16,* 313–336.

Lin, T. Y. (1982). Culture and psychiatry: A Chinese perspective. *Australian and New Zealand Journal of Psychiatry, 16,* 313–336.

Lin, T. Y. (1989). Neurasthenia in Asian cultures [Special issue]. *Culture, Medicine and Psychiatry, 13.*

Lipowski, Z. J. (1988). Somatization: The concept and its clinical application. *American Journal of Psychiatry, 145,* 1358–1368.

Mathew, R. J., Weinman, M. L., & Mirabi, M. (1981). Physical symptoms of depression. *British Journal of Psychiatry, 139,* 293–296.

McHugh, S., & Vallis, T. M. (1986). Illness behavior: Operationalization of the biopsychosocial model. In S. McHugh & T. M. Vallis (Eds.), *Illness behavior*. New York: Plenum Press.

Mechanic, D. (1972). Social psychologic factors affecting the presentation of bodily complaints. *The New England Journal of Medicine, 286,* 1132–1139.

Mechanic, D. (1979). Development of psychological distress among young adults. *Archives of General Psychiatry, 36,* 1233–1239.

Meichenbaum, D. (1976). Toward a cognitive theory of self-control. *Consciousness and Self-Regulation, 1,* 1–66.

Nguyen, S. D. (1982). Psychiatric and psychosomatic problems among southeast Asian refugees. *Psychiatric Journal of the University of Ottawa, 7,* 163–172.

Ong, P., & Hee, S. (1993). *Losses in the Los Angeles civil unrest, April 19-May 1, 1992: Lists of the damaged properties*. Los Angeles: UCLA Center for Pacific Rim Studies.

Raskin, A., Chien, C. P., & Lin, K. M. (1992). Elderly Chinese- and Caucasian-Americans compared on measures of psychic distress, somatic complaints and social competence. *International Journal of Geriatric Psychiatry, 7*, 191–198.

Rin, H., Schooler, C., & Caudill, W. A. (1973). Symptomatology and hospitalization. *Journal of Nervous and Mental Disease, 157*, 296–312.

Schepank, H. (1988). Psychoneuroses and psychophysiological disorders: Prevalence, courses and strategies for prevention. *Psychotherapy and Psychosomatics, 49*, 187–196.

Shepherd, M., Cooper, B., Brown, A. C., & Kalton, G. W. (1966). *Psychiatric illness in general practice*. London: Oxford University Press.

Simon, G. E. (1991). Somatization and psychiatric disorders. In L. J. Kirmayer & J. M. Robbins (Eds.), *Current concepts of somatization: Research and clinical perspectives* (pp. 37–62). Washington, DC: American Psychiatric Association.

Singer, K. (1975). Depressive disorders from a transcultural perspective. *Social Science & Medicine, 9*, 289–301.

Tongyonk, J. (1972). Depressions in Thailand in the perspective of comparative-transcultural psychiatry. *Journal of Psychiatric Association of Thailand, 17*, 44–50.

Tseng, W. S. (1975). The nature of somatic complaints among psychiatric patients: The Chinese case. *Comprehensive Psychiatry, 16*, 237–245.

Tseng, W. S., & Hsu, J. (1970). Chinese culture, personality formation and mental illness. *International Journal of Social Psychiatry, 16*, 5–14.

Uba, L. (1994). *Asian Americans: Personality patterns, identity, and mental health*. New York: Guilford Press.

U.S. Department of Commerce, Bureau of the Census (1988). *Asian and Pacific islander population in the United States: 1980* (Report No. PC80-2-IE). Washington, DC: Government Printing Office.

Ware, N. C., & Kleinman, A. (1992). Culture and somatic experience: The social course of illness in neurasthenia and chronic fatigue syndrome. *Psychosomatic Medicine, 54*, 546–566.

Woodruff, R., A., Murphy, G. E., & Herjanic, M. (1967). The natural history of affective disorders. 1. Symptoms of 72 patients at the time of index hospital admission. *Journal of Psychiatric Research, 5*, 255–263.

Zheng, Y., Xu, L., & Shen, Q. (1986). Styles of verbal expression of emotional and physical experiences: A study of depressed patients and normal controls in China. *Culture, Medicine and Psychiatry, 10*, 231–243.

CHAPTER 19

Behavioral Approaches to Illness Prevention for Native Americans

STEVEN SCHINKE

THE STATE OF NATIVE AMERICAN HEALTH

Much evidence suggests that the health of Native Americans is worse than the health of America's general population. In fact, Native American people suffer inordinately from cancers linked to both behavioral and lifestyle patterns (Beauvais, Oetting, Wolf, & Edwards, 1989; "Cancer hits all time high," 1991; Mao, Morrison, Semenciw, & Wigle, 1986; National Cancer Institute, 1986). Cancer is the third leading cause of death among Native Americans (Rhoades, Hammond, Welty, Hander, & Amler, 1987). Whereas cancer was a relatively rare problem for Native Americans in the earlier part of this century, deaths from cancer among Alaska Natives and Indians in the northern United States now exceed average U.S. rates (Lanier, 1993). In addition, the 5-year survival rate for Native American people with cancer is the lowest of any ethnic group in the United States (Stillman, 1992).

Lung cancer is the leading cause of cancer mortality among Native Americans (Department of Health and Human Services [DHHS], 1991). The most dramatic increase in lung cancer mortality has been among

STEVEN SCHINKE • Columbia University School of Social Work, New York, New York 10025.

Handbook of Diversity Issues in Health Psychology, edited by Pamela M. Kato and Traci Mann. Plenum Press, New York, 1996.

Native American females (DHHS). The rate of cervical cancer in American Indian women is twice that for all U.S. women of all races (Hampton, 1993). Yet much variability exists in cancer mortality among Native Americans from different regions. Between 1968 and 1987, Native Americans from Alaska, North Dakota, South Dakota, and Montana had overall cancer rates that were consistently at or greater than the overall U.S. cancer rates, whereas Native Americans from other regions had lower rates than the U.S. averages.

Chronic diseases, including end-stage renal disease (ESRD) and diabetes, are major public health problems for Native Americans. In the period 1983 through 1986, the diabetes-attributed incidence of ESRD among Native Americans was 5.8 times that for whites (Newman, Marfin, Eggers, & Helgerson, 1990). Chronic disease is a major cause of death among Native Americans (Jackson, 1986). Recent studies have discovered a high correlation between diabetes and heart disease among American Indians (Howard, 1992). Some American Indian populations are among the most obese in the world (Rhoades, 1992), and obesity is a risk factor for both diabetes and heart disease.

Although mortality rates for cardiovascular disease are lower in Native Americans than in the U.S. population as a whole, cardiovascular disease remains the leading cause of death for Native Americans. Moreover, cardiovascular morbidity rates are increasing in some tribes (Howard, 1992; Rhoades, 1992). In addition, Native Americans suffer from tuberculosis 6 times more often than the general population (Rhoades). There is also a greater prevalence of pneumonia, influenza, and meningitis among Native Americans than in the general population (Rhoades).

Native Americans have the highest rate of death from unintentional injuries of all minority groups (DHHS, 1985). Indeed, these "accidents" are the second leading cause of death among Native Americans (Indian Health Service, 1984). Most of these accidents, both fatal and nonfatal, have been attributed to alcoholism or other self-destructive behavior (Blum, 1992).

BEHAVIORAL PRACTICES ASSOCIATED WITH CANCER RISKS

The unhealthy lifestyle patterns followed by Native Americans account for the higher rates of cancers and other health problems. According to the Centers for Disease Control and Prevention, almost half of all factors that influence a person's chance of surviving to age 65 are related to lifestyle behaviors (Cunningham-Sabo & Davis, 1993). For example, about 30% of cancer incidence is related to tobacco use, and about 50% of all cancer deaths are related to diet (Cunningham-Sabo & Davis).

Poverty is also a contributing factor to health problems among Native American people. According to the Indian Health Service's (1990) data, more than 28% of the Native American population falls below the poverty line, compared to less than 13% of the general population. The percentage of high school and college graduates among Native Americans is also lower than the percentage among the general population (55% vs. 66% and 7% vs. 16%, respectively). In the following sections, lifestyle factors that affect Native American health will be discussed.

Nutritional Factors

Cancer research suggests an association between food intake and the risk of developing certain types of cancer (American Cancer Society, 1991). A diet high in fat, for example, has been associated with breast, colon, and prostate cancer. Salt-cured, smoked, and nitrite-cured foods have been similarly linked to esophageal and stomach cancer. In contrast, high-fiber foods and a varied diet of vegetables and fruits rich in vitamins A and C may reduce risk for a wide range of cancers.

In addition to cancers, nutritional factors contribute to 3 more of the 10 leading causes of death in the Native American population: heart disease, cirrhosis, and diabetes (Blum, 1992). As Native Americans adopt values and behaviors of mainstream culture, they are consuming less traditional foods and are becoming more dependent on prepackaged staples. Many Native Americans living in poverty rely on government commodities as their sole source of food. These food commodities (canned meats, cheese, butter), distributed on reservations, are typically high in fat. Thus, among some Native Americans, the intake of high-fat foods is widespread, whereas consumption of the grains, fresh vegetables, and fruit more common in their traditional diet is infrequent (Blum; Singer & Schinke, in press). These changes in dietary behavior partially account for the life-threatening illnesses found among Native Americans (Blum; Singer & Schinke).

Tobacco Use

Cigarette smoking has a proven association with cardiovascular disease (DHHS, 1983), cancer (DHHS, 1982), and chronic obstructive lung disease (DHHS, 1984). Ingestion of tobacco through the lungs, when smoked, or through buccal and oral mucosa tissue, when chewed or sniffed, is not only dangerous to those tissues but is also addictive. Cancers of the lung, oral cavity, larynx, esophagus, bladder, pancreas, kidney, stomach, and uterus are also associated with habitual cigarette use (Office on Smoking and Health, 1982, 1983, 1984).

Combined with alcohol use, tobacco use places Native Americans at risk for throat cancer and for injuries related to fire (Bobo & Gilchrist, 1983; Bobo, Gilchrist, Schilling, Noach, & Schinke, 1987). According to a survey and 14,000 adolescents from both rural areas and reservations,

Native American youth are more likely to have tried more substances than any other group of adolescents (Blum, 1992). By seventh grade, 28% of Indian youth report at least one episode of getting drunk, 44% have tried marijuana, and 72% have tried cigarettes. From these statistics, it appears that Native American youth begin abusing substances at a younger age than their Anglo counterparts. Moreover, 15% of the surveyed Native American high school students smoke daily, and even more females smoke than males. These results compare with previous studies documenting that, compared with adolescents of other American ethnic–racial groups, Native American youth not only use alcohol, tobacco, and other drugs earlier but also use them at higher rates and with more severe lifelong health, social, and economic consequences (Beauvais & La-Boueff, 1985; Hall & Dexter, 1988; Oetting et al., 1983; Okwumabua & Duryea, 1987; Schinke et al., 1986).

The use of smokeless tobacco is often a precursor to the use of other substances among adolescents and young adults (Schinke et al., 1989a). Studies have noted a progressive increase of substance use as adolescents move into young adulthood (Schinke, Botvin, & Orlandi, 1991). Many youth judge smokeless tobacco use as less harmful or less risky than smoked tobacco; only nonusers routinely described all tobacco use as harmful. Relative to nonusers, smokers and smokeless tobacco users do not see the products they use as harmful (Schinke, Gilchrist, Schilling, & Senechal, 1986).

Other findings indicate that snuff and chewing tobacco are used frequently, heavily, and at an early age by Native-American youth (Schinke et al., 1986a; Schinke, Schilling, Gilchrist, Ashby, & Kitajima, 1987, 1989). Indeed, one-sixth of male Native American high school students use smokeless tobacco products daily (Blum, 1992).

Alcohol Abuse

Alcohol abuse is a contributor to the poor health of the Native American population. Native Americans lead the nation in rates of alcohol-related cirrhoses, diabetes, fetal abnormalities, accident fatalities, and homicides (Pedigo, 1983; Ward, 1984). Moreover, the rate of alcoholism among Native Americans is 332% greater than that for all other ethnic groups (Indian Health Service, 1990). Alcohol abuse has proven refractory to treatment efforts (Pedigo; Topper, 1985). Half of the Native American junior high school students and two-thirds of the senior high school students surveyed by Blum (1992) had tried alcohol. By the 12th grade, 25% of the male students and 14% of the female students consumed alcohol at least weekly (Blum, 1992). In most age categories, national figures indicate higher rates of alcohol-related deaths for Native Americans than for the general U.S. population. In the age group 25 to 34, for example, Native American males die 2.8 times more frequently than U.S.

averages from motor-vehicle crashes, 2.7 times more than U.S. averages from other accidents, 2.0 times more than U.S. averages from suicide, 1.9 times more than U.S. averages from homicide, and 6.8 times more frequently than U.S. averages from alcoholism (May, in press). Female drinking is high in some tribes and growing rapidly in others (May, 1989; May & Smith, 1988; Whittaker, 1982). Finally, when compared with majority culture adolescents, Native American youth progress into and sustain excessive use of alcohol and illegal drugs more often (Red Horse, 1982; Trimble, Padilla, & Bryan, 1985).

Psychosocial Factors

Several psychosocial factors influence the health behaviors of Native Americans. Cultural influences, gender-specific influences, and social influences all affect the behavior of American Indian populations (Schinke et al., 1990). Some of these factors are the same for Native Americans and members of the majority culture, whereas others are unique to Native Americans. For example, Native Americans and members of the majority culture may drink or smoke because of peer pressure toward substance use, or because of the recreational value of drinking and drug taking. Explanations for substance abuse that are unique to Native Americans, however, include the spiritual meaning of intoxication, the view that smokeless tobacco is a rite of passage into adulthood (Beauvais & La-Boueff, 1985), and cultural conflicts between Native Americans and the majority society (Austin, 1988; Jones-Saumty, Hochhaus, Dru, & Zeiner, 1983; Lewis, 1982; Pedigo, 1983; Schinke et al., 1985a; Schinke et al., 1985b; Walker & Kivlahan, 1984). These psychosocial factors will be discussed in the following sections.

Cultural Influences

Acculturation is a possible explanation for Native American substance use (Walker & Kivlahan, 1984). Acculturation affects every Native American tribe, yet varies both individually and regionally. Native Americans, whether living on reservations or in cities, may feel multiple pressures related to conflicts between their own culture and the dominant society. Such pressures demand a coping response. Some researchers believe that Native Americans adopt tobacco use or alcohol use as a coping mechanism against acculturation stress (Moncher, Holden, & Schinke, 1991; Schinke, Moncher, Holden, Orlandi, & Botvin, 1992; Schinke et al., 1990).

Historical and tribal factors may also partially explain substance use patterns and dietary behavior. Tobacco and psychoactive substances have spiritual value among Native American people (Weibel-Orlando, 1985). Because of its consciousness-altering effects, substance use is associated with positive attributes among some North American tribal groups. Native American history also plays a role in Native American people's dietary choices. For example, contrary to the belief that fried bread is a traditional Native American food, it actually grew out of the government rations of white flour, baking powder, and lard that were imposed on Native Americans who lived on reservations (Jackson, 1990).

Gender-Specific Influences

Similar to other minority and majority culture youth, Native American adolescents confirm gender-specific styles of tobacco use (Brunswick & Messeri, 1984; Dembroski, 1984). Like their non-Native American counterparts, Native American females may use tobacco to control their weight. Young Native American women, however, use smokeless tobacco at higher rates and more heavily than young women in majority and minority cultures. Lacking traditional male role models, young Native American men may use tobacco as a sign of masculinity (Beauvais & LaBoueff, 1985; Lewis, 1982).

Social Influences

Peer pressure and other interpersonal influences (such as adult modeling) offer explanations for substance use relevant not only to the Native American youth population but also to non-Indian youth. Peer pressure, however, has special meaning for Native American people (Beauvais, 1980). Among Native Americans, to refuse drugs or alcohol can be seen as rude and confrontational. Native American adolescents may also see smoked (and smokeless) tobacco use as rites of passage into adulthood (Schinke et al., 1985b). Smokeless tobacco use may be further explained by such influences as advertising and the absence of laws governing its sale and labeling.

Understanding the history and acculturation challenges of the Native American people as well as gender-specific and social influences toward health risk behavior increases the cultural sensitivity of prevention interventions. Cultural sensitivity may be the key to the success of behavioral prevention approaches with Native American youth.

BEHAVIORAL APPROACH TO PREVENTION INTERVENTION

Prevention interventions urging Native Americans to abstain from alcohol and tobacco use, decrease consumption of dietary fat, and increase consumption of foods rich in carotene, fiber, and other nutrients are long overdue (Hiatt, Klatsky, & Armstrong, 1988; Shoenborn & Benson, 1988; Wallace, Watson, & Watson, 1988). Approaches to cancer risk reduction, however, need to be tailored specifically for Native American youth. These interventions are imperative not only for reducing the incidence of cancers but also for helping Native American adolescents promote their health and social functioning in positive and lasting ways.

Despite the success of prevention strategies to reduce the use of tobacco and alcohol and to modify diet in the mainstream population (Schinke, in press), these efforts have not been incorporated into the lives of most Native Americans. Few studies have focused exclusively on the Native American population. Because of the ability of children and adolescents to make early lifestyle changes, Native American youth have much to gain from culturally focused prevention interventions (Blum, 1992; Office of Minority Health, 1989). Reaching children and adolescents before they begin to experiment with substances or other unhealthy behaviors is essential. The remainder of this chapter will discuss a behavioral approach to prevention that holds promise for preventing tobacco and alcohol abuse and for modifying dietary habits among Native American youth.

Considerable research has been conducted to test the efficacy of substance abuse prevention strategies (Botvin, Schinke, & Orlandi, in press; Gilchrist & Schinke, 1985; Schinke, Orlandi, & Cole, 1992). The most promising prevention interventions focus on the psychosocial factors promoting substance-use initiation (Botvin & Wills, 1985; Flay, 1985). These strategies focus primarily on social influences believed to promote substance use or on the enhancement of personal and social competence by teaching broader coping skills (Biglan et al., 1987; Botvin, Baker, Renick, Filazzola & Botvin, 1984; Flay et al., 1985; Pentz, 1983; Schinke & Gilchrist, 1983). The behavioral prevention approach is rooted in social learning theory (Bandura, 1977) and problem behavior theory (Jessor & Jessor, 1977). This approach conceptualizes substance use as a socially learned and functional behavior that is adopted from influential role models and is further affected by acquired knowledge, attitudes, and beliefs. The intent of the behavioral health approach is to teach a broad range of general skills for coping with typical pressures encountered in adolescence, including pressures to use substances. These approaches are geared toward helping adolescents gain control over their lives, and more specifically, over their interactions with peers and family members.

Many studies testing personal and social skills training have demonstrated significant behavioral effects (Botvin & Dusenbury, 1989; Moncher & Schinke, 1994; Schinke et al., 1988; Schinke, Schilling, & Gilchrist, 1986). These studies have demonstrated that generic skills approaches to smoking prevention can reduce youths' smoking by 42% to 75%. An important objective for both types of skills training (personal and social) is to move adolescents from merely understanding skills to actually adopting the skills in their everyday lives. To that end, skills training combines instruction, demonstration, behavioral rehearsal, feedback, and reinforcement to support subjects' experiences for the behaviors they are learning.

Intervention Development

Our research on tobacco use prevention and dietary modification among Native American adolescents is designed to provide adolescents with the personal and social skills needed to avoid unhealthy behaviors. The following discussion outlines the stages of intervention development that we follow, including designing the relevant curriculum, the importance of collaboration, and the selection of an intervention team to assist researchers in developing relevant prevention interventions.

Assessment

The first step in developing a targeted behavioral intervention for preventing cancer risks among Native American adolescents is gathering information about cancer risk factors in the Native American population. Baseline data should empirically document the nature and extent of cancer risk factors among the Native American youth population. Assessment instruments to quantify youths' tobacco use and dietary habits must be developed and administered. The data must then be analyzed to determine the psychological and behavioral correlates of cancer-related dietary habits and of tobacco use. In our research, we use measurement instruments that have been field tested and revised in our own and others' research with this population (Gilchrist, Schinke, Trimble, & Cvetkovich, 1987; Oetting et al., 1983; Schinke et al., 1988; Schinke et al., 1986a; Schinke et al., 1989; Singer & Schinke, in press). Formative testing with focus groups of target subjects refines and adds precision to each measurement instrument and scale. Focus group data, however, can be marred by participants' biases or by the investigator's use of leading questions. Conducting multiple sessions with a random selection of community participants and using carefully constructed questions help to guard against these biases.

Content for focus groups comes from our own and others' questionnaires on the variables of interest and related behavioral risks. Focus groups may involve subjects representing both genders, substantial ethnic-racial minority and majority culture groups, and both urban and suburban settings within the study region. Focus group leaders follow guidelines for convening, executing, and recording the sessions (Krueger, 1988), and we analyze and interpret focus group data according to conventional procedures (Patton, 1980).

Once focus group data have informed changes to the format, ordering, and language of each instrument, we psychometrically test the measures. Psychometric tests involve stratified samples of another group of subjects from each gender, minority and majority culture group (if relevant), and urban and suburban community site. Psychometric tests determine the reliability of each instrument and scale through test-retest and split-half procedures. Whenever feasible, we cross-validate our measures' scores with data from parallel instruments. For example, data from a new or adapted measure can be compared with findings from extant measures on the same variables.

The initial phase of the cancer risk reduction curriculum that we administered, called FACETS (Singer & Schinke, in press), involved designing a brief self-report questionnaire to assess the frequency of and types of Native American's food intake. Using the National Health and Nutrition Examination Survey (Block, Hartman, & Naughton, 1990), we revised a self-report survey consisting of 66 items. Commonly eaten foods and foods recommended for inclusion or omission for a cancer-prevention diet were listed. The survey asked parents to indicate how often their families ate grains, fresh vegetables and fruits, meats, dairy products, fats and oils, snack foods, and dried peas and beans. Parents were also asked to list their children's favorite foods, rate food intake frequencies, specify typical Native American foods their children ate, and report their most frequently used cooking methods.

Other self-report measures administered in this study were multiple-choice questions concerning the number of cigarettes, smokeless tobacco products, alcohol, and other drugs that have been consumed during the index reporting period (usually the most recent past day and week). Other questions gathered information about subjects' demographic profile, knowledge and attitudes about tobacco and diet, education level, self-esteem, communication skills, problem-solving skills, and other psychosocial determinants of tobacco use and diet.

Biochemical sampling is often used with self-report procedures to convince subjects that their tobacco use will be physiologically evident, which often corrects their tendency to underreport or overreport their recent tobacco use (Murray, O'Connell, Schmid, & Perry, 1987). Biochemical sampling is the collection of saliva, hair, blood, skin, and other bodily fluids to determine the veracity of the self-reported responses to questions about tobacco use. This sampling procedure can be carried out at the same time that subjects are completing the self-report questionnaires. Saliva and expired lung air are most often used for the measurements.

Initial Data Analysis

We obtained frequency counts for responses to the nutrition survey described in the previous self-report illustration. The targeted population's use of various foods was compared to data from a national sample.

Other items, such as food intake and cooking methods, were compared with urban versus reservation subjects.

Baseline information on psychological and behavioral correlates of youth's substance use is helpful for predicting the risk that an adolescent will or will not use tobacco in the future. Examples of psychological and behavioral factors relevant to cancer risk prevention are subjects' knowledge, attitudes, and preferences about tobacco use and diet, all of which are attainable through self-report measures.

Cultural Adaptation

Information concerning subjects' knowledge, attitudes, and beliefs about tobacco and diet shape the intervention program by guiding its level and complexity of instruction. Cultural and lifestyle aspects of tobacco use and dietary habits must be assessed as well. Information should be collected concerning subjects' awareness of their cultural background and its influence on their lives. This type of information helps inform investigators about the amount and nature of culturally relevant material to include in the intervention.

In the food survey mentioned previously, for example, we compared dietary data from a national sample with data from a survey of Native American parents who listed their children's favorite foods and the frequency of intake of various foods. Results revealed differing eating patterns for Native Americans and the mainstream population. We found that Native American children's reported favorite foods were higher in fat than their majority culture counterparts (Singer & Schinke, in press). These findings point to the relevance of sociocultural aspects of food selection. In our study, as in others, urbanization classification, geographical location, and cultural specificity influence eating patterns (Koehler, Harris, & Davis, 1989; Story, Bass, & Wakefield, 1986).

The cultural relevance of the intervention can be enhanced by incorporating information to increase Native American youth's awareness of their cultural background and its influence on their lives. For example, Native American children could be educated regarding their cultural culinary traditions. As discussed earlier in this chapter, even though fried bread is thought of as a traditional Native American food, it is actually an invention of Native Americans in response to government rations. At the turn of the century, when Native Americans were moved onto reservations, they became dependent on these federal government rations. Including a historic perspective in the curriculum design can reinforce healthy food choices among Native American youth.

Finally, to design a prevention intervention curriculum that is both theoretically sound and culturally relevant, researchers need to consider the body of prevention research found in the literature. Our past work with smoking cessation and nutrition in the Native American population, together with the expanding body of literature on psychosocial approaches to prevention, contributed to the development of our curriculum.

Collaboration

Designing a curriculum should be a collaborative effort. Parents, youth, tribal leaders, school staff, and human service workers can all take part in curriculum development. We have found that without the approval of collaborating reservation and tribal leaders, health promotion and cancer risk reduction efforts designed for Native American adolescents are less likely to succeed.

In our dietary modification and tobacco use prevention study, members of our research team contacted Native American reservation communities and urban organizations to invite their participation in the project (Singer & Schinke, in press). A collaboration meeting was held with key community figures to discuss effective ways to implement a cancer prevention project in the targeted community. We presented current prevention research and health promotion strategies for youth to the community. Community representatives then discussed their health concerns and their opinions about the strengths and weaknesses of current cancer prevention programs.

Community representatives can contribute to the intervention in several ways. Representatives can explain the significance of tobacco in the Native American society from both a ceremonial and cultural perspective. In our intervention, for example, they helped highlight how the commercialization of tobacco had overshadowed its traditional ceremonial use (Singer & Schinke, in press). Collaborating community representatives can also help emphasize cultural awareness. As a result of our collaboration effort, each curriculum lesson included cultural information.

Intervention Team

Working together, professionals and Native American community members can implement conceptually sound, culturally relevant, and empirically based cancer risk reduction programs. With the appropriate level of supervision, cancer prevention on an Indian reservation can be delivered by paraprofessionals (e.g., teachers). In our study, we hired indigenous Native American people who were at least 20 years old and who had 1 or more years of experience in health education. These staff were recruited on site and paid for their participation. Native American team members can help to ensure the credibility and integrity of each part of the intervention, help secure the trust of subjects for personal intervention, and serve as an important link to the greater Native American community.

CURRICULUM COMPONENTS AND IMPLEMENTATION

Our study to prevent cancer risks associated with diet and tobacco delivers three interventions: one to modify diet, one to prevent tobacco use, and one that is a combination of the two. Our intervention design thus addresses the separate and synergistic effects of tobacco use prevention and dietary modification interventions among Native American youths. Groups of 15 youths received the intervention in eighteen 50-minute sessions held after school at local community agencies.

The tobacco use prevention intervention is based on social learning theory (Bandura, 1977), problem behavior theory (Jessor & Jessor, 1977), and persuasive-communication theory (McGuire, 1964). Each of these theories illustrates how behavior is learned from and promoted by the social and family environment. Social learning theory proposes that social factors influence and are influenced by personal and behavioral determinants. For example, youths' perceptions that deviant behaviors are normative among their peers may promote deviance through the establishment of maladaptive beliefs. According to problem behavior theory, problem behavior results from an interaction of personal, physiological, genetic, and environmental factors. The theory suggests that some adolescents find deviant acts functional because the acts help them achieve personal goals. Also according to problem behavior theory, youths are more vulnerable to peer pressure when they have few effective coping strategies, few skills to handle social situations, and anxiety about social situations. Finally, persuasive-communication theory suggests how to frame messages aimed at convincing subjects of a different point of view (in this case, healthier habits) to enhance the persuasive effect of those messages. The Life Skills Training (LST) approach is also incorporated into the intervention (Botvin & Wills, 1985). This approach teaches pressure-resistance tactics within the framework of a program designed to enhance general, personal, and social competence.

The dietary-modification intervention is similar to the tobacco-use prevention intervention and incorporates the same theoretical principles. It covers such concepts as peer pressure, communication, problem solving, media pressures, and healthy choices. In addition, the dietary modification intervention emphasizes consuming fewer fatty foods and more high-fiber foods and maintaining a desirable weight.

The intervention is comprised of content areas and skills training. Primary content areas within the tobacco use prevention and dietary modification intervention are Native American heritage, the importance of role models, specific health information, positive self-image, and the influence of the media on behavior. These content areas will be discussed in turn in the following pages. Skills training consists of elements to promote bicultural competence and problem solving, coping, and interpersonal communication skills. The skills training component of the intervention will be described in the upcoming pages as well. Skills training and the content areas mentioned above are critical because studies indicate that Native Americans who have been exposed to the concept of bicultural competence are better adjusted and have a lower rate of tobacco and substance use than either Native Americans who adopted the mainstream culture or those who remained tied to Native American traditions (LaFramboise, 1982; LaFramboise & Rowe, 1983; Oetting, Goldstein, Beauvais, Edwards, & Velarde, 1980).

Primary Content Areas of the Intervention

Native American Heritage

Collaborative efforts between the community and investigators help to ensure that the regional and tribe-specific ethnic values are included in the curriculum. Folk tales, legends, and myths are used to promote healthy choices and to devalue risky behaviors.

Other studies conducted by our researchers have used computer software programs to share Native American folk tales and legends that support traditional values and healthful food choices (Schinke, Moncher, & Singer, in press). The software is based on a Seneca legend known as "The Boy Who Lived with Bears" and is presented in the context of an American Indian story (Bruchac, 1987). Within the software lesson, youth learn about the traditional advantages of sound nutrition and the non-habitual use of tobacco (Caduto & Bruchac, 1988). Nutritional content for the lesson is drawn from Native American customs and traditions regarding food choices and eating habits.

Native American arts and crafts, excerpts from Indian writings, and posters depicting Native American role models can help to create a feeling of pride. This pride in ethnic identity can be used as a stepping stone for discussing the strengths and positive attributes of Native people. In each instance, personal, familial, and community values can be related to Indian youth's choices concerning tobacco use and diet. For example, the group can obtain knowledge concerning the traditional use of the hallucinogen peyote during religious ceremonies. Youth can learn that the use of peyote has always severely excluded the secular and habitual use of the substance (Beauvais & LaBoueff, 1985). By emphasizing ethnic identity, the intervention encourages Native American youth to apply both the prevention skills they have learned and also information about their cultural heritage to promote health and avoid unhealthy behaviors.

Role Models

A second aspect of the intervention is to allow youth to learn from positive role models. Youth involved in our intervention participate in homework activities where they report on Native American people who abstain from tobacco and who project autonomy, independence, and sophistication. This information can be synthesized through a discussion in which a group leader emphasizes that these respected community figures successfully resisted media and peer pressure to use tobacco. Similarly, in the dietary-modification intervention, participants can discuss how others influence their behavior. Looking beyond their community, subjects can identify a media personality such as an athlete or dancer and investigate that person's diet and other health habits.

Health Information

In the intervention, health information is provided in various and interesting ways. Software programs, films, games, and peer testimonials can give subjects the knowledge they need concerning the consequences of smokeless and smoked tobacco. As with other intervention activities, games should be designed to be culturally relevant. We pattern intervention games after traditional Native American games. Health information included in the dietary modification intervention teaches youth how the body absorbs food and the role that food, exercise, sleep, and good hygiene play in maintaining a healthy body.

Positive Self-Image

To help subjects improve their self-image, group leaders can help subjects to deconstruct stereotypes of Native Americans. Group members can contrast stereotypes of Native Americans with Euro-American images of attractiveness, popularity, sophistication, and success. The stereotypes of Indian life portrayed on television, in print, and in films can also be discussed over the course of several sessions. Discussions on how the mass media sells the idea that people who use tobacco are more hip, trendy, and rich can help the group to understand the reality and the health consequences related to tobacco use. As a result of participation in these activities, subjects can begin to see the negative images and stereotypes of Native American people within society and can learn to discount them.

Advertisements

In sessions that focus on advertising, subjects can be taught how to read advertising messages critically. Participants can collect an assortment of magazine and newspaper advertisements for both smoked and smokeless tobacco and for food. Looking at the ads, group members can discuss the kinds of lifestyles being sold by the advertisements, the promises made by the company, and the motivation behind the ads. Another media exercise might teach subjects how to read food labels for nutritional content in various foods.

Skills Training

Problem-Solving Skills

Problem solving skills teach youth to discriminate among their options and to make reasoned decisions when faced with choices involving tobacco use, food, or other situations involving risk-taking behaviors. In our intervention, Native American youth learned how to use a decision-making model to practice effective responses to various pressures. Youth are taught to *Stop*, consider their *Options*, make a *Decision*, and to *Act* (SODAS). Self-praise, the final step in the SODAS model, encourages youth to reward their own behavior by praising themselves for thoughtful problem solving. Each step in the decision-making model can be explained by group leaders and then practiced by subjects in role plays.

Coping Skills

In our intervention, Native American subjects also learn coping strategies for problem situations. Subjects learn how to recognize situational, social, and emotional cues that may trigger tobacco use and poor food choices. Situational cues include personal and interpersonal events and settings associated with tobacco use and certain dietary choices. Social cues relate to personal and interpersonal actions that could precipitate tobacco use, such as seeing friends smoke or use smokeless tobacco. Emotional cues include urges and temptations to smoke or make poor food choices. With practice, subjects can learn how to cope with situational, social, and emotional cues.

Communication Skills

The communication skills component of the intervention illustrates ways in which young people communicate effectively and ineffectively. Cultural, gender, and individual differences in communication styles can be highlighted and discussed. Through role-playing activities, subjects model and practice styles of communication that can be used to help them resist unhealthy food choices or avoid tobacco use. Videotapes of Native American youth who are initially shy and then learn to interact competently with peers are one way to begin the communication sessions. Through modeling and seeing change, subjects learn skills to effectively interact with peers. These skills are essential for communicating individual needs and maintaining self-respect.

Concluding the Intervention

To conclude the intervention, youth can invite their families and community members to attend a special closing event. At this event, youth can share their intervention experiences and the knowledge they gained about themselves, their culture, and healthy choices. Youth participants can role play situations demonstrating what they learned through the intervention. In our work, we award "graduation" certificates to all subjects who have completed the program to acknowledge the importance of what they have learned.

CONCLUSION

Of all the means for remediating problems of tobacco use and poor nutrition among Native American adolescents, none offers more hope than behavioral approaches in prevention. Prevention interventions hold promise not only for reducing the lifetime incidence of drug use among Native Americans but also for helping Native American adolescents promote their health and social functioning in positive and lasting ways. This chapter describes a psychosocial and behavioral approach for reducing the risk of cancer among younger Native Americans. Our approach teaches Native American youth to have pride in their ethnicity; to look to role models for inspiration; to learn the facts and consequences related to tobacco use and unhealthy food choices; to practice skills such as decision making, coping, assertiveness and problem solving; and to interpret realistically media portrayals of tobacco use.

We have discussed how incorporating Native American heritage into prevention efforts through collaborations with tribes and organizations helps to build a curriculum that is meaningful for participating youth. Collaborating community members can help tailor tobacco-use prevention and nutrition curricula designed for mainstream populations. Not only are community members the best informed about their own lifestyle patterns, but they are also more likely to support the program if they feel a sense of ownership.

In this chapter, we also reviewed the relationship between behaviors and risk for disease, along with the need for prevention intervention at an early age. The processes of gathering and analyzing data, as well as developing a culturally sensitive curriculum, have also been described and illustrated.

Additional research on the prevention of health risk behaviors among Native American youth is sorely needed. In addition to intervention studies, epidemiological and correlational research should explore the nature of substance use by Native American youth and the progression of use with age. We hope that the behavioral intervention outlined in this chapter will strengthen future efforts to develop programs to enhance adaptive youth development and prevent the incidence of health problems associated with diet, tobacco, and alcohol abuse.

REFERENCES

American Cancer Society. (1991). *Cancer facts & figures—1991*. Atlanta, GA: Author.

Austin, G. (1988). *Substance abuse among minority youth: 1. Native Americans* (Prevention Research Update No. 2). Western Center for Drug-Free Schools.

Bandura, A. (1977). *Social learning theory*. Englewood Cliffs, NJ: Prentice-Hall.

Beauvais, F. (1980). *Preventing drug abuse among American Indian young people*. Fort Collins, CO: Western Behavior Studies.

Beauvais, F., & LaBoueff, S. (1985). Drug and alcohol abuse intervention in American Indian communities. *International Journal of the Addictions, 20*, 139–171.

Beauvais, F., Oetting, E. R., Wolf, W., & Edwards, R. W. (1989). American Indian youth and drugs, 1976–87: A continuing problem. *American Journal of Public Health, 79*, 634–636.

Biglan, A., Severson, H., Ary, D. V., Faller, C., Gallison, C., Thompson, R., Glasgow, R., & Lichtenstein, (1987). Do smoking prevention programs really work: Attrition and the internal and external validity of a refusal skills training program. *Journal of Behavioral Medicine, 10*, 159–171.

Block, G., Hartman, A. M., & Naughton, D. (1990). A reduced dietary questionnaire: Development and validation. *Epidemiology, 1*, 58–64.

Blum, R. (1992). *The state of Native American youth health*. Minneapolis, MN: University of Minnesota.

Bobo, J. K., & Gilchrist, L. D. (1983). Urging the alcoholic client to quit smoking cigarettes. *Addictive Behaviors, 8*, 297–305.

Bobo, J. K., Gilchrist, L. D., Schilling, R. F., Noach, B., & Schinke, S. P. (1987). Cigarette smoking attempts by recovering alcoholics. *Addictive Behaviors, 12*, 209–215.

Botvin, G. J, Baker, E., Renick, N., Filazzola, A. D., & Botvin, E. M. (1984). A cognitive behavioral approach to substance abuse prevention. *Addictive Behaviors, 9*, 137–147.

Botvin, G. J., & Dusenbury, L. (1989). Substance abuse prevention and the promotion of competence. In L. A. Bond & B. E. Compas (Eds.), *Primary prevention and promotion in the schools*. Newbury Park, CA: Sage.

Botvin, G. J., Schinke, S. P., & Orlandi, M. A. (Eds.). (in press). *Drug abuse prevention with multi-ethnic youth*. Newbury Park, CA: Sage.

Botvin, G. J., & Wills, T. A. (1985). Personal and social skills training: Cognitive behavioral approaches to substance abuse prevention. In C. Bell & R. Battjes (Eds.), *Prevention research: Deterring drug abuse among children and adolescents* (NIDA Research Monograph Series). Washington, DC: U.S. Government Printing Office.

Bruchac, J. (1987). *Iroquois stories, heroes and heroines, monsters and magic*. Syracuse, NY: Crossing Press.

Brunswick, A. G., & Messeri, P. (1984). Gender differences in the processes leading to cigarette smoking. *Journal of Psychosocial Oncology, 2*, 49–69.

Caduto, M. J., & Bruchac, J. (1988). *Keepers of the earth: Teacher's guide*. Golden, CO: Fulcrum.

Cancer hits all-time high for North Dakota natives. (1991, Nov. 27). *Lakota Times*.

Cunningham-Sabo, L., & Davis, S. (1993). Pathways to health: A health promotion and cancer prevention project for American Indian youth. *Alaska Medicine, 35*, 275–279.

Dembroski, T. M. (1984). Stress and substance interaction effects on risk factors and reactivity. *Behavioral Medicine Update, 6*, 16–20.

Department of Health and Human Services. (1982). *The health consequences of smoking: Cancer* (Public Health Service (OSH) Publication No. 82-50179). Washington, DC: U.S. Government Printing Office.

Department of Health and Human Services. (1983). *The health consequences of smoking: Cardiovascular disease.* (Public Health Service Publication (OSH) No. 82-50179). Washington, DC: U.S. Government Printing Office.

Department of Health and Human Services. (1984). *The health consequences of smoking: Chronic obstructive lung disease.* (Public Health Service Publication (OSH) No. 82-50205). Washington, DC: U.S. Government Printing Office.

Department of Health and Human Services. (1985). *Report of the secretary's Task Force on black and minority health. Volume II: Crosscutting issues in minority health.* Washington, DC: U.S. Government Printing Office.

Department of Health and Human Services. (1991). *Cancer mortality among Native Americans in the United States.* Washington, DC: U.S. Government Printing Office.

Flay, B. R. (1985). Psychosocial approaches to smoking prevention: A review of findings. *Health Psychology, 4,* 449–488.

Flay, B. R., Ryan, K. B., Best, J. A., Brown, K. S., Kersell, M. W., d'Avernas, J. R., & Zanna, M. P. (1985) Are social psychological smoking prevention programs effective? The Waterloo study. *Journal of Behavioral Medicine, 8,* 37–59.

Gilchrist, L. D., & Schinke, S. P. (Eds.). (1985). *Preventing social and health problems through life skills training.* Seattle: University of Washington Press.

Gilchrist, L. D., Schinke, S. P., Trimble, J. E., & Cvetkovich. G. T. (1987). Skills enhancement to prevent substance abuse among American Indian adolescents. *International Journal of the Addictions, 22,* 869–879.

Hall, R. L., & Dexter, D. (1988). Smokeless tobacco use among Native Americans and other adolescents in the northwest. *American Journal of Public Health, 78,* 1586–1588.

Hampton, J. W. (1993). Cancer in Indian country: Keynote address. *Alaska Medicine, 35,* 243–245.

Hiatt, R. A., Klatsky, A. L., & Armstrong, M. A. (1988). Alcohol consumption and the risk of breast cancer in a prepaid health plan. *Cancer Research, 48,* 2284–2287.

Howard, B. V. (1992). The strong heart study. *Diabetes, 41*(Suppl. 2), 4–11.

Indian Health Service. (1984). *A periodical of the mental health programs.* Washington, D.C.: U.S. Government Printing Office.

Indian Health Service. (1990). *Trends in Indian health.* Washington, DC: U.S. Government Printing Office.

Jackson, Y. M. (1986). Nutrition in American Indian health: Past, present, and future. *Journal of the American Diet Association, 86,* 1561.

Jackson, Y. M. (1990). *Diet, culture, and diabetes.* Unpublished manuscript.

Jessor, R., & Jessor, S. L. (1977). *Problem behavior and psychosocial development: A longitudinal study of youth.* New York: Academic Press.

Jones-Saumty, D., Hochhaus, L., Dru, R., & Zeiner, A. (1983). Psychosocial factors of familial alcoholism in American Indians and Caucasians. *Journal of Clinical Psychology, 39,* 783–790.

Koehler, K. M., Harris, M. B., & Davis, S. M. (1989). Core, secondary, and peripheral foods in the diets of Hispanic, Navajo, and Jemez Indian children. *Journal of the American Dietetic Association, 89,* 538–540.

Krueger, R. A. (1988). *Focus groups: A practical guide for applied research.* Newbury Park, CA: Sage.

LaFramboise, T. D. (1982). *Assertion training with American Indians: Cultural/behavioral issues for trainers.* Las Cruces, NM: New Mexico State University.

LaFramboise, T. D., & Rowe, W. (1983). Skills training for bicultural competence: Rationale and application. *Journal of Consulting Psychology, 30,* 589–595.

Lanier, A. (1993). Epidemiology of cancer in Alaska natives. *Alaska Medicine, 35*(4), 245–248.

Lewis, R. G. (1982). Alcoholism and the Native American: A review of the literature. *Alcohol and Health Monograph 4: Special Population Issues.* Washington, DC: U.S. Government Printing Office.

Mao, Y., Morrison, H., Semenciw, R., & Wigle, D. (1986). Mortality on Canadian Indian reserves. *Canadian Journal of Public Health, 77,* 263–268.

May, P. A. (1989). Alcohol abuse and alcoholism among American Indians: An overview. In T. D. Watts & R. Wright (Eds.), *Alcoholism in minority populations.* Springfield, IL: Charles C Thomas.

May, P. A. (in press). The prevention of alcohol and other substance abuse among American Indians: A review and analysis of the literature. *NIAAA Monographs.*

May, P. A., & Smith, M. B. (1988). Some Navajo Indian opinions about alcohol abuse and prohibition: A survey and recommendations for policy. *Journal of Studies on Alcohol, 49,* 324–334.

McGuire, W. J. (1964). Inducing resistance to persuasion: Some contemporary approaches. In L. Berkowitz (Ed.), *Advances in experimental social psychology* (Vol. 1). New York: Academic Press.

Moncher, M. S., Holden, G. W., & Schinke, S. P (1991). Psychosocial correlates of substance abuse among youth: A review of current etiological constructs. *International Journal of the Addictions, 26,* 377–414.

Moncher, M. S., & Schinke, S. P. (1994). Group intervention to prevent tobacco use among Native American youth. *Research on Social Work Practice, 4,* 160–171.

Murray, D. M., O'Connell, T. S., Schmid, L. S., & Perry, C. L. (1987). The validity of smoking self-reports by adolescents: A reexamination of the bogus pipeline procedure. *Addictive Behaviors, 12,* 7–15.

National Cancer Institute (1986). *Cancer in minorities: Report of the subcommittee on cancer, part I.* Washington, DC: U.S. Government Printing Office.

Newman, J. M., Marfin, A. A., Eggers, P. W., & Helgerson, S. D. (1990). End-state renal disease among Native Americans, 1983–1986. *American Journal of Public Health, 80,* 318–319.

Oetting, E. R., Beauvais, F., Edwards, R., Waters, M. R., Velarde, J., & Goldstein, G. S. (1983). *Drug use among Native American youth.* Fort Collins: Colorado State University.

Oetting, E. R., Goldstein, G. S., Beauvais, F., Edwards, R., & Velarde, J. (1980). *Drug abuse among Indian children.* Fort Collins: Colorado State University.

Office of Minority Health (1989). *Cancer and minorities.* Washington, DC: U.S. Government Printing Office.

Office on Smoking and Health. (1982). *The health consequences of smoking: Cancer: A report of the surgeon general.* Washington, DC: U.S. Government Printing Office.

Office on Smoking and Health. (1983). *The health consequences of smoking: Cardiovascular disease: A report of the surgeon general.* Washington, DC: U.S. Government Printing Office.

Office on Smoking and Health. (1984). *The health consequences of smoking: Chronic obstructive lung disease: A report of the surgeon general.* Washington, DC: U.S. Government Printing Office.

Okwumabua, J. O., & Duryea, E. J. (1987). Age of onset, periods of risk, and patterns of progression in drug use among American Indian high school students. *International Journal of Addictions, 22,* 1269–1276.

Patton, M. Q. (1980). *Qualitative evaluation methods.* Beverly Hills, CA: Sage.

Pedigo, J. (1983). Finding the "meaning" of Native American substance use: Implications for community prevention. *Personnel and Guidance Journal, 61,* 273–277.

Pentz, M. A. (1983). Prevention of adolescent substance abuse through social skills development. In T. J. Glynn, C. G. Leukefeld, & J. P. Ludford (Eds.), *Preventing adolescent drug abuse: Intervention strategies.* (NIDA Research Monograph No. 47, pp. 195–232). Washington, DC: NIDA.

Red Horse, Y. (1982). A cultural network model: Perspectives for adolescent services and para-professional training. In S. M. Manson (Ed.), *New directions in prevention among American Indian and Alaska Native communities* (pp. 173–188). Portland: Oregon Health Science University.

Rhoades, E. (1992, June). *Heart disease now ranked as number one killer of American Indians.* Paper presented at the 4th National Forum on Cardiovascular Health, Pulmonary Disorders, and Blood Resources, Washington, DC.

Rhoades, E. R., Hammond, J., Welty, T. K., Hander, A. O., & Amler, R. W. (1987). The Indian burden of illness and future health interventions. *Public Health Reports, 102*(4), 361–368.

Schinke, S. P. (in press). Prevention science and practice: An agenda for action. *Journal of Primary Prevention.*

Schinke, S. P., Botvin, G. J., & Orlandi, M. A. (1991). *Substance abuse in children and adolescents.* Newbury Park, CA: Sage.

Schinke, S. P., Botvin, G. J. Trimble, J. E., Orlandi, M. A., Gilchrist, L. D., & Locklear, V. S. (1988). Preventing substance abuse among American-Indian adolescents: A bicultural competence skills approach. *Journal of Counseling Psychology, 35,* 87–90.

Schinke, S. P., & Gilchrist, L. D. (1983). Primary prevention of tobacco smoking. *Journal of School Health, 53,* 416–419.

Schinke, S. P., Gilchrist, L. D., Schilling, R. F., & Senechal, V. A. (1986). Smoking and smokeless tobacco use among adolescents: Trends and intervention results. *Public Health Reports, 101,* 373–378.

Schinke, S. P., Gilchrist, L. D., Schilling, R. F., Walker, R. D., Kirkham, M. A., Bobo, J. K., Trimble, J. E., Cvetkovich, G. T., & Richardson, S. S. (1985). Strategies for preventing substance abuse with American Indian youth. *White Cloud Journal, 3,* 12–18.

Schinke, S. P., Gilchrist, L. D., Schilling, R. F., Walker, R. D., Locklear, V. S., Bobo, J. K., Maxwell, J. S., Trimble, J. E., & Cvetkovich, G. T. (1985b). Preventing substance abuse with American Indian youth. *Social Casework, 66,* 213–217.

Schinke, S. P., Gilchrist, L. D., Schilling, R. F., Walker, R. D., Locklear, V. S., & Kitajima, E. (1986a). Smokeless tobacco use among Native American adolescents. *New England Journal of Medicine, 314,* 1051–1052.

Schinke, S. P., Moncher, M. S., Holden, G. W., Botvin, G. J., & Orlandi, M. A. (1989). American Indian youth and substance abuse: Tobacco use problems, risk factors and preventive interventions. *Health Education Research, 4,* 137–144.

Schinke, S. P., Moncher, M. S., Holden, G. W., Orlandi, M. A., & Botvin, G. J. (1992). Preventing substance abuse among Native American youth. In C. W. LeCroy (Ed.), *Case studies in behavioral social work practice* (pp. 287–296). Homewood, IL: Dorsey Press.

Schinke, S. P., Moncher, M. S., & Singer, B. R. (in press). Native American youths and cancer risk reduction: Effects of software intervention. *Journal of Adolescent Health.*

Schinke, S. P., Orlandi, M. A., & Cole, K. C. (1992). boys and girls clubs in public housing developments: Prevention services for youth at risk. *Journal of Community Psychology, 28,* 118–128.

Schinke, S. P., Orlandi, M. A., Schilling, R. F., Botvin, G. J., Gilchrist, L. D., & Landers, C. (1990). Tobacco use by American Indian and Alaska Native people: Risks, psychosocial factors, and preventive intervention. *Journal of Alcohol and Drug Education, 35,* 1–12.

Schinke, S. P., Schilling, R. F., & Gilchrist, L. D. (1986c). Prevention of drug and alcohol abuse in American Indian youths. *Social Work Research and Abstracts, 22,* 18–19.

Schinke, S. P., Schilling, R. F., Gilchrist, L. D., Ashby, M. R., & Kitajima, E. (1987). Pacific northwest Native American youth and smokeless tobacco use. *International Journal of the Addictions, 9,* 881–884.

Schinke, S. P., Schilling, R. F., Gilchrist, L. D., Ashby, M. R., & Kitajima, E. (1989b). Native youth and smokeless tobacco: Prevalence rates, gender differences, and descriptive characteristics. *Journal of the National Cancer Institute, 8,* 39–42.

Schoenborn, C. A., & Benson, V. (1988). Relationships between smoking and other unhealthy habits: United States, 1985. *Advance Data, No. 154, Vital Statistics*. Hyattsville, MD: National Center for Health Statistics.

Singer, B. R., & Schinke, S. P. (in press). Reducing cancer risks among Native American adolescents: Cultural issues, intervention strategies, and baseline findings. *Preventive Medicine*.

Stillman, P. (1992). Racism, poverty contribute to high cancer death rates. *Lakota Times*.

Story, M., Bass, M. A., & Wakefield, L. (1986). Food preferences of Cherokee Indian teenagers in Cherokee, North Carolina. *Ecology of Food and Nutrition, 19*, 51–58.

Topper, M. D. (1985). Navajo "alcoholism": Drinking, alcohol abuse and treatment in a changing cultural environment. In L. A. Bennett & G. M. Ames (Eds.), *The American experience with alcohol*. New York: Plenum Press.

Trimble, J. E., Padilla, A. M., & Bryan, J. (1985). Drug abuse prevention research priorities for ethnic-minority populations. Unpublished manuscript.

Walker, R. D., & Kivlahan, D. R. (1984). Definitions, models, and methods in research on sociocultural factors in American Indian alcohol use. *Substance and Alcohol Actions/Misuse, 5*, 9–19.

Wallace, C. L., Watson, R. R., & Watson, A. A. (1988). Reducing cancer risks with vitamins C, E, and selenium. *American Journal of Health Promotion, 3*, 5–16.

Ward, J. A. (1984). Preventive implications of a Native Indian mental health program: Focus on suicide and violent death. *Journal of Preventive Psychiatry, 2*, 371–385.

Weibel-Orlando, J. (1985). Indians, ethnicity, and alcohol: Contrasting perceptions of the ethnic self and alcohol use. In L. A. Bennett and G. M Ames (Eds.), *The American experience with alcohol*. New York: Plenum Press.

Whittaker, J. O. (1982). Alcohol and the Standing Rock Sioux Tribe: A twenty-year follow-up study. *Journal of Studies on Alcohol, 43*, 191–200.

CHAPTER 20

A Biological, Environmental, and Cultural Basis for Ethnic Differences in Treatment

MICHAEL SMITH AND KEH-MING LIN

During the past half century, progress in pharmacotherapy has led to effective therapeutic regimens for a wide variety of medical conditions. At the same time, clinicians have become increasingly sophisticated at using pharmaceuticals and in minimizing their adverse side effects. Modern clinical pharmacology, however, has been based largely on research and clinical experiences with Caucasian patients and subjects. Relatively little is known about applying pharmacotherapy to ethnic minority populations in this country and to non-Western populations worldwide (Lawson, 1986), even though non-Caucasians comprise fully 25% of the U.S. population. According to the 1990 census, 12% of the U.S. population is African-American, 9% Hispanic-American, 3% Asian-American, and 1% Native Americans. These percentages are higher than in previous census reports and are expected to continue growing (Bureau of the Census, 1990).

MICHAEL SMITH and KEH-MING LIN • Research Center on the Psychobiology of Ethnicity, Harbor–UCLA Research and Education Institute, Torrance, California 90502.

Handbook of Diversity Issues in Health Psychology, edited by Pamela M. Kato and Traci Mann. Plenum Press, New York, 1996.

Recent research shows that response to psychopharmacological medications can depend upon ethnic and cultural factors. Understanding these results is crucial for American pharmacotherapists, who are prescribing medication to an increasingly diverse population. In this chapter we first review studies demonstrating differential drug responses based on ethnicity, followed by an examination of some of the basic mechanisms that mediate ethnic and cultural differences in the fate and effects of medications. These mechanisms include genetic differences, environmental factors, pharmacodynamic differences, and cultural factors.

ETHNIC VARIATION IN DRUG RESPONSE

Variations in drug response are classified as differences in the two processes that allow drugs to take effect: pharmacokinetics and pharmacodynamics. Pharmacokinetics describes the process by which a drug is metabolized and transported. Pharmacodynamics describes the process by which a drug affects the body. Recent research has uncovered significant differences in ethnic groups' responses to several classes of medications, including psychotropics (both neuroleptics and benzodiazepines), analgesics, and cardiovascular agents. This research is reviewed in the next sections.

Neuroleptics

Several carefully designed studies have demonstrated that Asians and Caucasians differ significantly in their responses to the neuroleptic haloperidol. Haloperidol is used in the treatment of schizophrenia and other medical disorders that have psychosis as a symptom. When Asian and Caucasian normal volunteers (Lin, Poland, Lau, & Rubin, 1988) and schizophrenic patients (Potkin et al., 1984) were given comparable doses of haloperidol, Asians had approximately a 50% higher concentration of the medication in their plasma. A series of recent studies indicated that the higher concentration was due to Asians' lower rate of haloperidol metabolism. Consequently, Asians showed more prominent effects of haloperidol than did Caucasians who were given equivalent doses (Chang, Chen, Lee, Hu, & Yeh, 1987; Jann et al., 1989; Jann, Lam, & Chang, 1993). The mechanisms responsible for these ethnic differences in pharmacokinetics have not been elucidated.

Pharmacodynamic differences between Asians and Caucasians were suggested by the larger prolactin responses to haloperidol in Asians noted in the above study (Lin et al., 1988b). These differences in response remained statistically significant after controlling for variations in haloperidol concentrations, suggesting the existence of ethnic differences at the drug receptor level. In a subsequent clinical treatment study (Lin et al., 1989), Asian schizophrenic patients responded optimally to significantly lower plasma haloperidol concentrations compared to their Caucasian counterparts, again suggesting that pharmacodynamic factors contribute to ethnic differences in response to haloperidol.

In a comparison study including four patient groups treated with therapeutic doses of haloperidol, researchers reported significantly different pharmacokinetic profiles for Chinese- and African-Americans compared to Caucasians and Hispanics (Jann et al., 1993). Other researchers, however, found no differences between Canadian blacks and Caucasians in the pharmacokinetics of two other neuroleptics (Midha, Hawes, Hubbard, Korchinski, & McKay, 1988a; 1988b).

Benzodiazepines

Earlier clinical reports demonstrated significant differences in the dosing and side effects of benzodiazepines between Asians and Caucasians (Lin, Poland, & Nakasaki, 1993; Rosenblat & Tang, 1987). These differences were recently confirmed by four separate pharmacokinetic studies (Ghoneim et al., 1981; Kumana, Lauder, Chan, Ko, & Lin, 1987; Lin, Lau, Smith, & Poland, 1988; Zhang, Reviriego, Lou, Sjoqvist, & Bertilsson, 1990). Diazepam was used in three of the studies, whereas alprazolam was used in the other study. The studies involved the administration of the drugs by oral routes, intravenous routes, or both. Importantly, the studies were conducted in Asians residing in a number of different sites around the world, including Los Angeles, St. Louis, Hong Kong, and Beijing. Given the diversity of sites, the consistent finding of a slower metabolism of benzodiazepines in Asians suggests that genetic factors are more important than environmental factors in the control of benzodiazepine metabolism.

In addition, a recent study of the effects of adinazolam, a benzodiazepine currently being investigated as an anxiolytic and antidepressant, found that African-Americans showed increased metabolism and greater drug effects on psychomotor performance than did Caucasians (Fleishaker, Smith, Friedman, & Hulst, 1992; Lin et al., 1993).

Analgesics

Several commonly used analgesics have been studied in regard to ethnic differences in their metabolism and effects. For example, Kalow (1992) reported that acetaminophen, a commonly used over-the-counter pain medication, displays a significantly slower rate of metabolism in Asian Indians than in Caucasians. Smoking, alcohol intake, and oral contraceptive use also significantly increased the metabolic rates, and together explained a portion of the variance in the metabolism of the drug.

However, after controlling for these factors, ethnic variation in metabolic rates still remained statistically significant.

In a series of elegantly conducted studies, researchers demonstrated that the conversion of codeine to morphine was slower in Chinese than in Swedish Caucasians (Yue et al., 1989a; Yue, Hasselstrom, Svensson, & Sawe, 1991a; Yue, Svensson, Alm, Sjoqvist, & Sawe, 1989b; Yue, Svensson, Sjoqvist, & Sawe, 1991b; Yue, VonBahr, Odar-Cederlof, & Sawe, 1990). Since the analgesic effect of codeine depends on its conversion to morphine (and subsequently to metabolites of morphine), one might expect the Chinese to be less sensitive to the effects of codeine. A slower overall metabolism of codeine, however, led to significantly higher concentrations of codeine in the Chinese, which overshadowed the influence of the slower conversion to morphine. Consequently, Chinese patients may require lower doses of codeine than do Caucasians for comparable analgesic effects.

Cardiovascular Drugs

In a review of studies on ethnic variation in response to different antihypertensives (Hall, 1990), African-Americans displayed improved responsiveness to therapy with calcium channel blockers or diuretics compared to some beta-blockers and ACE inhibitors (Goodman, Rosendorff, & Gould, 1985). Ethnic differences in response to beta-blockers are partially determined by pharmacodynamic mechanisms. These mechanisms will be discussed below. Other factors that could also contribute to the overall differences in responsivity include increased intracellular sodium and calcium, salt retention, volume expansion, and a low renin profile in African-American hypertensives.

In a recent study of the calcium channel blocker nifedepine, Asian Indians were noted to display slower metabolism of the drug than Caucasians. This resulted in a longer half-life of both the parent compound and its metabolite as well as a prolonged duration of clinical effects for the Asian subjects (Ahsan et al., 1993). The authors assumed that these differences were environmentally induced, since they noticed a major difference in the diets of the two groups. Changing the groups' diets, however, did not alter the pharmacokinetic profile of nifedepine.

THE MECHANISMS OF ETHNIC VARIATION IN DRUG RESPONSE

Research has uncovered several mechanisms that produce ethnic differences in drug response. Chief among these mechanisms are genetic differences in enzymes that control the metabolism of drugs. Genetic differences have also been postulated to be responsible for differences in the pharmacodynamics of certain drugs. Environmental and cultural factors also contribute to ethnic variations in response to pharmaco-therapy.

Below we first review several groups of polymorphic enzymes; variations in the structure of these enzymes are believed to be genetically based and to produce ethnic variations in the metabolism of a number of substances. Then we discuss environmental influences on the operation of these enzymes and review pharmacodynamic differences between ethnic groups. Finally, we discuss the role that cultural beliefs play in determining the effectiveness of pharmacotherapy.

Ethnicity and Pharmacogenetics

Pharmacogenetics, the study of the genetic control of enzymes responsible for drug metabolism, has been an active field of research in the past several decades. The development of modern pharmacogenetics is closely intertwined with observations of dramatic ethnic differences in response to medications. For example, the frequent occurrence of a rare blood disorder among African-American soldiers treated with an anti-malarial drug in World War II led to the discovery of an inborn enzyme deficiency (Kalow, 1991). People who lack this enzyme develop a blood disorder when exposed to certain foods and medications.

A second early case of genetic differences in pharmacokinetics arose in the 1950s soon after the introduction of the muscle relaxant suc-cinylcholine. Instead of the usual 2- to 6-hour duration of muscle relaxation followed by a rapid recovery, some patients were paralyzed for extended periods and often required mechanical ventilation. The mechanism for this variance is the existence in some patients of an atypical enzyme, which results in the patient's inability to metabolize the muscle relaxant.

P-450 Enzyme System

Recently, a primary focus of pharmacogenetic research has been a group of enzymes known as the cytochrome P-450 isozymes (Clark, Brater, & Johnson, 1988; Shen & Lin, 1990). These enzymes may be regarded as one of the most important defense systems that has evolved in animals to protect them against potentially harmful substances (Gonzalez & Nebert, 1990), which may enter their system either from their diet or through other means (e.g., exposure to pollens). These enzymes are also one of the major routes of metabolism for many commonly used pharmaceuticals; they are responsible for the metabolism of many commonly used medications, including cardiovascular, analgesic, and psychotropic agents (Bertilsson & Aberg-Wistedt, 1983; Bertilsson, Eichelbaum, & Mellstrom, 1980; Dahl-Puustinen, Liden, & Alm, 1989; Kupfer & Preisig,

1984; Mellstrom, Bertilsson, & Lou, 1983; Shaheen, Biollaz, & Koshakji, 1989; Skjelbo, Brosen, Hallas, & Gram, 1991; Ward, Walle, & Walle, 1989; Zhou, Koshakji, Siolberstein, Wilkinson, & Wood, 1989).

Individuals can be classified as either extensive metabolizers or poor metabolizers of the substances that are mediated by the P-450 enzymes (Gonzalez, 1989; Kalow, 1991; Meyer, 1990; Wilkinson, Guengerich, & Branch, 1989; Wood & Zhou, 1991). Specifically, two of these enzymes (debrisoquine hydroxylase and mephenytoin hydroxylase) are polymorphic in nature. Poor metabolizers lack a functional enzyme, which often results in slower drug metabolism and toxic blood levels with normal doses.

Substantial cross-ethnic differences in the frequency of poor metabolizers exist. For example, the frequency of poor metabolizers of debrisoquine varies from less than 3% in the Cuna Amerindians, Middle Easterners, and Asians (Du & Lou, 1990; Horai, Taga, Ishizaki, & Ishikawa, 1990; Ishizaki, Eichelbaum, & Horai, 1987; Islam, Idle, & Smith, 1980; Jorge, Arias, Inaba, & Jackson, 1990; Lee, Nam, & Hee, 1988; Lou, Ying, Bertilsson, & Sjoqvist, 1987; Mahgoub, Idle, & Smith, 1979; Nakamura, Goto, & Ray, 1985; Wanwimolruk, Patamasucon, & Lee, 1990; Xu & Jiang, 1990) to 10% in Caucasians and Hispanics in Europe and North America (Silver, Poland, & Lin, 1993). Among various groups of black Africans, there is a wide range of frequencies, with 0% to 8% of Saharan Africans, 4% of Venda in South Africa, 1.9% of African Americans, and 19% of Sans Bushmen being classified as poor metabolizers (Silver et al., 1993).

Recent genotyping studies further demonstrated that the majority of Caucasian poor metabolizers have additional genetic differences that cause mutations resulting in a completely inactive enzyme. In contrast, the same genetic differences, but without the mutations, are highly prevalent (34%) among Asians. Although the Asians with these genetic differences were classified phenotypically as extensive metabolizers, their metabolic capacity was significantly lower than Caucasian extensive metabolizers. It was also lower than that of Asian extensive metabolizers who do not have these genetic differences. This led to an overall lower metabolic activity in Asians as compared to Caucasians, although not low enough for the Asians to be considered poor metabolizers. A recent study with African-Americans found similar results with a high prevalence (33%) of the same genetic difference related to slower metabolism. Thus, care must be taken when comparing these classifications across ethnic groups (Meyer, 1992).

The frequency of poor metabolizers of mephenytoin hydroxylase also varies substantially across ethnic groups (Silver et al., 1993). While poor metabolizers of this enzyme are relatively rare among Caucasians, they are quite prevalent in Asian populations, with approximately 20% of Japanese and Chinese being classified as poor metabolizers. A recent study of African-Americans also reported a rate of poor metabolizers significantly higher than in Caucasians (Meyer, 1992).

Acetylation

Shortly after the antitubercular drug isoniazid was introduced, researchers noted that use of the drug resulted in ethnic differences in side-effect profiles (Weber, 1987). This awareness led to the discovery that polymorphic expression of the enzyme N-acetyl transferase results in individual differences that can be classified as either a slow acetylator or rapid acetylator phenotype. Distributions of these phenotypes also display large ethnic variations. For example, the frequency of slow acetylator status in Caucasians (52–67%; Grant, Morike, & Eichelbaum, 1990; Weber, 1987) is significantly higher than the frequencies for Japanese and Chinese people (10–22%; Dufour, Knight, & Harris, 1964; Grant, Tand, & Kalow, 1984), as well as for Cuna and Ngawbe Guaymi Amerindians (24% and 29%; Inaba & Arias, 1987).

Acetylation status is clinically important for several reasons. Acetylation is the major route of metabolism of several classes of commonly used medications, including antimicrobials and antihypertensives, as well as caffeine (Mendoza, Smith, Poland, Lin, & Strickland, 1991). In addition, slow acetylators are at higher risk of developing drug-induced systemic lupus erythematosus, hypersensitivity reactions, and isoniazid polyneuropathy (Rieder, Shear, Kanee, Tang, & Spielberg, 1991). Compared to rapid acetylators, slow acetylators are more likely to demonstrate improved responsiveness to phenelzine, hydralazine, and isoniazid at similar doses. Acetylation status, furthermore, is associated with the development of a number of disorders including Gilbert's disease; Grave's disease; silicosis; and colorectal, laryngeal, and bladder cancer (Weber, 1987).

Alcohol Metabolism

Two important alcohol-metabolizing enzymes, alcohol dehydrogenase (ADH) and aldehyde dehydrogenase (ALDH), also demonstrate polymorphic variation. The discovery of atypical alcohol dehydrogenase in 1965 and the genetic basis of aldehyde dehydrogenase deficiency in 1979 provided an explanation for earlier observations of large cross-ethnic variations in response to alcohol (Agarwal & Goedde, 1990; Yamamoto, Yeh, Le, & Lin, 1988; Yoshida, 1983). For example, the increased frequency of ALDH deficiency observed in Asians (8–53%) compared to Caucasians (0%; Mendoza et al., 1991) is thought to be an important factor in the low incidence of alcoholism in Asians (Shibuya & Yoshida, 1988). This may be caused by the adverse experience of the "flushing reaction" in

ALDH-deficient individuals when they consume alcohol. This reaction, which is similar to that seen with antabuse, results from the high levels of acetaldehyde that build up in the blood stream of ALDH-deficient individuals.

Ethnicity and Plasma Protein-Binding

Many pharmacoactive agents must rely on plasma proteins for their transportation to the target organ (Reidenberg & Erill, 1986). Variations in the concentration of these drug-binding proteins in the plasma can significantly influence the effect of the drug by changing the amount of the drug available to cross the blood–brain barrier (Levy & Moreland, 1984; Routledge, 1986). Alterations in the concentrations of these plasma proteins could have profound clinical significance (Baumann & Eap, 1991; Crabtree, Jann, & Pitts, 1991).

Of the various proteins and cells in the blood that provide binding sites for drugs, only one category of plasma proteins (*alpha*$_1$ acid glycoproteins) has been shown to display ethnic differences (Baumann & Eap, 1988; Kremer, Wilting, & Janssen, 1988). Ethnic variation is found in the absolute concentration of this protein, as well as the distribution of two variants of the protein (Fukuma, Kashimimura, Umetsu, Yuasa, & Suzuki, 1990; Juneja, Weitkamp, & Straitil, 1988; Umetsu, Yuasa, & Nishimura, 1988). One of the variants more readily binds to several drugs (including nortriptyline, amitriptyline, and methadone) and varies in frequency from 15% to 27% in Asians to 34% to 67% in Caucasians and African-Americans (Juneja et al.).

Thus far, very few cross-ethnic studies of plasma protein binding have been conducted (Mendoza et al., 1991). Available studies have reported conflicting findings, indicating the need for more vigorous and systematic research in this area.

Ethnicity and Environmental Factors

Environmental factors might also contribute to the observed ethnic differences in drug response. The activity of the cytochrome P-450 enzymes, for example, is not only controlled by genetics but can also be quite sensitive to environmental changes, including exposure to different diets, environmental toxins, and other drugs (Clark et al., 1988). Branch, Salih, and Homeida (1978) compared the rate of metabolism of antipyrine and found a significantly longer half-life of the drug among Sudanese living in their home villages compared with Sudanese residing in Britain or to white British subjects. The latter two groups metabolized the antipyrine at similar rates, suggesting that environmental factors such as diet were responsible for the pharmacokinetic differences.

Similar findings were reported in subsequent studies involving Asian Indians living in India, Asian Indian immigrants residing in Britain, and white British subjects (Dollery, Fraser, & Mucklow, 1979; Fraser et al., 1979). A follow-up study (Desai, Sheth, & Mucklow, 1980) found that the immigrants who retained their dietary habits as lactovegetarians metabolized the drug similarly to those living in their home country, whereas the pharmacokinetic profiles of those who became meat eaters were indistinguishable from the British whites.

Further work supports the environmental basis of these differences in pharmacokinetics. Recent studies found that the activities of many of the cytochrome P-450 isozymes can be inhibited as well as induced by a wide variety of substances (Meyer, 1992; Okey, 1992). These substances include not only some of the extremely potent drugs that have been used for research in this area, but also commonly used pharmaceutical agents (e.g., cimetidine and carbamazepine); herbal medicines; environmental toxins; steroid and sex hormones; constituents of tobacco, alcohol, and caffeine; substances in charcoal-broiled beef, brussels sprouts, and cabbage; and certain types of dietary compositions (see, for a review, Murray & Reidy, 1990; Okey, 1992).

A final possible source of environmentally caused differences in drug response is the concurrent use of herbal medications and prescribed pharmacotherapy. These have rarely been the focus of attention for research, despite recent evidence indicating that such interactions may be far more extensive than previously believed (Jones & Runikis, 1987; Liu, 1991; Shader & Greenblatt, 1988). For example, the properties inherent in some of these herbal medications may cause psychosis, particularly when ingested concomitantly with tricyclic antidepressants or low potency neuroleptics. In a recent study, several Chinese herbs (including Fructus Schizandrae, Corydalis bungeane Diels, Kopsia officinallis, Clausena lansium, muscone, ginseng, and glycyrrhiza) were found to have potent stimulating effects on enzymes responsible for the metabolism of many medications, including psychotropics (Liu, 1991). A substance contained in two Chinese herbs substantially inhibits the activities of these enzymes. Increased awareness and further clarification of these issues are important because patients frequently rely on these traditional herbs along with pharmacotherapeutic agents.

Ethnicity and Pharmacodynamics

In addition to ethnic differences in drug metabolism and distribution, reports indicate the existence of ethnic differences that are caused by pharmacodynamic factors. Whereas pharmacokinetics can be thought of as the effects of the body on the drug, pharmacodynamics can be thought of as the effects of the drug on the body. The effects of mydriatics (drugs used to dilate the eye for diagnostic procedures) and beta-blockers (drugs used for the treatment of high blood pressure) represent two of the most significant examples of ethnic differences in pharmacodynamics.

Ethnic differences in the responses to topical mydriatics were first reported in 1927 (Chen & Poth, 1927). Since then, "impaired" mydriasis has been repeatedly observed in blacks and Asians following standard doses of epinephrine, cocaine, and atropine (Angenent & Koelle, 1953; Garde, Aston, Endler, & Sison, 1978). This reduction in the mydriatic effect appears to be correlated with the degree of pigmentation of the irises, and is not seen among albino Africans. This pattern of data suggest that the difference is not pharmacokinetically mediated. Research further demonstrated that Blacks were also significantly less responsive to intramuscular atropine and scopolamine than Caucasians (Garde et al., 1978).

Soon after their introduction to the market, beta-blockers, such as propranolol, frequently were found to be ineffective in treating black hypertensives (Moser & Lunn, 1981). In contrast, the doses of propranolol required for the effective treatment of hypertension were substantially smaller in Asians than in Caucasians (Zhou et al., 1989). Subsequent studies objectively demonstrated that the effects of propranolol on blood pressure and heart rate are most prominent in Asians, and least apparent in blacks, with Caucasians falling in between (Dimsdale, Zeigler, & Graham, 1988). These differences could not be explained by pharmacokinetic factors (Rutledge, Steinberg, & Cardozo, 1989; Zhou et al., 1989). At the same time, several studies (Rutledge et al., 1989; Stein, O'Malley, & Kilfeather, 1990; Venter, Daya, Joubert, & Strydom, 1985) have demonstrated that blacks have a higher degree of $beta_2$-adrenoreceptor sensitivity to certain medications. These studies together provide support for the hypothesis that differences in the sensitivity of drug receptors may be the major cause of the differential effects of propranolol and other beta-blockers in people of various ethnic groups (Kalow, 1989).

Observations of the ethnic differences in therapeutic concentrations of various psychotropics (Chang, Pandey, Yang, Yeh, & Davis, 1985; Hu, Lee, Yang, & Tseng, 1983; Takahashi, 1979; Yamashita & Asano, 1979) and their neurohormonal effects (Lin et al., 1988b) have led to speculation about the existence of ethnic differences in the pharmacodynamics of these drugs as well.

Cultural Factors

Culturally determined health beliefs and practices exert profound influences on the assessment of the efficacy and toxicity of medication, placebo response, and compliance behavior. Pharmacologic agents possess powerful symbolic and social meanings that are strongly influenced by sociocultural factors (Moerman, 1979). A large number of ethnic minority (as well as nonminority) patients are significantly influenced by indigenous or alternative medical concepts (Kleinman, 1980), even in the presence of modern Western medical services. For example, a belief held by some minority patients in the United States is that Western medicines are highly potent but often deal only with the superficial manifestations of the illness, instead of dealing with the underlying conditions of the diseases. At the same time, the medicines are believed to be more likely to cause serious untoward effects than non-Western therapies (Smith, Lin, & Mendoza, 1993).

These beliefs, probably passed down from early cultural experiences with antipyretic and antibacterial agents, can be especially troublesome in the case of psychotropic agents. Patients sharing these beliefs often will not understand the need for maintenance therapy in psychiatric conditions unless it is carefully explained and emphasized. Furthermore, the lack of immediate therapeutic effect for most psychotropics (especially tricyclic antidepressants) is incongruent with these preconceptions about Western medicine. In addition, when side effects occur, they can easily be taken as proof that Western medicines are indeed too strong. Therefore, taking into account patients' indigenous health beliefs and eliciting their expectations regarding Western medicines are important when psychotropic agents are prescribed. Only through such inquiries can misunderstandings and inconsistencies in expectations be determined and minimized.

Compliance is a significant problem in the treatment of chronic medical conditions (Sackett & Haynes, 1976), and especially in psychopharmacotherapies, because treatment is typically long term. Several recent studies have found that compliance to psychotropics may be more problematic among non-Western populations than among Caucasians (see, for example, Smith et al., 1993). Discrepancies between patients' and clinicians' beliefs, coupled with problems in communication, have been regarded as the major reasons for the ethnic differences in compliance. Unless clinicians routinely make an effort to elicit these indigenous beliefs and to provide medication education in an individualized and culturally congruent manner, noncompliance will continue to present a major problem in clinical settings.

Placebo effects are mediated through symbolic rather than instrumental mechanisms and are expected to be influenced a great deal by culture (Moerman, 1979). At present there is very little specific information regarding how placebo responses might differ cross-culturally. Clinical lore has long suggested that Asians often express excessive concerns about the side effects of psychotropics (Lin & Shen, 1991), which may lead to placebo side effects and to subsequent discontinuation or lowering of the drug dosage. Carefully controlled research on placebo effects and compliance is needed.

A recent study of 57 Chinese psychiatric patients treated with lithium demonstrates the importance of cultural beliefs in patients' interpretations and perceptions of side effects (Lee, 1993). In contrast to Western patients, Chinese patients rarely complained of "missing highs," loss of creativity, weight gain, or metallic taste. Although excessive thirst and urination were present in the majority of these patients, these side effects were positively, not negatively, interpreted. Complaints such as lethargy, poor memory, and drowsiness appeared to be related to patients' fears of not being able to work and actually occurred at a similar frequency in age- and sex-matched healthy controls.

CONCLUSION

As is evident from the literature reviewed above, a wide variety of pharmacokinetic, pharmacodynamic, and sociocultural factors could lead to significant cross-ethnic as well as interindividual variations in response to pharmacoactive agents. Because of the phenomenal progress of research methodology in recent years, it has become increasingly feasible to examine in detail the nature and extent of these differences as well as the mechanisms responsible for the variations. As a result, knowledge regarding ethnic influences on the metabolism and effects of medications used in clinical settings has been expanding. Because this is a fairly new field of investigation, however, much remains to be explored, and many of the reported findings are still awaiting replication. Despite the need for further research, the information reviewed above clearly indicates that ethnicity and culture are important factors that should be routinely considered in the practice of all fields of medicine.

A number of experts in the field believe that evolutionary pressure may be the driving force for the pervasiveness of cross-ethnic variations in drug responses, although this belief is highly speculative. The genetic basis of the glucose-6-dehydrogenase deficiency discussed at the beginning of the chapter is an excellent example for such a thesis. This trait is associated with an increased resistance to malaria infection. The ancestors of most carriers of this trait originally came from malaria-infested areas, including central Africa, and the selective survival value of such an attribute is evident (Kalow, 1991). The evolutionary origins of the ethnic variation of other enzymes are not as easily discernible. However, it is quite possible that they reflect differences in diet and other environmental factors that groups were exposed to for hundreds of years. In addition, Kalow (1993) recently argued that just as genetic variability in susceptibility to infectious diseases has been shown to be conducive to the survival of populations, so does pharmacogenetic variability help to ensure the survival of a population facing an onslaught of toxic chemicals in the environment.

Regardless of the heuristic value of such speculations, ethnic variations in drug responses is an issue that is becoming increasingly important for clinicians and researchers as the populations throughout the world continue to diversify. Progress in this field of investigation is crucial for the provision of rational and appropriate care for patients of all ethnic and cultural backgrounds.

REFERENCES

Agarwal, D., & Goedde, H. (1990). *Alcohol metabolism, alcohol intolerance and alcoholism: Biochemical and pharmacogenetic approaches.* Berlin: Springer-Verlag.

Ahsan, C., Renwick, A., Waller, D., Challenor, V., George, C., & Amanullah, M. (1993). The influences of dose and ethnic origins on the pharmacokinetics of nifedipine. *Clinical Pharmacology and Therapeutics, 54,* 329–338.

Angenent, W., & Koelle, G. (1953). A possible enzymatic basis for the differential action of mydriatics on light and dark irises. *Journal of Physiology, 119,* 102–117.

Baumann, P., & Eap, C. (1988). *Alpha-acid glycoprotein genetics, biochemistry, physiological functions and pharmacology.* New York: Alan R. Liss.

Baumann, P., & Eap, C. (1991). Plasma monitoring of antidepressants: clinical relevance of the pharmacogenetics of metabolism and of acid glycoprotein binding. *Biological Psychiatry, 29,* 75–95.

Bertilsson, L., & Aberg-Wistedt, A. (1983). The debrisoquine hydroxylation test predicts steady-state plasma levels of desipramine. *British Journal of Clinical Pharmacology, 15,* 388–390.

Bertilsson, L., Eichelbaum, M., & Mellstrom, B. (1980). Nortriptyline and antipyrine clearance in relation to debrisoquine hydroxylation in man. *Life Sciences, 27,* 1673–1677.

Branch, R., Salih, S., & Homeida, M. (1978). Racial differences in drug metabolizing ability: A study with antipyrine in the Sudan. *Clinical Pharmacology and Therapeutics, 24,* 283–286.

Bureau of the Census. (1990). *Statistical abstracts of the United States: 1990* (110th ed.). Washington, DC: Author.

Chang, W. H., Chen, T. Y., Lee, C. F., Hu, W. H., & Yeh, E. K. (1987). Low plasma reduced haloperidol/haloperidol ratios in Chinese patients. *Biological Psychiatry, 22,* 1406–1408.

Chang, S., Pandey, G., Yang, Y., Yeh, E., & Davis, J. (1985). *Lithium pharmacokinetics: Interracial comparison.* Paper presented at the 138th Annual Meeting of the American Psychiatric Association, Dallas, TX.

Chen, K. K., & Poth, E. J. (1927). The racial difference of the mydriatic action of ephedrine, cocaine, and euphthalmine. *Proceedings of the Society for Experimental Biology and Medicine, 25,* 150–151.

Clark, W., Brater, D., & Johnson, A. (1988). *Goth's Medical Pharmacology* (12th ed.). St. Louis: C. V. Mosby.

Crabtree, B., Jann, M., & Pitts, W. (1991). Alpha acid glycoprotein levels in patients with schizophrenia: Effect of treatment with haloperidol. *Biological Psychiatry, 29,* 18A–43A.

Dahl-Puustinen, M. L., Liden, A., & Alm, C. (1989). Disposition of perphenazine is related to polymorphic debrisoquine hydroxylation in human beings. *Clinical Pharmacology and Therapeutics, 46,* 78–81.

Desai, N. K., Sheth, U. K., & Mucklow, J. C. (1980). Antipyrine clearance in Indian villagers. *British Journal of Clinical Pharmacology, 9,* 387–394.

Dimsdale, J., Zeigler, M., and Graham, R. (1988). The effect of hypertension, sodium, and race on isoproterenol sensitivity. *Clinical and Experimental Hypertension: Theory and Practice,* A10, 747–756.

Dollery, C., Fraser, H., & Mucklow, J. (1979). Contribution of environmental factors to variability in human drug metabolism. *Drug Metabolism Review, 9,* 207–220.

Du, Y., & Lou, Y. (1990). Polymorphism of debrisoquine 4-hydroxylation and family studies of poor metabolizers in Chinese population. *Acta Pharmacologica Sinica, 11,* 7–10.

Dufour, A. P., Knight, R. A., & Harris, H. W. (1964). Genetics of isoniazid metabolism in Caucasians, Negroes, and Japanese populations. *Science, 145*, 391.

Fleishaker, J., Smith, T., Friedman, H., & Hulst, L. (1992). Separation of the pharmacokinetic/pharmacodynamic properties of oral and IV adinazolam mesylate and N-desmethyladinazolam mesylate in health volunteers. *Drug Investigations, 4*, 155–165.

Fraser, H., Mucklow, J., Bulpitt, C., Kahn, C., Mould, G., & Dollery, C. (1979). Environmental factors affecting antipyrine metabolism in London factory and office workers. *British Journal of Clinical Pharmacology, 7*, 237–243.

Fukuma, Y., Kashimimura, S., Umetsu, K., Yuasa, I., & Suzuki, T. (1990). Genetic variation of alpha-2-HS-glycoprotein in the Kyushu district of Japan: Description of three new rare variants. *Human Heredity, 40*, 49–51.

Garde, J., Aston, R., Endler, G., & Sison, O. (1978). Racial mydriatic response to belladonna premedication. *Anesthesia and Analgesia, 57*, 572–576.

Ghoneim, M., Korttila, K., Chiang, C., Jacobs, L., Schoenwald, R., Newaldt, S., & Lauaba, K. (1981). Diazepam effects and kinetics in Caucasians and Orientals. *Clinical Pharmacology and Therapeutics, 29*, 749–746.

Gonzalez, F. (1989). The molecular biology of cytochrome P450s. *Pharmacological Reviews, 40*, 243–288.

Gonzalez, F., & Nebert, D. (1990). Evolution of the P450 gene superfamily: Animal-plant "warfare," molecular drive, and human genetic differences in drug oxidation. *Trends in Genetics, 6*, 182–186.

Goodman, C., Rosendorff, C., & Gould, A. (1985). Comparison of the antihypertensive effect of enalipril and propanalol in black South Africans. *South African Medical Journal, 67*, 672–6.

Grant, D., Morike, K., & Eichelbaum, M. (1990). Acetylation pharmacogenetics. *Journal of Clinical Investigation, 85*, 968–972.

Grant, D., Tand, B., & Kalow, W. (1984). A simple test for acetylator phenotype using caffeine. *British Journal of Clinical Pharmacology, 17*, 459–464.

Hall, D. H. (1990). Pathophysiology of hypertension in blacks. *American Journal of Hypertension, 3*, 366S–371S.

Horai, Y., Taga, J., Ishizaki, T., & Ishikawa, K. (1990). Correlations among the metabolic ratios of three test probes (metoprolol, debrisoquine, sparteine) for genetically determined oxidation polymorphism in a Japanese population. *British Journal of Clinical Pharmacology, 29*, 111–115.

Hu, W., Lee, C., Yang, Y., & Tseng, Y. (1983). Imipramine plasma levels and clinical response. *Bulletin of Chinese Society of Neurology and Psychiatry, 9*, 40–49.

Inaba, T., & Arias, T. D. (1987). On phenotyping with isoniazid: The use of urinary acetylation ratio and the uniqueness of antimodes. Study of two Amerindian populations. *Clinical Pharmacology and Therapeutics, 42*, 493–497.

Ishizaki, T., Eichelbaum, M., & Horai, Y. (1987). Evidence for polymorphic oxidation of sparteine in Japanese subjects. *British Journal of Clinical Pharmacology, 23*, 482–485.

Islam, S. I., Idle, J. R., & Smith, R. L. (1980). The polymorphic 4-hydroxylation of debrisoquine in a Saudi Arab population. *Xenobiotica, 10*, 819–825.

Jann, M., Chang, W., Davis, C., Chen, T., Deng, H., Lung, F., Ereshefsky, L., Saklad, S., & Richards, A. (1989). Haloperidol and reduced haloperidol plasma levels in Chinese vs. non-Chinese psychiatric patients. *Psychiatry Research, 30*, 45–52.

Jann, M., Lam, Y., & Chang, W. (1993). Haloperidol and reduced haloperidol plasma concentrations in different ethnic populations and interindividual variabilities in haloperidol metabolism. In K. Lin, R. Poland, & G. Nakasaki (Eds.), *Psychopharmacology and psychobiology of ethnicity* (pp. 133–152). Washington, DC: American Psychiatric Press.

Jones, B., & Runikis, A. (1987). Interaction of ginseng with phenelzine. *Journal of Clinical Psychopharmacology*, 201–202.

Jorge, L. F., Arias, T. D., Inaba, T., & Jackson, P. R. (1990). Unimodal distribution of the metabolic ratio for debrisoquine in Cuna Amerindians of Panama. *British Journal of Clinical Pharmacology, 30*, 281–285.

Juneja, R., Weitkamp, L., & Straitil, A. (1988). Further studies of the plasma, Alpha B-glycoprotein polymorphism: Two new alleles and allele frequencies in Caucasians and in American Blacks. *Human Heredity, 38*, 267–272.

Kalow, W. (1989). Race and therapeutic drug response. *New England Journal of Medicine, 320*, 588–589.

Kalow, W. (1991). Interethnic variation of drug metabolism. *Trends in Pharmacological Science, 12*, 102–107.

Kalow, W. (Ed.). (1992). *Pharmacogenetics of Drug Metabolism.* New York: Pergamon Press.

Kalow, W. (1993). Pharmacogenetics: Its biologic roots and the medical challenge. *Clinical Pharmacology and Therapeutics, 54*, 235–241.

Kleinman, A. (1980). *Patients and healers in the context of culture.* Berkeley: University of California.

Kremer, J., Wilting, J., & Janssen, L. (1988). Drug binding to human alpha-1-acid glycoprotein in health and disease. *Pharmacological Review, 40*, 1–45.

Kumana, C., Lauder, I., Chan, M., Ko, W., & Lin, H. (1987). Differences in diazepam pharmacokinetics in Chinese and white Caucasians: Relation to body lipid stores. *European Journal of Clinical Pharmacology, 32*, 211–215.

Kupfer, A., & Preisig, R. (1984). Pharmacogenetics of mephenytoin: A new drug hydroxylation polymorphism in man. *European Journal of Clinical Pharmacology, 26*, 753–759.

Lawson, W. (1986). Racial and ethnic factors in psychiatric research. *Hospital and Community Psychiatry, 37*, 50–54.

Lee, E. J., Nam, Y. P., & Hee, G. N. (1988). Oxidation phenotyping in Chinese and Malay populations. *Clinical and Experimental Pharmacology and Physiology, 15*, 889–891.

Lee, S. (1993). Side effects of chronic lithium therapy in Hong Kong Chinese: An ethnopsychiatric perspective. *Culture, Medicine, and Psychiatry, 17*, 301–320.

Levy, R., & Moreland, T. (1984). Rationale for monitoring free drug levels. *Clinical Pharmacokinetics (Suppl. I)*, 1–9.

Lin, K., Lau, J., Smith, R., & Poland, R. (1988a). Comparison of alprazolam plasma levels and behavioral effects in normal Asian and Caucasian male volunteers. *Psychopharmacology, 96*, 365–369.

Lin, K., Poland, R., Lau, J., & Rubin, R. (1988b). Haloperidol and prolactin concentrations in Asians and Caucasians. *Journal of Clinical Psychopharmacology, 8*, 195–201.

Lin, K., Poland, R., & Nakasaki, G. (Eds.). (1993). *Psychopharmacology and psychobiology of ethnicity.* Washington, DC: American Psychiatric Press.

Lin, K., Poland, R., Nuccio, I., Matsuda, K., Hathuc, N., Su, T., & Fu, P. (1989). Longitudinal assessment of haloperidol dosage and serum concentration in Asian and Caucasian schizophrenic patients. *American Journal of Psychiatry, 146*, 1307–1311.

Lin, K., & Shen, W. (1991). Pharmacotherapy for southeast Asian psychiatric patients. *Journal of Nervous and Mental Disease, 179*, 346–50.

Liu, G. (1991). Effects of some compounds isolated from Chinese medicinal herbs on hepatic microsomal cytochrome P-450 and their potential biological consequences. *Drug Metabolism Review, 23*, 439–465.

Lou, Y., Ying, L., Bertilsson, L., & Sjoqvist. (1987). Low frequency of slow debrisoquine hydroxylation in a native Chinese population. *Clinical Pharmacology and Therapeutics, 15*, 443–450.

Mahgoub, A., Idle, J. R., & Smith, R. L. (1979). A population and familial study of the defective alicyclic hydroxylation of debrisoquine among Egyptians. *Xenobiotica, 9*, 51–56.

Mellstrom, B., Bertilsson, L., & Lou, Y. C. (1983). Amitriptyline metabolism: Relationship to polymorphic debrisoquine hydroxylation. *Clinical Pharmacology and Therapeutics, 34*, 516–520.

Mendoza, R., Smith, M., Poland, R., Lin, K., & Strickland, T. (1991). Ethnic psychophar-
    macology: The Hispanic and Native American perspective. *Psychopharmacology Bulle-*
    tin, 27, 449–461.

Meyer, U. (1990). Genetic polymorphisms of drug metabolism. *Fundamental and Clinical*
    Pharmacology, 4, 595–616.

Meyer, U. (1992). Molecular genetics and the future of pharmacogenetics. In W. Kalow (Ed.),
    Pharmacogenetics of Drug Metabolism (pp. 879–888). New York: Pergamon Press.

Midha, K., Hawes, E., Hubbard, J., Korchinski, E., & McKay, G. (1988a). A pharmacokinetic
    study of trifluoperazine in two ethnic populations. *Psychopharmacology, 95,* 333–338.

Midha, K., Hawes, E., Hubbard, J., Korchinski, E., & McKay, G. (1988b). Variation in the
    single dose pharmacokinetics of fluphenazine in psychiatric patients. *Psychophar-*
    macology, 96, 206–211.

Moerman, D. (1979). Anthropology of symbolic healing. *Currents in Anthropology, 20,*
    59–80.

Moser, M., & Lunn, J. (1981). Comparative effects of pindolol and hydrochlorothiazide in
    black hypertensive patients. *Angiology, 32,* 561–566.

Murray, M., & Reidy, G. (1990). Selectivity in the inhibition of mammalian cytochromes
    P-450 by chemical agents. *Pharmacology Review, 42,* 85–101.

Nakamura, K., Goto, F., & Ray, W. A. (1985). Interethnic differences in genetic polymor-
    phism of debrisoquine and mephenytoin hydroxylation between Japanese and Cauca-
    sian populations. *Clinical Pharmacology and Therapeutics, 38,* 402–408.

Okey, A. (1992). *Enzyme induction in the cytochrome P-450 system.* New York: Pergamon
    Press.

Potkin, S., Shen, Y., Pardes, H., Phelps, B., Zhou, D., Shu, L., Korpi, E., & Wyatt, R. (1984).
    Haloperidol concentrations elevated in Chinese patients. *Psychiatry Research, 12,*
    167–172.

Reidenberg, M., & Erill, S. (1986). *Drug-protein binding.* New York: Oxford University Press.

Rieder, M. J., Shear, N. H., Kanee, A., Tang, B. K., & Spielberg, S. P. (1991). Prominence of
    slow acetylator phenotype among patients with sulfonamide hypersensitivity reactions.
    Clinical Pharmacology and Therapeutics, 49, 13–17.

Rosenblat, R., & Tang, S. (1987). Do Oriental psychiatric patients receive different dosages
    of psychotropic medication when compared with Occidentals? *Canadian Journal of*
    Psychiatry, 32, 270–274.

Routledge, P. (1986). The plasma protein binding of basic drugs. *British Journal of Clinical*
    Pharmacology, 22, 499–506.

Rutledge, D., Steinberg, M., & Cardozo, L. (1989). Racial differences in drug response:
    Isoproterenol effects on heart rate following intervenous metoprolol. *Clinical Pharmacol-*
    ogy and Therapeutics, 45, 380–386.

Sackett, D., & Haynes, R. (1976). *Compliance with therapeutic regimens.* Baltimore: The
    Johns Hopkins Press.

Shader, R., & Greenblatt, D. (1988). Bees, ginseng and MAOI's revisited. *Journal of Clinical*
    Psychopharmacology, 8, 325.

Shaheen, O., Biollaz, J., & Koshakji, R. P. (1989). Influence of debrisoquine phenotype on
    the inducibility of propranolol metabolism. *Clinical Pharmacology and Therapeutics, 45,*
    439–443.

Shen, W., & Lin, K. (1990). Cytochrome P-450 monooxygenases and interactions of psycho-
    tropic drugs. *International Journal of Psychiatry in Medicine, 21,* 21–30.

Shibuya, A., & Yoshida, A. (1988). Frequency of the atypical aldehyde dehydrogenase-2 gene
    (ALDH2/2) in Japanese and Caucasians. *American Journal of Human Genetics, 43,*
    744–748.

Silver, B., Poland, R., & Lin, K. (1993). Ethnicity and the pharmacology of tricyclic anti-
    depressants. In K. Lin, R. Poland, & G. Nakasaki (Eds.), *Psychopharmacology and*
    psychobiology of ethnicity (pp. 61–89). Washington, DC: American Psychiatric Press.

Skjelbo, E., Brosen, K., Hallas, J., & Gram, L. (1991). The mephenytoin oxidation polymorphism is partially responsible for the N-demethylation of imipramine. *Clinical Pharmacology and Therapeutics, 49*, 18–23.

Smith, M., Lin, K., & Mendoza, R. (1993). "Non-biological" issues affecting psychopharmacotherapy: Cultural considerations. In K. Lin, R. Poland, & G. Nakasaki (Eds.), *Psychopharmacology and psychobiology of ethnicity* (pp. 37–58). Washington, DC: American Psychiatric Press.

Stein, M., O'Malley, K., & Kilfeather, S. (1990). Ethnic differences in cyclic AMP accumulation: Effect on alpha, beta, and prostanoid receptor responses. *Clinical Pharmacology and Therapeutics, 47*, 360–365.

Takahashi, R. (1979). Lithium treatment in affective disorders: Therapeutic plasma level. *Psychopharmacology Bulletin, 15*, 32–35.

Umetsu, K., Yuasa, I., & Nishimura, H. (1988). Genetic polymorphisms of orosomucoid and alpha-2-HS-glycoprotein in a Philippine population. *Human Heredity, 38*, 287–290.

Venter, C. P., Daya, S., Joubert, P. H., & Strydom, W. J. (1985). Ethnic differences in human lymphocytic cyclic AMP production after isoprenaline stimulation and propranolol blockade. *British Journal of Clinical Pharmacology, 19*, 187–190.

Wanwimolruk, S., Patamasucon, P., & Lee, E. J. D. (1990). Evidence for the polymorphic oxidation of debrisoquine in the Thai population. *British Journal of Pharmacology, 29*, 244–247.

Ward, S., Walle, T., & Walle, U. (1989). Propranolol's metabolism is determined by both mephenytoin and debrisoquin hydroxylase activities. *Clinical Pharmacology and Therapeutics, 45*, 75–79.

Weber, W. W. (1987). *The acetylator genes and drug responses.* New York: Oxford University Press.

Wilkinson, G. R., Guengerich, F. P., & Branch, R. A. (1989). Genetic polymorphism of S-mephenytoin hydroxylation. *Clinical Pharmacology and Therapeutics, 43*, 53–76.

Wood, A., & Zhou, H. (1991). Ethnic differences in drug disposition and responsiveness. *Clinical Pharmacokinetics, 20*, 1–24.

Xu, X., & Jiang, W. (1990). Debrisoquine hydroxylation and sulfamethazine acetylation in a Chinese population. *Acta Pharmacologica Sinica, 11*, 387–388.

Yamamoto, J., Yeh, E. K., Le, C. K., & Lin, K. M. (1988). Alcohol abuse among Koreans and Taiwanese. In L. Towle & T. Harford (Eds.), *Cultural influences and drinking patterns: A focus in Hispanic and Japanese populations* (Research Monograph No. 19). Rockville, MD: National Institute on Alcohol Abuse and Alcoholism.

Yamashita, I., & Asano, Y. (1979). Tricyclic antidepressants: Therapeutic plasma level. *Psychopharmacology Bulletin, 15*, 40–41.

Yoshida, A. (1983). *Differences in the isozymes involved in alcohol metabolism between Caucasions and Orientals.* New York: Alan R. Liss.

Yue, Q. Y., Bertilsson, L., Dahl-Puustinen, M. L., Sawe, J., Sjoqvist, F., Johansson, I., & Ingelman-Sundberg, M. (1989a). Disassociation between debrisoquine hydroxylation phenotype and genotype among Chinese. *Lancet, 2*, 870.

Yue, Q. Y., Hasselstrom, J., Sevensson, J. O. & Sawe, J. (1991a). Pharmacokinetics of codeine and its metabolites in Caucasian healthy volunteers: Comparisons between extensive and poor hydroxylators of debrisoquine. *British Journal of Clinical Pharmacology, 31*, 635–642.

Yue, Q. Y., Svensson, J. O., Alm, C., Sjoqvist, F., & Sawe, J. (1989b). Interindividual and interethnic differences in the demethylation and glucuronidation of codeine. *British Journal of Clinical Pharmacology, 28*, 629–637.

Yue, Q. Y., Svensson, J. O., Sjoqvist, F., & Sawe, J. (1991b). A comparison of the pharmacokinetics of codeine and its metabolites in healthy Chinese and Caucasian extensive hydroxylators of debrisoquine. *British Journal of Clinical Pharmacology, 31*, 643–647.

Yue, Q. Y., VanBahr, C., Odar-Cederlof, I., & Sawe, J. (1990). Glucuronidation of codeine and morphine in human liver and kidney microsomes: Effect of inhibitors. *Pharmacology and Toxicology, 66,* 221–226.

Zhang, Y., Reviriego, J., Lou, Y., Sjoqvist, F., & Bertilsson, L. (1990). Diazepam metabolism in native Chinese poor and extensive hydroxylators of S-mephenytoin: interethnic differences in comparison with white subjects. *Clinical Pharmacology and Therapeutics, 48,* 496–502.

Zhou, H., Koshakji, R., Siolberstein, D., Wilkinson, G., & Wood, A. (1989). Altered sensitivity to and clearance of propranolol in men of Chinses descent as compared with American white. *New England Journal of Medicine, 320,* 565–570.

CHAPTER 21

Socioeconomic Status and the Health of Racial Minority Populations

DAVID R. WILLIAMS AND TONI RUCKER

INTRODUCTION

This chapter considers the role that socioeconomic status (SES) plays in racial and ethnic variations in health status in the United States. The Office of Management and Budget's standard for federal statistics recognizes four racial groups (black, white, American Indian or Alaskan Native, and Asian/Pacific Islander) and one ethnic category (Hispanic). However, because this directive is without scientific basis, because race and ethnicity are socially constructed categories, and because the distinctions between race and ethnicity are unclear in health research, we treat all of these categories as "racial" groups.

We begin by considering data on the magnitude of racial differences in health and argue that these variations must be understood within the context of the well-documented association between SES and health. Next we show that there is a strong relationship between race and SES, with SES variations accounting for a large part of racial differences in health status. The complexities of the association between race and SES

DAVID R. WILLIAMS • Department of Sociology and Survey Research Center, Institute for Social Research, University of Michigan, Ann Arbor, Michigan 48106.   TONI RUCKER • Department of Sociology, University of Michigan, Ann Arbor, Michigan 48109.

Handbook of Diversity Issues in Health Psychology, edited by Pamela M. Kato and Traci Mann. Plenum Press, New York, 1996.

are discussed. We show that SES shapes the distribution of risk factors and resources that affect health, including health attitudes and behavior. Directions for research and interventions are also addressed.

RACIAL DIFFERENCES IN HEALTH

There are racial variations in health across a broad range of health outcomes. This pattern is well documented for the black (or African-American) population, with blacks having higher rates of death, disease, and disability than whites (Braithwaite & Taylor, 1992; Livingston, 1994). This pattern has existed from our earliest health data. A growing body of evidence documents a widening of the racial disparity due to less rapid gains in the improvement of health for blacks compared to whites and worsening health status of the African-American population (Williams & Collins, 1995). All of the other major racial minority populations have lower overall death rates than whites (National Center for Health Statistics, 1994), but they also have elevated rates of morbidity and mortality for select health indicators. Recent reviews of the health of Hispanics (or Latinos) indicate that although they have lower death rates for the two leading causes of death in the United States (heart disease and cancer), they have higher death rates than non-Hispanics for some causes of death, such as cirrhosis of the liver, diabetes, tuberculosis, and homicide (Furino, 1992; Sorlie, Backlund, Johnson, & Rogot, 1993; Vega & Amaro, 1994). Latinos also have elevated rates of infectious diseases such as measles, tetanus, and AIDS, and higher rates of obesity and glucose intolerance. There is also considerable variation within the Hispanic population with a general tendency for Puerto Ricans to report poorer health status than the other Hispanic groups.

Selected subgroups of the Asian and Pacific Islander American population (APIA) also have elevated rates of disease (Zane, Takeuchi, & Young, 1994). For example, high rates of death for cancer and heart disease are evident for Native Hawaiians; Japanese-Americans have high rates of stomach cancer; Chinese-Americans have rates of liver cancer that are four times higher than that of the white population. The mortality rates for Native Americans served by the Indian Health Service are considerably higher than the national average for tuberculosis (520% higher), alcoholism (433% higher), diabetes (188% higher), accidents (166% higher), homicides (71% higher), suicides (54% higher), and pneumonia and influenza (44% higher). Death rates from suicide are particularly high for American Indians in young adulthood (Fingerhut & Makuc, 1992).

Racial variations in health reflect the unique historical experiences and the current social conditions of racial groups. An adequate understanding of racial differences in health must consider these larger social structures and processes and identify the ways in which they affect health status. Health behaviors and other risk factors for disease must be understood within the context of the living and working conditions that facilitate their initiation and maintenance. Socioeconomic status is one such structural characteristic that is critical to understanding racial variations in health.

SES AND HEALTH

Whether measured by poverty, earnings, wealth, education, occupation, or a composite index of these factors, SES is one of the strongest determinants of health, with persons of higher SES enjoying better health status than their lower SES counterparts (Adler, Boyce, Chesney, Cohen, & Folkman, 1994; Bunker, Gomby, & Kehrer, 1989; Krieger, Rowley, Herman, Avery, & Phillips, 1993; Williams, 1990; Williams & Collins, 1995). Across a broad range of health indicators, persons of lower SES are disadvantaged in terms of health. Some of the most impressive findings come from studies of mortality, which continue to reveal a positive association between SES and length of life (Haan, Kaplan, & Camacho, 1987; Pappas, Queen, Hadden, & Fisher, 1993). National surveys reveal consistently that morbidity, impairments, and disability are most prevalent among the poorer social groups (Lerner, 1975; Newacheck, Butler, Harper, Prontokowski, & Franks, 1980). Measures of deprivation based on neighborhood characteristics are also associated with mortality independent of individual socioeconomic status indicators (Haan et al., 1987; Krieger, 1991). SES is also a powerful predictor of variations in mental health status. For example, the Epidemiologic Catchment Area Study (ECA), the largest study of psychiatric disorders ever conducted in the United States, found that low SES predicted elevated rates of a broad range of psychiatric conditions (Holzer, Shea, Swanson, Leaf, & Myers, 1986; Robins & Reiger, 1991).

This inverse association between SES and health status is evident cross-nationally and has persisted across time. Elevated levels of disease and death among low SES populations is a universal phenomenon and is evident in data from the developing and industrialized world (Marmot, Kogevinas, & Elston, 1987; Williams, Wilson, & Chung, 1992). Trends in the social distribution of certain diseases indicate that even when a particular illness initially was more prevalent among the higher SES groups, over time it became more common among the poor (Williams, 1990). Heart disease and AIDS illustrate this pattern in U.S. data.

RACE AND SES

Race is strongly related to SES, and SES differences between racial groups play a major role in accounting for racial variations in health. For example, nearly one-half of all black children live below the poverty line

(Shulman, 1990). National data reveal that there are large disparities in poverty rates between the white population and other racial groups. Compared to 12% of whites, 33% of blacks and 29% of Hispanics are poor (NCHS, 1994). Fourteen out of 17 major subgroups of the APIA population have rates of poverty that are higher than the national average, and three of these groups (Laotians, Cambodians, and Hmong) have rates of poverty that exceed 45% (Takeuchi & Young, 1994).

Racial differences in economic status are also readily evident in national income data. Table 1 indicates that nearly 43% of blacks and 33% of Hispanics have annual household incomes of less than $15,000, compared to 22% of whites. Whites are more than twice as likely as blacks and Hispanics to earn over $75,000. This overall pattern of differences may be even more pronounced for some demographic groups, such as the elderly. In a study of persons who retired in 1980–81, Snyder (1989) found that the median income was $11,000 for black couples compared to $18,000 for white couples. In spite of some progress over time, the racial gap in income persists. For example, the adjusted mean personal income for African-Americans increased from 85% of that for whites in 1968 to 90% in 1988 (Thomas, 1993).

Table 2 provides national data on racial differences in educational attainment. With the exception of Asian and Pacific Islanders, minority racial groups fall significantly behind whites in educational attainment. High school completion rates are similar for whites (80%) and APIAs (82%), but these groups are much more likely to complete 4 years of high school than blacks (67%) or Hispanics (51%). The overall number for Hispanics conceals the variation for subpopulations within that category. The high school completion rate is 44% for Mexicans, 58% for Puerto Ricans, and 61% for Cubans. The racial gap in years of education attained is even greater at higher levels of education. Twenty-two percent of whites completed 4 years of college or more compared to 11% of blacks, 6% of Mexicans, 10% of Puerto Ricans, and 19% of Cubans. The APIA numbers are high and in some instances reflect even higher educational achievement than whites. However, it is important to recognize that APIAs are overrepresented at both ends of the educational distribution. Compared

TABLE 1. Money Income of Households: Percent Distribution by Income Level, Race, and Hispanic Origin in Constant Dollars, 1992

	<$14,999	$15–24,999	$25–34,999	$35–49,999	$50–74,999	$75,000+
White	21.6	16.7	15.1	17.7	17.0	11.9
Black	42.2	18.3	13.2	12.8	8.8	4.2
Hispanic	33.0	20.8	16.3	14.5	10.5	5.0

Source: *Statistical Abstracts 1994*.

TABLE 2. Educational Attainment by Race, 1991

	Completed four or more years of high school	Completed four or more years of college
White	79.9	22.2
Black	66.7	11.5
Asian and Pacific Islander	81.8	39.1
Hispanic	51.3	9.7

Source: *Statistical Abstracts 1994.*

to the national average, APIAs are twice as likely (and APIA women three times as likely) to have completed only 0 to 4 years of elementary education (Lin-Fu, 1993).

RACE, SES, AND HEALTH

Given the magnitude of racial differences in SES, it is not surprising that statistically adjusting black–white differences in health for SES has a dramatic effect. Researchers have found that racial disparities in health status are sometimes eliminated and always substantially reduced when adjusted for SES (Cooper, 1993; Krieger et al., 1993; Krieger & Fee, 1994; Williams & Collins, 1995). In fact, it is not generally recognized that SES differences in health in the United States are much larger than racial differences in health (Navarro, 1990).

What is puzzling to some researchers is the persistence of racial differences in health status after controlling for SES. That is, research frequently finds that within each level of SES, blacks have worse health status than whites. For example, one recent study found higher infant mortality rates among college educated black women than among their similarly situated white peers (Schoendorf, Hogue, Kleinman, & Rowley, 1992). In some studies the black–white mortality ratio increases with rising SES (Krieger et al., 1993).

Several researchers have recently emphasized that the failure of the traditionally utilized SES indicators to completely explain racial differences in health reflects the interactive and incremental role of racism as a determinant of health (Cooper, 1993; Krieger et al., 1993; Williams, Lavizzo-Mourey, & Warren, 1994). The construct racism incorporates ideologies of superiority, negative attitudes and beliefs toward racial and ethnic outgroups, and differential treatment of members of these groups by both individuals and societal institutions (Williams & Collins, 1995). The unequal distribution of income, education, and occupational status reflects the manipulation of institutions and social processes by those with greater power and resources to create and perpetuate inequalities based on race.

Historically, attitudes and beliefs about racial groups have been translated into policies and societal arrangements that limited the opportunities and life chances of groups regarded as inferior. Race is thus more than an abstract, ideological concept, but has been a fundamental organizing principle of society (Omi & Winant, 1986; Winant, 1994). Minority populations' disproportionate representation in the lower segments of social stratification reflects the successful implementation of social processes that were designed to relegate groups with undesirable physical characteristics such as skin color to positions and roles consistent with the dominant society's evaluation of them.

Discrimination is a facet of social life that leads to differential treatment and access for racial and ethnic groups. It would follow, then, that these social groups are not fully brought into the fabric of social life and face types of unfair treatment that may adversely affect health outcomes on a daily basis. Constant exposure to these obstacles, hassles, and indignities based on race may adversely affect physiological processes (Williams & Collins, 1995).

Racism may most dramatically affect health status by creating differential opportunity such that the commonly used SES indicators do not fully capture the differences in social and economic circumstances between households of different races (Williams & Collins, 1995). For example, racial differences in income do not fully capture racial differences in the economic resources available to a household. A comprehensive accounting of household economic resources requires an assessment not only of revenues but also of the availability of financial reserves. In this regard it is instructive that racial differences in wealth are larger than those for income. Whereas white households have a median net worth of $44,408, the net worth is $4,604 for black households and $5,345 for Hispanic households (Eller, 1994). Moreover, racial differences in wealth exist at all income levels. For example, for the poorest 20% of the U.S. population (where Africans and Hispanics are overrepresented), white households have a net worth of $10,000 compared to $1 for blacks and $575 for Hispanics. Thus even at equivalent levels of income, minority populations are distinctly disadvantaged compared to whites in terms of economic security and the ability to cushion a shortfall of income.

Racial differences are also evident for the average level of income earned for a given level of education. Whites with high school diplomas have higher income returns on their investment in education than their black counterparts (Ashraf, 1994). A given level of education also represents different socioeconomic realities for members of different racial groups. Residential segregation has concentrated African-Americans in the least desirable neighborhoods. Because of the strong relationship between place of residence and school attendance, whites are more likely than blacks to attend safe, high-quality schools. Equality in educational attainment is important for reducing racial inequality in earnings, but even when minority group members achieve the same level of education as whites, they receive lower levels of income.

A growing body of evidence indicates that the goods and services available to whites are not only better in quality but also lower in price compared to those available to blacks. Minority populations are often concentrated in neighborhoods where there are deteriorating structures and an overall lack of quality goods and services. For example, studies reveal that compared to whites, African-Americans pay higher prices for new cars (Ayres 1991), higher property taxes on homes of similar value (Schemo 1994), and higher costs for food (Alexis, Haines, & Simon, 1980) and mortgages (Pol, Guy, & Bush, 1982). These purchasing power differences by race mean that a given level of income differs across race in its ability to procure goods and services in society.

Employment discrimination is also a mechanism by which racism can affect health. First, systematic racial bias in hiring workers can lead minority populations to have high levels of unemployment and underemployment and thus lower levels of economic resources. Second, even after adjusting for education and job experience, black workers are more likely than their white peers to hold jobs where they are exposed to hazardous conditions. The average black worker is 37% to 52% more likely to be in an occupation that results in a serious injury or illness than the average white worker (Robinson, 1984). Thus across racial lines, a given level of occupational status reflects different risks of exposure to adverse working conditions.

In addition to racism, differences in early life SES and health conditions between the races can also contribute to the failure of controls for SES to completely account for racial and ethnic differences in disease patterns. An adult's health status is a function not only of current SES but also of the SES conditions experienced over the life course (Williams & Collins, 1995). Some evidence suggests that the quality of the early childhood environment has a profound and lasting effect on health, well-being, and competence (Hertzman, 1994). Some diseases acquired in childhood, such as tuberculosis and typhoid, can be harbored for decades and manifest themselves later in life. SES in early life reflects not only early exposure to adverse conditions but also can set in place patterns and conditions that perpetuate a life characterized by low SES. Health status in infancy and childhood can influence SES differences in later health either through the maintenance of these SES differences in health problems over the life course or through selective social mobility (Power, Manor, Fox, & Fogelman, 1990). The material conditions and life quality of a person or community in childhood may be crucial to determining health status throughout the life span.

A growing body of empirical evidence documents the long-term consequences of early life conditions. For instance, the risk of death from heart disease in the 5th decade of life is strongly associated with the size of an individual's placenta at birth and weight gain during the 1st year of life (Barker & Osmond, 1986; Barker, Osmond, Di, & Wadsworth, 1989). Similarly, Lundberg (1991) found that exposure to economic hardship during childhood is associated with a higher risk of both physical and mental illness in adulthood, even after controlling for age, sex, class of destination, and class of origin.

WHAT IS SES?

SES is more than an abstract concept. SES indicates the social location of an individual or group in the structure of society. One's position in social structure determines access to power, privilege, desirable resources, and rewards, including those that facilitate the maintenance and enhancement of health. In concrete and pervasive ways SES structures everyday life. Social location can importantly shape life's successes, opportunities, and adversities, thus facilitating exposure to the resources and avenues that will either enhance or adversely affect life outcomes, including health. An individual's position in the social stratification system will determine not only the status and power that she or he wields in relation to external structures and processes but also the degree of control to manage and influence the events in one's life and the larger community. The disproportionate representation of minority racial groups at lower levels of social stratification reflects a relative lack of power and control over their lives and community.

Persons lower in SES are more likely than their higher SES counterparts to be entangled in a life of uncertainty in which obtaining the basic necessities of life is more likely to be a challenge. Low SES means that there is a greater likelihood of a struggle for quality, safe housing; difficulties in securing employment; inadequate educational systems for one's children; and lack of access to quality health care. Dealing with economic deprivation and discrimination may not be an unfamiliar experience. Frequently, there is worry and strain about being able to pay bills, provide for daily needs, and protect one's own.

Low SES can also place a strain on relationships. Although low SES persons have networks of support that facilitate survival, these social ties are also likely to generate considerable stress (Belle, 1990). Everyday social experiences not only determine the quality of life that one is able to enjoy but may also impact basic psychological and physiological processes and shape behavior patterns in ways that affect health.

A growing body of evidence from animal studies indicates that social ranking influences how animals respond to stress. In particular, studies of baboons in the wild reveal that the functioning of major physiological systems differs for dominant compared to subordinate animals in ways that enhance the subordinate animals' risk of stress-related disease (Sapolsky, 1990). This program of research indicates that the healthier physiological profile of dominant animals is a result of the security and control that comes from being at the top of a stable hierarchy. In addition, having outlets for tension and being able to control and predict the outcomes of social interaction appear to reduce the adverse effects of stress. These animal studies reveal that social ranking so strongly determines the activities of everyday life and the responses of others that these researchers define social rank as how often animals get what they want.

THE SOCIAL DISTRIBUTION OF PSYCHOSOCIAL FACTORS

A growing body of evidence suggests that SES determines both the exposure to and impact of psychosocial variables (Mirowsky & Ross 1986; Williams & House, 1991). Risk factors and resources that affect health are not randomly distributed in the population but are consequences of social organization. Thus a broad range of dispositional and behavioral factors that are related to health outcomes can be viewed as intervening mechanisms between social position and health status (Williams, 1990). Health psychologists and other social and behavioral scientists study these variables as risk factors or resources for health outcomes but typically give inadequate attention to their social distribution.

Health-enhancing resources vary by SES. For example, the quantity and quality of social ties have emerged as major psychosocial factors that appear to affect a broad range of health outcomes (House, Umberson, & Landis, 1988). Social support is embedded in the larger socioeconomic context, and low SES persons report lower levels of the frequency of social contact with friends and relatives, as well as lower levels of organizational involvement and support (Williams, 1990). In addition, the quality of social ties also seems to vary by SES. That is, although some of the poor are enmeshed in a supportive network of relatives and friends that facilitates survival (Liebow, 1967; Stack, 1975), the social networks of the poor appear to be less emotionally supportive than those of higher SES persons. In fact, because of the broader economic challenges of the poor, social networks of lower SES persons may provide both stress and support (Belle, 1990). Psychological resources such as a sense of mastery and control also vary by SES (Mirowsky & Ross, 1986; Williams, 1990).

Low SES residential environments usually involve high rates of exposure to a broad range of stressors (Harburg et al., 1973). Life in poor urban environments frequently includes inadequate nutrition, substandard education, crime, traffic hazards, poor and overcrowded housing, marital instability, unemployment and underemployment, and a lack of health insurance and access to basic health services. Lower SES persons also have higher exposure to environmental risk factors such as water pollution, pesticides, industrial chemicals, and hazardous waste (Bryant & Mohai, 1990).

There is an interaction between race and SES in terms of exposure to stressful conditions in urban environments. The black urban poor encounter adverse living conditions more frequently than their white counterparts. The African-American poor have been increasingly concentrated in depressed central city neighborhoods with poor living conditions, whereas the white urban poor are more evenly dispersed throughout the city, with many residing in relatively safe and comfortable neighborhoods away from the inner city (Wilson, 1987). Lower SES blacks in the United States experience higher rates of some stressors, such as unemployment, than lower SES whites (Williams & House, 1991). Research on John Henryism illustrates that the interactions between race and SES may be complex (James, 1994). The John Henryism scale measures an active orientation to master stress. The research to date indicates that high scores on this scale are predictive of increased risk of high blood pressure for low SES blacks but not for whites or high-SES blacks.

The determinants of health are embedded in the structural conditions that shape the life experiences of social groups. Health practices such as nutrition and eating habits, exercise, tobacco, alcohol, and drug abuse are associated with SES (Schoenborn, 1986). In Alameda County, for example, lower SES persons were three to four times more likely to report poorer health habits than their higher SES counterparts (Berkman & Breslow, 1983).

The social distribution of high-risk behaviors are frequently produced by the cooperative efforts of large-scale societal institutions. For example, women, teenagers, the poor, and members of minority groups are special targets of the tobacco and alcohol industries (Davis, 1987; Singer, 1986). These industries are part of a larger social structure that exploits underprivileged social groups and benefits from their hardships. Hacker, Collins, and Jacobson (1987) have provided a detailed description of how the alcohol industry has tied itself to the black community and linked alcohol consumption to the music, sports, and cultural events that are integral to the values and tastes of blacks. Some alcohol products, such as malt liquors (beer with higher alcohol content) are marketed almost exclusively to blacks. In addition to the pervasive presence of commercial enticement, alcoholic beverages are also more readily available to the poor and minorities. Retail outlets for alcohol are more prevalent in low-income and minority neighborhoods than in more affluent communities (Rabow & Watt, 1982). The location of liquor stores reflects cooperative efforts of the state and economic interests because state licensing boards control when and where alcoholic beverages are sold.

Researchers must therefore give greater attention to the structural influences on the distribution of risk behaviors and the role that external forces play in the everyday lives of lower SES persons. What is often viewed as uninformed decisions and behaviors on the part of racial and ethnic group members may in reality illustrate the adaptation of these groups to the constraints that they face. How an individual spends his or her leisure time and what relaxing activities they engage in directly depend upon the resources and the larger external environment.

Changes in health behavior are also associated with SES. A review of the evidence on SES and health-behavior change indicates that across a broad range of behaviors, including quitting smoking, initiating breast-feeding, eating nutritiously, or engaging in physical activity, health education campaigns are more effective in improving the behavior of higher SES groups than of lower SES groups (Williams, 1990). For example, in recent decades the prevalence of cigarette smoking in the United States has declined five times more rapidly among college graduates than among persons with less than a high school education (Pierce, Fiore, Novotny, Hatziandreau, & Davis, 1989). Higher SES persons are both more likely to quit smoking and less likely to start than their low-SES counterparts. People with more education are more aware of health risks and more likely to take action to reduce those risks.

Some evidence suggests that even the effectiveness of behavioral interventions vary by SES. Relaxation techniques, for example, have been shown to be relatively effective in the treatment of mild to moderate hypertension, but the efficacy of those procedures are linked to the social context. The amount of stress in an individual's life affects the effectiveness of stress-reduction techniques. The effectiveness of these techniques is enhanced in populations of highly motivated patients in favorable social circumstances (Patel & Marmot, 1988).

It is no surprise that SES is a factor when examining the likelihood of behavioral changes. Persons with higher levels of education are more attentive to health information, more trusting of the claims of science, and have greater knowledge of health. However, the greater propensity of higher SES persons to engage in actions to improve their health is not simply due to having more health knowledge (Williams, 1990). Instead, it reflects the reality that health behaviors are induced and constrained by the social and material context. Lower SES persons face more stress and have fewer resources to cope with it than their higher SES peers (Mirowsky & Ross, 1986). Preoccupation with daily survival is often foremost in the minds of low-SES persons because the poor cannot take meeting their basic needs for granted. Behaviors that may be detrimental to health outcomes in the long run may provide sustenance and relief from structural impediments in the short term. Cigarette smoking, for example, is the single most important source of preventable deaths in the United States, but smoking is widely used to alleviate stress and tension. Smoking can be a useful strategy to break up the drudgery of life and bring diversion and at least temporary relief from chronic irritations and hassles. Higher SES persons may have alternatives to the use of cigarettes, whereas lower SES persons who face different structural constraints and truncated options may perceive that cigarette smoking is their only viable stress-reduction option.

Preventive health behaviors are higher on the hierarchy of need than the more basic needs of food, clothing, and shelter. Accordingly, until these primary needs are met, low-SES persons will (appropriately) focus on addressing basic needs and confronting their most immediate dangers before worrying about health concerns that are distant, uncertain, and less relevant to the daily struggles of basic survival (Williams, 1990).

IMPLICATIONS FOR RESEARCH AND INTERVENTION

The evidence reviewed clearly indicates that health-enhancing and pathogenic factors cannot be viewed as autonomous individual characteristics unrelated to living and working conditions and independent of the broader social and political order. Researchers must give renewed attention to identifying why populations, as opposed to individuals, vary in their level of risk factors. Researchers must also give more attention to identifying the ways in which the lives of participants in studies are constrained by broader social, economic, and political forces. Studies should also attend to the ways in which SES shapes both the subjective reality and the objective conditions of life. Dorn's (1980) study of alcohol use among teenagers illustrates the utility of this approach and the extent to which researchers who take social structure seriously may have to go beyond the conventional ways of conducting their studies. In addition to interviewing teenagers, Dorn also interviewed guidance counselors, teachers, and local employers and studied the local labor market by researching documentary evidence and visiting local workplaces. He was thus able to understand the use of alcohol within the context of the teenagers' lives and elucidate the ways in which their occupational experiences and structure of their community shaped their values and behavior and gave rise to the observed patterns of alcohol use. Future research must seek to identify the pathways through which multiple components of social structure create healthy or pathogenic socioenvironmental conditions and combine additively or interactively with individual characteristics to produce particular patterns of disease (Williams, 1990).

Some researchers are intimidated by the prospect of creating interventions that might make a difference given the power of social structure. However, the literature provides examples of relatively small changes that have had dramatic impact in terms of outcome for lower SES persons. Syme's (1978) study of 244 low SES hypertensive patients illustrates how addressing underlying social and economic conditions can enhance the management of hypertension and improve the effectiveness of antihypertensive therapy. The patients in this study were matched by age, race, gender, and blood pressure history and randomly assigned to one of three groups. The first group received routine hypertensive care from a physician. In addition to receiving routine care, the second group also attended weekly clinic meetings that were run by a health educator and nurse practitioner for 12 weeks. These didactic sessions provided health education with regard to hypertension. The third group received routine care and was visited by community health workers who had been recruited from the immediate community and had received 1 month of training to address the diverse social and medical needs of persons with hypertension. These outreach lay workers provided information on hypertension but also discussed family difficulties, financial strain, employment opportunities, and as appropriate, provided support, advice, referral, and direct assistance.

After 7 months of follow-up, the hypertensive patients in all groups were evaluated by the clinic medical staff. Patients in the third group were more likely to have their blood pressure controlled than patients in the other two groups. In addition, those in the third group knew twice as much about blood pressure and were more compliant with taking their hypertensive medication than patients in the other two groups. Interestingly, the good compliers in the third group were twice as successful in controlling their blood pressure as good compliers in the health-education-intervention group. Thus even the effectiveness of the pharmacological treatment appeared to be enhanced in the group that also addressed the underlying stressful conditions in the lives of these hypertensive persons. This study dramatically illustrates that reducing stress and helping patients deal with the challenges of their socioeconomic context can have important effects on the outcomes of interventions.

A study by Buescher, Smith, Holliday, and Levine (1987) further illustrates how addressing underlying economic and social issues can improve the impact of medical care. This study compared the effectiveness of two approaches in the delivery of prenatal care in a population of predominantly black, low-SES women in Guilford County, North Carolina. One group received prenatal care at the county health department, and the other group received prenatal care from private-practice physicians. Women who received care from the community-based physicians were twice as likely to have a low-birthweight baby compared to women who visited the health department. The health department's prenatal care program attempted to comprehensively address the medical and social needs of the pregnant mothers. Prenatal care was provided by nurse practitioners, instead of by physicians. During prenatal care visits time was devoted to counseling the women about nutrition and other aspects of personal care. As appropriate, referrals were made to the

Women, Infants, and Children Program that provides nutritional supplements to poor women. These referrals, as well as missed clinic appointments, were aggressively followed up. It appears that the advantage of the county health department's program was that it offered low-income women an extended network of social support, capable of meeting their needs in much the same way that older more knowledgeable women have traditionally guided and supported young inexperienced mothers (James, 1993).

Lieberson's (1985) distinctions between basic causes and surface causes is one that behavioral researchers should constantly grapple with. Basic causes are those forces responsible for generating a particular outcome. Changes in these factors in turn produce changes in the outcome. On the other hand, surface causes are related to the outcome. The changes in these causes do not produce corresponding change in the outcome. That is, as long as the underlying basic causal mechanisms are intact, changes in surface causes will lead to the emergence of new intervening mechanisms to maintain the same outcome. The patterns of SES differences in health status over the course of this century is consistent with this interpretation. That is, the leading causes of death and the major risk factors associated with them have changed from the turn of the century to the present, but we have witnessed the maintenance of the SES gradient in health. The more privileged groups control a disproportionate level of the goods and resources that promote good health. Whatever the intermediary links are, high-SES groups are more likely to have the available information and are better equipped socially, economically, and politically to capitalize on new information and translate it into tangible health benefits. The available evidence is clear that reductions in inequalities in health depend on reductions of societal inequality (Williams & Collins, 1995).

McKinlay (1975) warns that efforts to change the lifestyle of the poor without also altering social structure and life chances may not only be ineffective but also may do more harm than good. Telling people that they and their treasured practices are somewhat deviant and harmful but not giving them the means to change the immediate and larger environment that fosters such behaviors can be counterproductive. Syme (1994) argues that it is difficult to change high-risk behaviors even when the targeted social group really wants to change, and every effort is made to help, if little is being done to alter the societal forces that caused the problem in the first place.

ACKNOWLEDGMENTS

Preparation of this chapter was supported by Grant AG-07904 from the National Institute of Aging. We wish to thank Car Nosel for her assistance in preparing the manuscript.

REFERENCES

Adler, N. E., Boyce, T., Chesney, M. A., Cohen, S., & Folkman, S. (1994). Socioeconomic status and health: The challenge of the gradient. *American Psychologist, 49*, 15–24.

Alexis, M., Haines, G. H., & Simon, L. S. (1980). *Black consumer profiles*. Ann Arbor, MI: Division of Research, Graduate School of Business Administration, University of Michigan.

Ashraf, J. (1994). Differences in returns to education: An analysis by race. *American Journal of Economics and Sociology, 53*(3), 281–290.

Ayres, I. (1991). Fair driving: Gender and race discrimination in retail car negotiations. *Harvard Law Review, 104*(4), 817–872.

Barker, D., & Osmond, C. (1986). Infant mortality, childhood nutrition, and ischaemic heart disease in England and Wales. *The Lancet, 10*, 1077–1081.

Barker, D., Osmond, J. G., Di, K., & Wadsworth, M. (1989). Growth in utero, blood pressure in childhood and adult life, and mortality from cardiovascular disease. *British Medical Journal, 298*, 564–567.

Belle, D. (1990). Poverty and women's mental health. *American Psychologist, 45*, 385–389.

Berkman, L. F., & Breslow, L. (1983). *Health and ways of living*. Oxford, UK: Oxford University Press.

Braithwaite, R. L., & Taylor, S. E. (Eds.). (1992). *Health issues in the black community*. San Francisco: Jossey-Bass.

Bryant, B., & Mohai, P. (1990). *The proceedings of the Michigan conference on race and the incidence of environmental hazards*. Ann Arbor: University of Michigan School of Natural Resources.

Buescher, P. A., Smith, C., Holliday, J. L., & Levine, R. H. (1987). Source of prenatal care and infant birth weight: The case of a North Carolina county. *American Journal of Obstetrics and Gynecology, 53*, 204–210.

Bunker, J. P., Gomby, D. S., & Kehrer, B. H. (1989). *Pathways to health: The role of social factors*. Menlo Park, CA: Kaiser Family Foundation.

Cooper, R. S. (1993). Health and the social status of blacks in the United States. *Annals of Epidemiology, 3*, 137–144.

Davis, R. M. (1987). Current trends in cigarette advertising and marketing. *New England Journal of Medicine, 316*, 725–732.

Dorn, N. (1980). Alcohol in teenage cultures: A materialist approach to youth cultures, drinking and health education. *Health Education Journal, 39*, 67–73.

Eller, T. J. (1994). *Household wealth and asset ownership: 1991* (US Bureau of the Census, Current Population Reports, P70-34). Washington, DC: U.S. Government Printing Office.

Fingerhut, L. A., & Makuc, D. M. (1992). Mortality among minority populations in the United States. *American Journal of Public Health, 82*, 1168–1170.

Furino, A. (1992). *Health policy and the Hispanic*. Boulder, CO: Westview.

Haan, M. N., Kaplan, G., & Camacho, T. (1987). Poverty and health: Prospective evidence from the Alameda County study. *American Journal of Epidemiology, 125*, 989–998.

Hacker, A. G., Collins, R., & Jacobson, M. (1987). *Marketing booze to blacks*. Washington, DC: Center for Science in the Public Interest.

Harburg, E., Erfurt, J., Chape, C., Habenstein, L., Scholl, W., & Schork M. A. (1973). Socioecological stressor areas of black-white blood pressure: Detroit. *Journal of Chronic Disease, 26*, 595–611.

Hertzman, C. (1994). The lifelong impact of childhood experiences: A population health perspective. *Daedalus, 123*, 4, 167–180.

Holzer, C., Shea, B., Swanson, J., Leaf, P., & Myers, J. (1986). The increased risk for specific psychiatric disorders among persons of low socioeconomic status. *American Journal of Social Psychiatry, 6*, 259–271.

House, J. S., Umberson, D., & Landis, K. (1988). Structures and processes of social support. *Annual Review of Sociology*, *14*, 293–318.

James, S. A. (1993). Racial and ethnic differences in infant mortality and low birth weight. *Annals of Epidemiology*, *3*(2), 131–136.

James, S. A. (1994). John Henryism and the health of African-Americans. *Culture of Medicine and Psychiatry*, *18*, 163–182.

Krieger, N. (1991). Women and social class: A methodological study comparing individual, household, and census measures as predictors of black/white differences in reproductive history. *Journal of Epidemiology and Community Health*, *45*, 35–42.

Krieger, N., & Fee, E. (1994). Social class: The missing link in U.S. health data, *Journal of Health Services*, *24*, 25–44.

Krieger, N., Rowley, D. L., Herman, A. A., Avery, B., & Phillips, M. T. (1993). Racism, sexism, and social class: Implications for studies of health, disease, and well-being. *American Journal of Preventive Medicine*, *9* (Suppl.), 82 –122.

Lerner, M. (1975). Social differences in physical health. In J. Kosa & I. K. Zola (Eds.), *Poverty and health: A sociological analysis* (rev. ed., pp. 80–134). Cambridge: Harvard University Press.

Lieberson, S. (1985). *Making it count: The improvement of social research and theory*. Berkeley: University of California Press.

Liebow, E. (1967). *Tally's corner*. Boston: Little, Brown.

Lin-Fu, J. S. (1993). Asian and Pacific Islander Americans: An overview of demographic characteristics and health care issues. *Asian American and Pacific Islander Journal of Health*, *1*(1), 20–36.

Livingston, I. L. (1994). *Handbook of black american health: The mosaic of conditions, issues, and prospects*. Westport, CT: Greenwood.

Lundberg, O. (1991). Causal explanations for class inequality in health—an empirical analysis. *Social Science Medicine*, *32*, 385–393.

Marmot, M. G., Kogevinas, M., & Elston, M. A. (1987). Social/economic status and disease. *Annual Review of Public Health*, *8*, 111–135.

McKinlay, J. B. (1975). The help-seeking behavior of the poor. In J. Kosa, I. K. Zola (Eds.), *Poverty and health: A sociological analysis* (rev. ed., pp. 224–273). Cambridge: Harvard University Press.

Mirowsky, J., & Ross, C. E. (1986). Social patterns of distress. *Annual Review of Sociology*, *12*, 23–45.

National Center for Health Statistics. (1994). *Health United States 1993*. Hyattsville, MD: USDHHS.

Navarro, V. (1990). Race or class versus race and class: Mortality differentials in the United States. *Lancet*, *336*, 1238–1240.

Newacheck, P. W., Butler, L. H., Harper, A. K., Prontokowski, D. L., & Franks, P. E. (1980). Income and illness. *Medical Care*, *18*, 1165–1176.

Omi, M., & Winant, H. (1986). *Racial formation in the United States: From the 1960s to 1980s*. New York: Routledge.

Pappas, G., Queen, S., Hadden, W., & Fisher, G. (1993). The increasing disparity in mortality between socioeconomic groups in the United States, 1960 and 1986. *New England Journal of Medicine*, *329*, 103–115.

Patel, C., & Marmot, M. G. (1988). Efficacy versus effectiveness of relaxation therapy in hypertension. *Stress Medicine*, *4*, 283–289.

Pierce, J. P., Fiore, M., Novotny, T. E., Hatziandreau, E., & Davis, R. (1989). Trends in cigarette smoking in the United States: Educational differences are increasing. *Journal of the American Medical Association*, *261*, 56–65.

Pol, L. G., Guy, R. F., & Bush, A. J. (1982). Discrimination in the home lending market: A macro perspective. *Social Science Quarterly*, *63*, 716–728.

Power, C., Manor, O., Fox, A. J., & Fogelman, K. (1990). Health in childhood and social inequalities in health in young adults. *Journal of the Royal Statistical Society, 153*(1), 17–28.

Rabow, J., & Watt, R. (1982). Alcohol availability, alcohol beverage sales and alcohol-related problems. *Journal of Studies on Alcohol, 43,* 767–801.

Robins, L. N., & Reiger, D. A., (1991). *Psychiatric disorders in America: The epidemiologic catchment area study.* New York: Free Press.

Robinson, J. C. (1984). Racial inequality and the probability of occupation-related injury or illness. *Milbank Quarterly, 63*(4), 567–593.

Sapolsky, R. M. (1990). Stress in the wild. *Scientific American, 262,* 116–123.

Schemo, D. (1994, August 17). Suburban taxes are higher for blacks, analysis shows. *New York Times,* p. A/6.

Schoenborn, C. A. (1986). Health habits of U.S. adults, 1985: The "Alameda 7" revisited. *Public Health Reports, 101,* 571–580.

Schoendorf, K. C., Hogue, C. J. R., Kleinman, J. C., & Rowley, D. (1992). Mortality among infants of black as compared with white college-educated persons. *New England Journal of Medicine, 326,* 1522–1526.

Shulman, S. (1990). The causes of black poverty: Evidence and interpretation. *Journal of Economic Issues, 4,* 995–1016.

Singer, M. (1986). Toward a political economy of alcoholism. *Social Science Medicine, 23,* 113–130.

Snyder, D. C. (1989). A database with income and assets of new retirees by race and Hispanic origin. *Review of the Black Political Economy, 17,* 73–81.

Sorlie, P. D., Backlund, E., Johnson, N. J., & Rogot, E. (1993). Mortality by Hispanic status in the United States. *Journal of the American Medical Association 278,* 2464–2468.

Stack, C. B. (1975). *All our kin: Strategies for survival in a black community.* New York: Harper and Row.

Syme, S. L. (1978). Drug treatment of mild hypertension: Social and psychological considerations. *Annals New York Academy of Science, 304,* 99–106.

Takeuchi, D. T., & Young, K. N. J. (1994). Overview of Asian and Pacific Islander Americans. In N. W. S. Zane, D. T. Takeuchi, & K. N. J. Young (Eds.), *Confronting Critical Health Issues of Asian and Pacific Islander Americans* (pp. 3–21). Thousand Oaks, CA: Sage.

Thomas, M. E. (1993). Race, class, and personal income: An empirical test of the declining significance of race thesis, 1968–1988. *Social Problems, 40,* 328–342.

U.S. Bureau of the Census. (1994) *Statistical Abstract of the United States: 1994 (114th ed.).* Washington, DC: Bureau of the Census.

Vega, W. A., & Amaro, H. (1994). Latino outlook: Good health, uncertain prognosis. *Annual Review of Public Health, 15,* 39–67.

Williams, D. R. (1990). Socioeconomic differentials in health: A review and redirection. *Social Psychology Quarterly, 53,* 81–99.

Williams, D. R., & Collins, C. (1995). US socioeconomic and racial differences in health: Patterns and explanations. *Annual Review of Sociology, 21,* 349–86.

Williams, D. R., & House, J. S. (1991). Stress, social support, control, and coping: A social epidemiological view. In B. Badura & I. Kickbusch (Eds.), *Health promotion research: Towards a new social epidemiology* (pp. 147–172). Copenhagen: World Health Organization.

Williams, D. R., Lavizzo-Mourey, R., & Warren, R. C. (1994) The concept of race and health status in America. *Public Health Reports, 109*(1), 26–41.

Williams, D. R., Wilson, L., & Chung, A. M. (1992). Socioeconomic status, psychosocial factors and health in urban Guyana. *Sociological Focus, 25*(4), 279–294.

Wilson, W. J. (1987). *The truly disadvantaged.* Chicago: University of Chicago Press.

Winant, H. (1994). *Racial conditions: politics, theory, comparisons.* Minneapolis: University of Minnesota Press.

Zane, N. W. S., Takeuchi, D. T., & Young, K. N. S. (1994). *Confronting critical health issues of Asian and Pacific Islander Americans.* Thousand Oaks, CA: Sage.

Index

425